FUNCTIONAL MAGNETIC RESONANCE IMAGING – ADVANCED NEUROIMAGING APPLICATIONS

Edited by **Rakesh Sharma**

Functional Magnetic Resonance Imaging – Advanced Neuroimaging Applications
Edited by Rakesh Sharma

Published by InTech

Janeza Trdine 9, 51000 Rijeka, Croatia

Publishing Process Manager Jana Sertic

Technical Editor Teodora Smiljanic

Cover Designer InTech Design Team

Additional hard copies can be obtained from orders@intechopen.com

Functional Magnetic Resonance Imaging – Advanced Neuroimaging Applications, Edited by Rakesh Sharma
p. cm.
ISBN 978-953-51-0541-1

For EU product safety concerns:
IN TECH d.o.o., Prolaz Marije Krucifikse Kozulić 3, 51000 Rijeka, Croatia,
info@intechopen.com or visit our website at intechopen.com.

Meet the editor

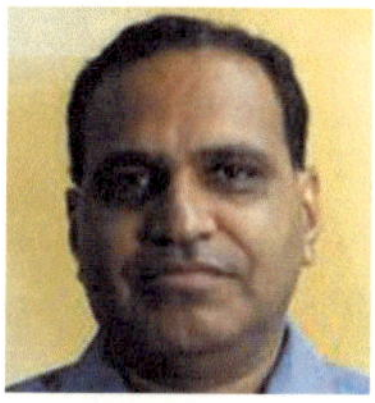

Dr Rakesh Sharma, Ph.D Biochemistry with second Ph.D Magnetic Resonance Imaging is professor at Amity University. He was employed at Center of Nanobiotechnology at Florida State University, Tallahassee, Florida since 2004. He is a scientist affiliated with department of Medicine, Columbia University, New York since 2000. His research interests are development of molecular imaging methods by MRI, PET and nanoparticles design. He authored seven books including four eBooks on line, 125 peer-reviewed research papers and articles, three US patents, 15 lecture series online in the fields of applied MRI, MR spectroscopy, biochemistry, nanotechnology and experimental research in atherosclerosis, cancer, liver diseases. He is CEO at Innovations And Solutions Inc. USA.

Contents

Preface

Functional Magnetic Resonance Imaging of brain is typically called fMRI. It has become a fundamental modality of imaging at any MRI suite of service center or hospital. Our book has been compiled with the aim of incorporating a wide range of applied neuropsychological evaluation methods. It is aimed at those who are embarking on neuropsychological research projects, as well as relatively experienced psychologists and neuroscientists who might wish to further develop their experiments. While it is not possible to detail every possible technique related to functional evaluation of brain in activation by using fMRI, the book attempts to provide working tips with examples and analysis to a wide range of the more commonly available techniques.

The methods described in this book are aimed at giving the reader a glimpse of some existing methods with the context in which each analytical fMRI method is applied, as well as providing some basis of familiarizing oneself with these techniques. While fMRI has been used in the study of cognition and neuroscience over the last two decades, it was only in the later part of 20th century that it has become an integral part of many psychological, behavioral and neuroscience research environments. This is, at least in part, due to the continued development of new statistical analysis methods, new fMRI hardware with scanning and monitoring accessories, better physio-compatible MRI suites, robust and fast acquisition techniques such as EPI-fMRI, GE-fMRI, etc., thanks to the continued joint efforts of governmental, industrial and academic institutions globally. Regardless of the MRI systems and the brands used, one should always be able to understand and justify the use of the right imaging fMRI protocol, designed for a specific study. With this aim, different approaches of fMRI methods of neuropsychological evaluation are presented in separate chapters. For learners, basic knowledge, safety issues, limitations and skepticism in fMRI data analysis and interpretation is presented with a working fMRI protocol for morphological MRI, MRSI data acquisition and analysis of neuronal dysfunction in multiple sclerosis.

In chapter 1, the author emphasized the basic concepts of fMRI, the need for quantitative calibration using gold standard, selection of correct paradigm, fMRI parameters, accrued experience in study design including design type, Blocked, Event-Related stimulus or mixed events, number of subjects, data size for each subject, stimulus conditions, and image acquisition parameters: repetitions for each condition, applied stimulus, TR/TE, and Number of slices. In chapter 2, authors introduced the physiological basis of neuroactivation in the brain during different motor-sensory actions with technical aspects of BOLD signal generation and interpretation. Imaging processing methods are discussed, with limitations and future prospects. fMRI technique and applications are reviewed with several examples. In chapter 3, we can read about the use of functional magnetic resonance imaging (fMRI) to obtain a biomarker in motor processing pathways in order to indicate the relationship between internal adaptation (influenced by conscious and non-conscious filtering and decision-making networks) and external environmental changes through the eye. The author claims that the clinical applications of fMRI biomarkers could include assessments of functional breakdowns in disease states, e.g., seizure disorders, memory deficits and visuo-cognitive abilities in patients with Alzheimer's disease, and eye movement control and balance in patients with traumatic brain injuries or Parkinson's disease. In chapter 4, authors hypothesized the performance of the hand-gesture task under the guidance of multiple rules for games such as rock–paper–scissors or null–two–five, using a balanced rule-guided behavioral system with the mirror system to overcome a covert and automatic tendency to imitate observed hand postures. Authors concluded that two different brain regions, for perception and motor-sensory, act under the guidance of behavioral rules in order to perform rule-guided behaviors and activities in rule-selective brain regions. In chapter 5, authors explored the application of Constraint-induced movement therapy in brain plasticity to evaluate the recovery after stroke and identify the specific correlations between movement recovery clinical endpoints and the fMRI data. Furthermore, the authors highlighted the needs such as common methodology of analysis and reporting the fMRI data for better comparison and interpretation of the results between studies, a comparison of different therapeutic techniques on the brain cortex reorganization and upper extremity recovery, and the establishment of optimal time for their application after stroke, with an aim to understand the treatment programs. In chapter 6, authors presented the potential of fMRI to evaluate the Reliability analysis required for the assessment of data to be structured in similar events or replicates performing the same task in different days under multiple experimental conditions. Authors emphasized the significance of reliability maps in detection of local infringements and selection of ROIs, along with temporal response functions into GLM for testing stimulus and task effects in the brain for each individual patient. In chapter 7, authors emphasized the precise analysis of different series in diagnosis and management of refractory SMA epilepsy in long-term follow-up. Conceptually, surgical approaches of the fontal lobe (frontopolar, of the convexity, central, orbitofrontal and SMA) must be considered separately and not as one sole group. In chapter 8, the author emphasizes that brain supports language processing via complex and sophisticated networks in Broca's and Wernicke's areas. Furthermore, the author speculates with skepticism on the growing number of fMRI studies on language in neurologically intact and injured brains to support relevant linguistic generalizations and explore a better neural organization of language, post-lesional neuroplasticity and recovery processes in support of rigorous investigations on issues of linguistic computations, bilingual language functionality, non-dominant hemisphere in brain. In chapter 9, authors reviewed the application of multimodal use of fMRI combined with magnetic resonance spectroscopy (MRS) in dyslexia of brain. Non-invasive technique was used to measure the neurochemicals distribution and N-acetylaspartate (NAA) and Choline (Cho) ratio within cerebellum to compare Western vs. Eastern data. Chemical shift imaging and logographic writing, linguistics testing in dyslexia demonstrated left vs. right cerebellar hemisphere differences. However, the fMRI-MR spectroscopy multimodal approach is in infancy but has a high potential in defining neuro disorders.

Functional MRI as imaging and evaluation modality

fMRI has become a very 'fashionable' technique and is often chosen as a research method, rather than for its suitability to a particular research question or population. Functional MRI serves as imaging and evaluation modality in basic sensory and perceptual processing in cognition states such as vegetative state (VS) and minimal conscious state (MCS). Wide applications of fMRI have been cited in useful auditory signals from auditory complex in speech sound discrimination, signals from visual cortex and tactile stimulation in a single vegetative conscious or severely injured patient. From a functional anatomy standpoint, temporal, parietal and frontal gyri in superior or inferior dimensions, occipital pole, and central sulcus regions in brain clearly show distinct BOLD signal responses in task performance or use of multisensory paradigm in neuroimaging. In the last decade, tremendous advancements have been made in the applied science of fMRI, such as functional connectivity, communication, emotion, familiarity, self-reference processing, conscious awareness, and hippocampus regional differences in BOLD signals. Findings from fMRI studies of cognition and consciousness all have one thing in common, but enormous variability between subjects, even within the same diagnostic category. One can wonder if this variability tells us anything about a patient's likely outcome. Clinically, it would be one of the most useful pieces of information fMRI could extract, while most studies state prognosis as one of the main goals of fMRI research in disorders of consciousness. In this direction, multimodal fMRI-PET, fMRI-MRS, fMRI-EEG, fMRI-MEG have evolved for analysis of neurochemicals, oxygen rich regions, regional electrophysiology etc. to classify the data from patients according to whether they showed no activation; typical, low-level activation of primary sensory cortices; or higher-level activation of associative cortices; atypical, higher-level associative cortex activation to make decision on recovery of consciousness and other neuro dysfunctions.

Limit of resolution and detection by fMRI

fMRI has contributed immensely to our understanding of disorders of consciousness and highlighted the need for brain-based tools to assess cognition and awareness in patients in vegetative and minimally conscious states but is clearly not the most practical solution to the problem by itself. Over the past few decades, improvements in emergency and intensive care medicine have resulted in an increased number of patients who survive severe brain injury. Some patients, unrecovered from coma, may remain in a vegetative or minimally conscious state. The diagnosis of coma, locked-in-syndrome and conscious state poses a challenge in accurate assessment of consciousness by some verbal or behavioral sign. Functional MRI serves to differentiate VS and MCS to generate verbal or motor responses by fMRI to indicate sensory or perceptual impairments, motor impairments, and subclinical seizure activity. However, fMRI does not allow inferring on patient's level of awareness or cognitive ability, but fMRI findings are crucial in the interpretation of data from higher-order cognitive tasks, particularly negative findings. Assessment of cognition function by fMRI BOLD activation patterns provides an opportunity to eliminate the need of behavioral responses to cognitive tasks. However, there are many reasons to fail to observe expected activations: a patient's neuroanatomy may have been severely altered and functional remapping may have occurred; a relevant sensory system (e.g., the auditory system for a speech recognition task) may have been damaged; the coupling between neuronal firing and hemodynamic response may differ substantially from that of healthy brains. Thus, proponents of fMRI argue that functional neuroimaging assessments of cognition in patients with disorders of consciousness should proceed in a hierarchical fashion, from basic sensory processing to high-level cognition similar with EEG and evoked potentials were done over decades.

Major limitations in performing fMRI on patients with disorders of consciousness are patient safety issues. Implanted devices such as neurostimulators, CSF shunts, aneurysm clips, and bone flap fixation wires and clamps are of particular concern for brain injury patients. Many of these devices have now been tested and deemed MR-safe at specific fields, but many are still contra-indicated or restricted. Some aneurysm clips are ferromagnetic and may displace and cause serious injury or death. Some shunt valves use magnetic components and exposure to the MRI's magnetic field may change the valve settings and lead to increase intracranial CSF pressure. Neurostimulators may malfunction, overheat, or be displaced causing injury or death. History of implanted devices and any other surgical hardware, patient background regarding previous surgeries, implants, as well as possible embedded shrapnel or bullets are some of the concerns. The Safety Committee of the Society for Magnetic Resonance Imaging recommends that all patients who are unable to communicate should be physiologically monitored. fMRI now becomes a more standard form of evaluation in patients with disorders of consciousness in hospitals.

Choice of the fMRI protocol

Choice of fMRI method and task-paradigm chosen is a crucial issue. Once a patient has passed through all the necessary safety screening steps, there are still many hurdles to overcome in order to collect fMRI data from an unconsciousness patient. As a researcher, one should consider whether the chosen MRI protocol is the most effective and practical way to answer his/her research question. Since fMRI was introduced in the early 90's, it has had an immense impact on cognitive neuroscience research and its use has grown exponentially. Once at the scanning facility, many difficulties may be encountered in physical positioning of the patient in the scanner due to muscle contractures or injuries that prevent them from performing a task after stimulus delivery. fMRI studies in patients with disorders of consciousness are mostly conducted in the auditory modality to circumvent difficulties with the delivery of visual stimuli. However, auditory stimulation in the very noisy scanner environment presents its own set of challenges. Without a doubt, the most problematic source of artifact in patients is motion. Large, involuntary movements of the head or body are common, and movement cannot be entirely prevented from occurring in the scanner. Another source of artifact in brain-injured patients comes from devices implanted in the head, such as aneurysm clips, shunts, and neurostimulators. Even when these devices have been deemed non-ferromagnetic and completely MRI-safe, they are still foreign, usually metallic objects with significantly different magnetic susceptibility than the surrounding brain tissue. They can create significant artifacts, loss of signal, and/or distortion of the image surrounding the object. Short-time event related tasks, multi-sensory paradigms, and saccades are routinely used in prescribing fMRI protocols. Echo planar EPI-fMRI and gradient-echo GE-fMRI are rapid acquisition techniques. fMRI-DTI/PWI, fMRI-MPRAGE are variants in functional imaging. In order for an assessment fMRI technique to be readily adopted into standard clinical practice, it must be inexpensive, easily accessible, have few limitations in terms of patient compatibility, and be relatively simple to administer (preferably at the bedside). fMRI and patients with severe brain injuries can rarely or not at all combine to meet these criteria. There are still many significant logistical and methodological considerations that will in all likelihood prevent fMRI from becoming a part of routine diagnostic assessments in standard clinical practice.

Image processing and interpretation

Several issues arise when analyzing both structural and functional MRI data from patients with severe brain injuries. Most obvious is the issue of normalization. For example, patients with traumatic injury may have abnormal or deformed brain structures as a result of focal hemorrhages, hydrocephalus, shifting, craniotomy, swelling, dilated ventricles, atrophy, etc. This complicates the co-registration of functional data to anatomical data, as well as transformation into stereotaxic space (e.g., Talairach space or MNI space) for comparisons between patients, or between patients and controls. The heterogeneity of etiologies also complicates any between-subjects comparisons. In my opinion, even if normalization can be performed, it must be considered that, depending on the injury, a great deal of functional remapping should have taken place, so that functional areas may no longer correspond to the coordinates of the same functional areas in healthy controls or other patients. Better software for image processing is now becoming available. For more details, see Appendix 1 at the end of book.

BOLD signal is a measure of hemodynamic response, not a direct measure of neural activity. Neurovascular coupling is the relationship between neural activity and the hemodynamic response reflected by the BOLD signal. It is dependent on intact signaling between neurons and blood vessels, and on the various components of vascular reactivity such as changes to metabolic or neurotransmitter signaling, vascular tone, cerebral blood volume, blood flow, blood oxygenation, or oxygen consumption (see chapter two). It is now established that many diseases and pathologies, including brain injuries, alter neurovascular coupling and change the BOLD signal without necessarily affecting the neuronal function. The good part is that one can attribute changes in the BOLD signal to changes in neural activity if, and only if, signaling and vascular reactivity are not altered; and one can compare between groups (e.g., patients and controls) only if these properties are the same in both groups. Therefore, utmost caution must be used when interpreting the BOLD signal in brain-injured patients, and the potential confounds in the intermediate steps of neurovascular coupling must be considered. Several types of analysis software is available now. For more details, see Appendix 1 at the end of book.

A working example of growing science in fMRI of motor activity in multiple sclerosis

Over the years, we focused on neurochemical changes in multiple sclerosis with casual observations of reduction in functional activity in the ipsilateral sensorimotor cortex. Activation changes in ipsilateral motor areas correlated inversely with age, extent and progression of T1 lesion load, and occurrence of a new relapse in support of evolved brain plastic changes. It is now established that functional changes in the brain may not be correlated with slow tissue injury or neuro dysfunction appearing as lesions, sometimes normal-appearing brain tissue. Longitudinal fMRI studies on motor activity suggest cortical motor organization as dynamic changes evolved with time as a clinical correlate.

An example of fMRI study design and protocol is presented here for interested neuroscientists on morphological MRSI and fMRI data using a 1.5 T magnet with echo planar capabilities and a head volume radio frequency coil. Each subject lay supine in the scanner with eyes closed with minimum head movements on foam padding and a restraining strap. Data acquisition conditions: 1. localizer protocol- multiplanar T1-weighted localizer at slice orientation (parallel to the bi-commissural plane) and the same brain volume acquisition (last slice tangent to the cortical mantle surface) as standard for different fMRI sessions; 2. T2*-weighted echo planar imaging (64 • 64 matrix over a 24-cm field of view) to get 25 consecutive, 4-mm thick axial sections, TR/TE (repetition time/echo time) = 3000/50 ms, a 90_ flip angle and one excitation in total time of functional study = 225 s, to acquire total of 75 consecutive dynamics. 3. Motor task paradigm during fMRI acquisition, when both patients and healthy subjects perform a self-paced sequential finger opposition task (thumb repeatedly touched the other four fingers in a sequential order with the right hand). Seven periods of hand movement and seven periods of rest were alternated (each period lasting for 15 s) as 'start' and 'stop' acoustic signals were given during the acquisition under supervision by an operator who remains present to record the rate of hand movements for both patients and controls.

fMRI data analysis is done by SPM99 software to realign, normalize and spatially smoothen the images using a Gaussian kernel of 8 mm. Step-by-step method is followed. First, analysis of the time series of functional MR image from each subject is done to estimate the effects of experimental paradigm on a voxel-by-voxel basis using the principles of the general linear model. Second, data modeling is used for a boxcar design, convolved with the hemodynamic response function chosen to represent the relationship between the neuronal activation and blood flow changes. Four contrast images are generated in two steps: (I) task-related activation at fMRI1; (II) task-related activation at fMRI2; (III) task-related activity increase between the two fMRI studies (fMR1 < fMRI2); and (IV) task-related activity decrease between the two fMRI studies (fMR1 > fMRI2). These contrast images are then used for a second-level random effect analysis, according to a 2 × 2 design with time (fMR1 and fMRI2) and group (patients and controls) as factors. Next step is the analysis of main effects, interactions and simple main effects using subject specific contrasts as the response variable and one or two sample t-tests, presuming that clusters of voxels (corrected $P < 0.05$) have a peak Z score >3.7 to show significant changes.

Multiple regression analysis provides the extent of activations by clinical and radiological variables up to 11 or more within group to look at the effects of age and disease progression. Regression analysis calculates the correlation; for example, clusters of voxels (corrected $P < 0.05$) with peak Z score >2.4 are significantly correlated. Within each region of statistical significance, local maxima of signal increase (the voxels of maximum significance) and their location can be expressed in terms of x, y, and z coordinates, and those can be converted to the Talairach space using linear transformation (www.mrc-cbu.cam.ac.uk/Imaging/mnispace.html). Activations in the brain are seen as Talairach coordinates in different brain regions in x-, y-, and z- directions of left (L) and right (right) lobes in L-sensorimotor cortex (BA 1–4), L-inferior parietal lobule (BA 40), L-lateral premotor cortex (BA 6), L-supplementary motor area (BA 6), L-lentiform nucleus, L-thalamus, L-insula, L-cerebellum, R-sensorimotor cortex (BA 1–4), R- inferior parietal lobule (BA 40), R-lateral premotor cortex (BA 6), R-superior parietal cortex (BA 7), R-lentiform nucleus, R-thalamus, R-insula, R-cerebellum and Vermis.

Morphological fMRI acquisition and morphological MRI protocols are commonly used for proton density weighted PWI images (n=40 contiguous axial slices with 4-mm thickness, 256 × 256 matrix and 24-cm field of view) and T2-weighted spin-echo images (T2-WI) (TR = 2000 ms; TE = 20/90 ms), and T1-weighted spin-echo images (T1-WI) (TR = 550 ms; TE = 12 ms) before and after injection of an intravenous bolus of 0.3 mmoles/kg gadolinium diethyltriamine penta-acetic acid (Gd-DTPA). For MRSI, chemical shift imaging (CHESS) protocol at selective frequencies is prescribed, covering the whole brain for water suppressed metabolite mapping and metabolite ratio in two dimensions. For more details, readers are welcome to read chapters 2 and 10. By supervised automated segmentation, hyperintense T2 and hypointense T1 lesion loads (LL) can be calculated for each patient, using the display program MRIAP or Dispunc (D.L. Plummer, University College London, London, UK) with a semi-automated contouring technique. Various software is available for metabolite mapping and neurochemical analysis, SID, APSIP, and NMR2. However, fMRI-neurochemical imaging multimodal techniques are still in infancy.

Present state of art on fMRI and future prospects

Present concerns on fast, safe, robust inexpensive and reproducible fMRI do not mean that fMRI is incapable of solving the problem of diagnosis in disorders of unconscious patient with severe brain injury. On the contrary, Electroencephalography (EEG), for instance, is widely available, inexpensive, easy to administer at the bedside, robust to many artifacts that can cause fMRI data to be unusable (e.g., motion), and has virtually no restrictions regarding the patient compatibility and safety. Combined with fMRI, some of the data interpretation problems inherent in fMRI could be easily solved with EEG. For instance, periods of low arousal or sleep are common and complicate the interpretation of negative findings unless arousal can be closely monitored during scanning. EEG, particularly event-related potentials (ERPs) have a long history in cognitive neuroscience research and many well-established 'signature' patterns related to specific cognitive processes, to an even greater extent than does the fMRI. The use of ERPs with fMRI seems promising for assessment of cognition in non-communicative patients. Extensive, engineering-oriented literature on the classification of mental imagery for the purposes of brain-computer interfacing using EEG already exists, as a shift away from fMRI towards the use of EEG and ERPs for detecting covert awareness. MR spectroscopy is emerging as yet another chemical fMRI option in terms of neurochemical imaging.

In hope of wider acceptance of fMRI as a major clinical modality for neuropsychological analysis, this book is a concise text source to introduce the intricacies of fMRI, safety issues, recent applications in evaluation of behavioral and neurological disorders beginning with the basic science, to applications in noninvasive evaluation of disabilities in learning, linguistics, and surgery. In the end, the appendix is a handful resource for software useful in fMRI, MRI methods, presently available online. This book will be useful to learners, neuroscientists, and researchers dedicated to experimental fMRI applied in cognitive science.

Rakesh Sharma, PhD,
MS-PhD, ABR II
Professor (Nanotechnology)
Amity University,
India

Research Professor, Center of Nano-Biotechnology,
Florida State University, Tallahassee, FL
USA

Section 1

Basic Concepts of fMRI

1

Current Trends of fMRI in Vision Science: A Review

Nasser H. Kashou
Department of Radiology, Children's Radiological Institute, Nationwide Children's Hospital
Department of Radiology, Department of Ophthalmology, The Ohio State University Medical Center
Department of Biomedical, Industrial and Human Factors Engineering, Wright State University
USA

1. Introduction

Studying brain functional activities is an area that is experiencing rapid interest in the field of neuroimaging. Functional magnetic resonance imaging (fMRI) has provided vision science researchers a powerful and noninvasive tool to understand eye function and correlate it with brain activities. In this chapter, we focus on the physiological aspects followed by a literature review. More specifically, to motivate and appreciate the complexity of the visual system, we will begin with a description of specific stages the visual pathway, beginning from the distal stimulus and ending in the visual cortex. More importantly, the development of ascending visual pathway will be discussed in order to help in understanding various disorders associated with it such as monochromacy, albinism, amblyopia (refractive, strabismic). In doing so we will divide the first half into two main sections, the visual pathway and the development of the ascending pathway. The first of these sections will be mostly an anatomy review and the latter will discuss the development of this anatomy with specific examples of disorders as a result of abnormal development. We will then discuss fMRI studies with focus on vision science applications. The remaining sections of this chapter will be highlighting the work done on mainly oculomotor function, some perception and visual dysfunction with fMRI and investigate the differences and similarities in their findings. We will then conclude with a discussion on how this relates to neurologists, neuroscientists, ophthalmologists and other specialists.

2. Background

To motivate the discussion we begin by asking, what is the problem in visual perception? This will be answered briefly. In visual perception, we have both a distal and a proximal stimulus. The distal stimulus is what the subject is looking at, usually at a distance. In the case of vision, it determines the pattern of light arriving at the cornea. The proximal stimulus hits the sense organs directly. In the case of vision, it is the pattern of light arriving at the retina, for instance as a result of looking at the distal stimulus. There are several features that distinguish the distal and proximal stimuli. The distal stimulus is 3-dimensional, independent of point of view, upright, and has no lens blur or filter. An example of the latter two is that when we look at a person their head is on top and their feet are on the bottom and the physical person does not get blurred. The proximal on the other hand is 2-dimensional, depends on point of view, inverted, blurred and filtered by the lens. So the main problem in visual perception becomes clearer; that is to retrieve information about the distal stimulus with only the proximal stimulus to work with. This is important because it affects the perceptual representation which is the endpoint of the perceptual process. Perceptual representation is the state of the visually-guided motor behavior (keeps us from bumping into things), visual pattern recognition, visual understanding, and memory. Basically, as the subject sees an object (distal stimulus), the input falls on the retina (proximal stimulus) and an output of the distal stimulus is perceived via perceptual representations. Note, that this is not the same as the distal stimulus, because there are two kinds of perception, veridical and illusory. There are many examples of visual illusions, in which the perceptual representation suggests an incorrect distal stimulus. That is, the apparent distal stimulus differs from the veridical distal stimulus. With this concept, we can now refine the problem in visual perception, as trying to understand how the visual system creates a perceptual representation of the distal stimulus with only the proximal stimulus as an input. Why is this a problem? Because the relationship of distal to proximal is not one to one, that is a distal stimulus can be seen as many proximal stimuli and proximal stimuli can be many distal stimuli. This leads to the inverse problem of trying to recover a visual representation from the input, even when many representations are consistent with the proximal stimulus. Thus, this is a motivation to begin discussing the visual pathway and understand the retinal (proximal) input to the brain.

3. Visual pathway

The visual pathway consists of many stages. We will focus on the ganglion cells, lateral geniculate nucleus (LGN), and the primary visual cortex (V1). The ascending visual pathway begins when light hits the back of the retina and stimulates the photoreceptors (rods and cones). These photoreceptors transform radiant energy into electrical activity, which is transmitted to retinal bipolar cells and then into retinal ganglion cells. The retina has several layers and sub-layers with corresponding cells, such as ganglion, amacrine, bipolar and horizontal. Each of these cells play a role in the visual system and have their own receptive fields. Again, in this chapter we choose to focus and discuss the ganglion cells.

3.1 Ganglion cells

There are two major classes of ganglion cells. The smaller midget, or parvo, cells comprise about 80 percent of these cells and the larger parasol, or magno, cells about 10 percent (Lennie et al., 1990). As with other cells in the retina, these ganglion cells have their own receptive fields known as center surround with either on-center (off-surround) or off-center (on-surround). There are several differences between these two types of cells. Parvo cells are dominant in the fovea as opposed to the magno cells, which are dominant in the periphery. The parvo cells are also characterized as having a sustained response while the magno have a transient response (Purpura et al., 1990; Schiller & Malpeli, 1978). At any given eccentricity, parvo cells have a higher spatial resolution, lower contrast sensitivity, slower conduction velocity, and a more sustained response than do magno cells (Shapley et al., 1981). The parvo cells have low contrast sensitivity and detect color and form, while the magno have high contrast sensitivity and detect motion. Parvo cells rarely respond well to luminance contrasts below 10%, whereas magno cells often respond to stimuli with contrasts as low as 2% (Purpura et al., 1988; Sclar et al., 1990; Shapley et al., 1981). In addition to these two, there are other types of ganglion axons that exist; the more common of these are the konio cells which are small bistratified cells (Kaas et al., 1978). They are common in the parafovea, have low contrast sensitivity, and detect color. The major difference between the konio cells and the other two is that the konio have a uniform receptive field and thus have no spatial opponency. To many investigators the term konio has become synonymous with the blue-yellow pathway, just as parvo is now equated, too simplistically, with the red-green pathway (Sincich & Horton, 2005). But this is not always the case because, konio cells constitute a heterogeneous population of cells, some lacking blue-yellow color opponency (Hendry & Reid, 2000). The axons of all these ganglion cells exit the eye, forming the optic nerve and synapse in the midbrain. Since the diameter of the optic nerve and the number of the ganglion cell axons it contains are limited by the structure of the skull, not all the information that falls upon the retina is transmitted to the brain proper (Schwartz, 2004). Although there are more than 100 million photoreceptors within the retina, there are only 1 million ganglion cells, revealing an extensive degree of neural convergence (Curcio & Allen, 1990; Osterberg, 1935). At the optic chiasm, ganglion cell fibers from the nasal retina of each eye cross over to join the temporal fibers of the fellow eye to form the optic tract (Schwartz, 2004). The long axons of the retinal ganglion cells leave the eye, form the second cranial nerve (the optic nerve), and synapse in the dorsal lateral geniculate nucleus (dLGN), a midbrain structure (Schwartz, 2004). We will now discuss the LGN.

3.2 Lateral geniculate nucleus (LGN)

The primary target of the optic tract is the dorsal lateral geniculate nucleus (dLGN), a thalamic nucleus. In higher vertebrates, such as carnivores and primates, axons from the two eyes converge onto their primary target, the dorsal lateral geniculate nucleus (dLGN), but occupy distinct regions (the eye-specific layers) within this target (Guillery, 1970; Kaas et al., 1972; Linden et al., 1981). In primates (Rakic, 1976; 1977), the axonal terminals of ganglion cells of the two eyes initially share common territories within the dLGN, but through a process that eliminates inappropriately placed branches, projections from the two eyes become restricted to their appropriate layer. Most, but not all, retinal ganglion cells synapse in the six-layered structure. Layers 2, 3, and 5 receive input from the ipsilateral eye, whereas layers 1, 4, and 6 receive input from the contralateral eye, Fig. 1. The dorsal four layers, which are constituted of comparatively small neurons called parvo, or P-cells, are the parvocellular layers (layers 3,4,5,6). Larger neurons, commonly called magno or M-cells, comprise the two ventral magnocellular layers (layers 1,2). Axons from midget ganglion cells synapse on P-cells in the dLGN to form the parvo pathway, while axons from the parasol cells synapse on dLGN M-cells to form the magno pathway. The layers between the parvocellular and magnocellular layers contain very small neurons (konio cells). Studies have shown that konio cells provide the only direct geniculate input to layers 1-3 (Hendry & Yoshioka, 1994). The subcortical projection from the retina to cerebral cortex is strongly dominated by the two pathways (M and P pathways) the magnocellular and parvocellular subdivisions of the lateral geniculate nucleus (Shapley & Perry, 1986). The parvo layers receive input from color-opponent midget ganglion cells, whereas the magno layers are supplied by broadband parasol ganglion cells (Perry et al., 1984). Parvo pathway neurons show color opponency of either the red/green or blue/yellow type, which means that they respond to color change regardless of the relative luminance of the colors (Derrington & Lennie, 1984). The blue-yellow ganglion cells project to the konio layers just ventral to the third and fourth parvocellular layers (Calkins & Hendry, 1996). Layers 5 and 6 have on-center receptive fields, and layers 3 and 4 have off-center receptive fields. Layers 1 and 2 have both on- and off- center receptive fields. These projections from the retina to the LGN then lead to the visual cortex.

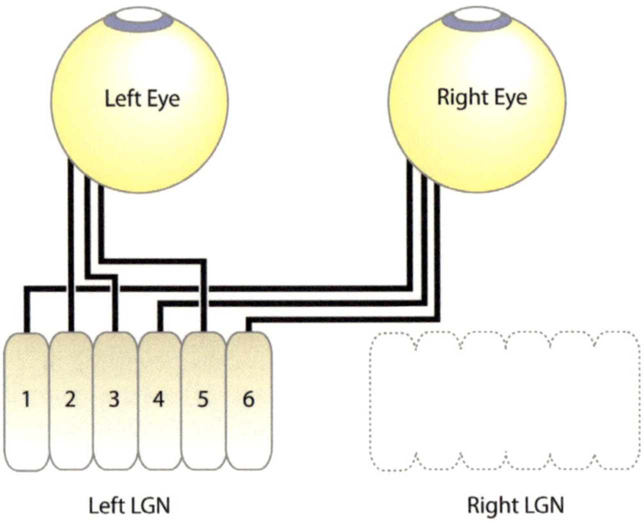

Fig. 1. Retinal ganglion cell projections to the lateral geniculate nucleus (LGN) of the thalamus. Note that layers 1,4, and 6 of the LGN receive visual information from the contralateral retina, whereas layers 2,3, and 5 receive visual information from the ipsilateral retina.

3.3 Primary visual cortex (V1)

The cells of dLGN send most of their axons to the cerebral cortex, specifically, the primary visual cortex (V1) along with the visual field representation in the retina and primary cortex. Inputs to V1, which are stratified by magno, parvo, and konio, become thoroughly intermingled by passage through the elaborate circuitry of V1 (Sincich & Horton, 2005). There are about 8 or 9 layers in V1. Layer 4 consists of three sublayers, 4A, 4B, and 4C. Layer 4C also is subdivided into 4Cα, and 4Cβ. The projections from the LGN go specifically to layer 4C and the information flows up and down from there (Merigan & Maunsell, 1993). The projections from parvocellular layers terminate primarily in layers 4A and 4Cβ, whereas those from magnocellular geniculate terminate in layer 4Cα (Fitzpatrick et al., 1985). Layer 4B receives direct input from 4Cα (M pathway), but not 4Cβ (P pathway) (Lund & Boothe, 1975; Lund et al., 1979). Layer 4Cβ projects to the blobs and interblobs (Horton & Hubel, 1981; Humphrey & Hendrickson, 1980). The blobs also receive major inputs from the M pathway by way of layers 4B and 4Cα (Blasdel et al., 1985; Fitzpatrick et al., 1985; Lachica et al., 1992; Lund, 1988). Fig. 2 gives the details of these connections.

More recently, Yazar et al. (2004) have found that some geniculate fibers terminate in both layers 4Cβ and 4A, implying either a direct parvo input to 4A or a konio input to 4Cβ. In layer 3B the cells in blobs and interblobs receive input from parvo (4Cβ), magno (4Cα), konio (4A), or mixed (4B) layers, in a range of relative synaptic strengths (Sawatari & Callaway, 2000). Cells in both 4Cα and 4Cβ project to layers 5 and 6 (Callaway & Wiser, 1996; Lund & Boothe, 1975). Feedback from layer 6 to the LGN is segregated only partially with respect to magno

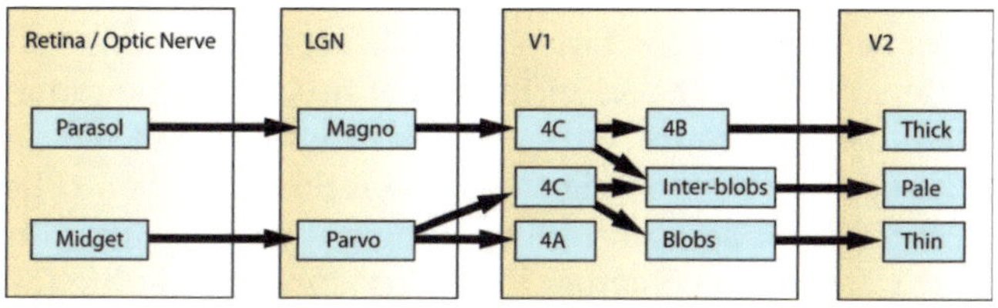

Fig. 2. Block diagram of ganglion cell mapping from retina through LGN, V1, and other cortical areas.

and parvo, thus mixing the geniculate channels (Fitzpatrick et al., 1994). There are two main types of cells in V1, stellate and pyramidal. The stellate cells are small interneurons found in layers 2-6 and the pyramidal cells are large relay neurons found in layers 2, 3, 5, and 6. The stellate cells are simple cells because of their receptive fields. The pyramidal cells are complex cells. The simple cells' receptive fields are of a certain size, are oriented in a certain way, and are sensitive to phase. They increase their rate of firing when stimulated in some places, and reduce it when stimulated in other places. The simple cells respond to a single spot of light and are additive and linear. The complex cells do not respond to a single spot of light, rather they respond to edges and bars, and are not sensitive to spatial phase. Many of the complex cells respond best to stimuli that move in one direction. So, if the stimulus is stationary, in the opposite direction, or a spot of light then the complex cells' receptive field will have no response. The complex cells are non-additive and are non-linear. Both the simple and complex cells respond to most proximal stimuli. All together, these cortical cells are tuned for spatial frequency, position, and orientation. This distinction is important in designing visual stimuli for fMRI studies to understand normal and abnormal visual function.

4. Development of the ascending pathway

We now describe how the visual pathway develops and the effects of abnormal development. During development anatomical projection patterns are restructured and functional reorganization takes place (Campbell & Shatz, 1992; Hubel & Wiesel, 1977; Shatz & Kirkwood, 1984; Wiesel, 1982). There are at least two ways by which neurons can be wired up accurately: connections may be specified from the outset, or synapse formation may initially follow an approximate wiring diagram, with precision achieved by the elimination of inappropriate inputs and the stabilization and growth of appropriate connections (Goodman & Shatz, 1993; Purves & Lichtman, 1985). The ganglion cells, LGN, and V1 are all wired up in a "retinotopic" fashion; meaning that the order of points on the retina (proximal stimulus) are preserved. In this mapping, the points that are further away from each other on the retina will be further away on the brain. It is easy to see that the proximal image is retinotopically related to the distal stimulus, simply because of the optics of the eye. However the retinotopic mapping from the retina to the LGN and from the LGN to V1 is harder to appreciate. Studies of patients with localized cortical damage showed that the receptive fields of neurons within area V1 are retinotopically organized (Holmes, 1918; 1944; Horton & Hoyt, 1991). As a matter of fact, the development of the retinotopic map is a general process for the central nervous system. Cell bodies are born early in embryogenisis; axons and dendrites come later. The nerve growth is then guided mechanically, probably by glial cells, to their overall destination. The patterns of activity of the neurons themselves determine the exact position of the synapses that are formed. Ganglion cells travel up the concentration gradient to the LGN. Target cells send guiding chemical messages, giving crude directions to the cells' overall destination by their concentration gradient. These chemical signposts act like beacons that attract the cells to project to approximately the correct part of the target tissue. At the same time the chemical signposts repel growth cones from the wrong axons. These guidance molecules also govern the decussation at the optic chiasm by signaling the retinal ganglion cells to either cross or not to to cross. The activity of adjacent retinal ganglion cells is correlated (Galli & Maffei, 1988), and "waves" of activity sweep across the retina during early life (Meister et al., 1991). Although the waves could potentially underlie the refinement of many retinal projection patterns, activity may not be required for establishing the M and P pathways of the primate retina that develop prenatally, and which show no apparent gross structural refinement with ensuing development (Meissirel et al., 1997). The immature and light-insensitive retina spontaneously generates a pattern of rhythmic bursting activity during the period when the connectivity patterns of retinal ganglion cells are shaped (Wong, 1999.). After the cells find a region, the wave then enforces precise ordering at the target. Thus the retinotopic map is finalized via the wave. Prenatal refinement of the retinotopic projections is achieved by these spontaneous waves of activation that propagate across the retina. Here ganglion cells are linked together by means of electrical synapses in a rough network and charge fluctuates randomly. The random response of one cell starts a wave of activity and the cells that fire together will eventually wire together. These spontaneous waves cause neighboring retinal regions to fire at about the same time. In fact, the correlation between the responses of cells is directly related to their separation on the retina (Wong, 1999.). So, the first principle of refinement is that cells that are neighbors tend to respond together. The second principle of refinement is that cells that fire together wire together. If there are two cells, 1 and 2, that are close to each other on the retina then when they fire together they will form neighboring synapses at the LGN. But cell 3, which is far from the first two on the retina will fire separately and thus synapse at the LGN separately. This is how the LGN is retinotopically wired up at birth along with V1 and other retinotopic cortical areas. Hence, the waves in the prenatal retina setup the relation between retina and brain. As for the postnatal retina, responses to stimuli set up the relation between the proximal stimulus and the brain. The postnatal wave may help guide the formation of synapses and determine which erroneous synapses are cut out for the normal mapping. When they arrive at their destinations, each process synapses over a relatively large area. Since target cells have lots of cells synapsing onto them, there are a lot more synapses present in V1 at 6 months and 1 year than in an adult. The process of the synapse starts as each axon from different cell bodies tries to take over a large piece of visual cortex and inevitably overlap occurs. At these regions of overlap a competition occurs, and the cell with the most or strongest synapse claims that region and the other synapses pull back. This synaptic elimination is a key element in the refinement of connectivity in both the central and peripheral nervous systems (Cowan et al., 1984; Goodman & Shatz, 1993; Lichtman et al., 1999; Nguyen & Lichtman, 1996; Purves & Lichtman, 1985). This produces a retinotopic map that has less overlap than before, and has many fewer synapses. If there is a vacant area then other nearby cells synapse onto it without meeting any competition and in turn increase their synaptic field. This process of being able to change as a result of experience is called plasticity, and is required for normal development. It determines how the visual system is wired up during normal development. The synaptic development occurs at different time scales across the brain. For V1 the development ends from about 8 to 16 years and culling happens at about 1-2 years. If there is any difficulty or blur in one eye or an eye turn while these synapses are being formed and refined, the subject will develop a visual disorder. This leads us into the next section.

4.1 Disorders of the ascending pathway

We will now discuss several visual disorders associated with the ascending pathway before reviewing fMRI research in vision science. The disorders are: rod monochromacy, albinism, refractive amblyopia, and strabismic amblyopia.

4.1.1 Rod monochromat

Rod monochromat, also known as complete achromatopsia, is an autosomal recessive disease. The rod vision is normal but cone vision is completely absent, meaning there is no fovea. In a normal subject, the fovea is what projects to V1, so what happens to the foveal representation in this case? In a rod monochromat, the visual acuity is about 20/200 and the spectral sensitivity is that of rhodopsin, meaning there are big losses in the red compared to normal. As a result of not having cones, there is no color vision and the patient has photophobia and severe visual impairment due to glare. The fovea is grossly abnormal with no reflex and may have a few cones which may contain rhodopsin. As a result of this abnormality, pendular nystagmus forms. With respect to the ascending pathway, the vacant space of the part of V1 that normally receives signals from the fovea is occupied during the synaptic development stage by synapses originating in the parafoveal retina of the achromat.

4.1.2 Albinism

Albinism is characterized by a systematic misrouting of the connections between the retina and the visual cortex. The ascending projection in an albino is almost entirely crossed. Note the normal projection that is crossed is about 55%. This miswiring can produce nystagmus and strabismus. The clinical features of albinism include hypopigmentation of the fundus, and iris. There are variable degrees of pigmentation of the iris, hair, skin. Tyrosinase negative albino (oculocutaneous) individuals may be completely white with a visual acuity range from 20/60 - 20/400, but is usually worst than 20/200. Tyrosinase positive albino may look hypopigmented or even essentially normal with visual acuity range from 20/60 - 20/400, but is usually better than 20/200. More clinical features related to the eye include a very light fundus because there is no melanin in the retinal pigment epithelium (RPE). There is little differentiation of the fovea from the surrounding retina. Albinos also have high myopia or high hyperopia. In the albino system there is more than 90% decussation at the optic chiasm. This means that the guidance molecules during development failed to stop the neurons from going the opposite direction. For a better understanding of the ascending pathway abnormalities in albinos we will do a comparison with normals. If a distal stimulus is presented on the right hand side of a normal subject then the expected pathway from the right eye nasal retina would cross the optic chiasm and end up in the contralateral visual cortex (left visual cortex). For the same stimulus on an albino subject, the resulting signal would be the same as the normal. If the distal stimulus is changed to the left hand side for the normal, and looking at the right eye temporal retina, then the signal would not cross the optic chiasm and would end up in ipsilateral visual cortex (right visual cortex). The same repeated for the albino reveals the opposite since the majority of the neurons cross the optic chiasm and end up in the contralateral visual cortex again. The primary lesion in albinism is a genetically determined lack of melanin or melanosomes as mentioned earlier. As a side point, melanin is very important for many aspects of neurological development. For instance, the neural crests pigment and its location on the embryo is determined by melanin. Melanin is also involved in production of dopamine and serotonin and many other neurotransmitters related to neuroendocrine function.

4.1.3 Refractive amblyopia

Refractive/deprivation amblyopia is a result of the receptive fields not being used early in life. Thus, the culling at about 1 year postnatal removes their synaptic connections because lack of function. Specifically, the proximal stimulus is blurred during the critical period, meaning the high spatial frequencies are reduced or eliminated from the visual image, causing high spatial frequency tuned channels to either never develop, or be lost. In this case, the low spatial frequencies pass unattenuated, so the low spatial frequency tuned channels develop normally. The effect of this blur in refractive amblyopia is the direct loss of contrast sensitivity at high spatial frequencies, which is equivalent to a loss of visual resolution acuity. As for the remaining spatial frequency channels, they stay relatively normal because they are stimulated normally during the critical period. This illustrates the principle that the receptive fields must be used if they are to be maintained. If the proximal stimuli do not stimulate the receptive fields effectively, the cells tend to stop responding to the intended stimulus even if it is presented occasionally. The cell may begin to respond to other stimuli, and therefore develop a new receptive field. The input from the other eye is likely to grab the synapse area because of competition. As a result there is anisometropia, an unequal refractive error in the two eyes. Thus, the eye with the larger refractive error continues to experience chronic blur. Dominance of the good eye becomes exaggerated during development, because of competition between incoming signals. Most cells in the primary visual cortex come to have predominant input from the good eye. If one eye is handicapped during the competition, it tends to lose its synaptic connections. Thus, the development of ocular dominance columns in amblyopia is distorted, and depends on the age at which deprivation begins. The most dangerous periods of refractive amblyopia are in the first 6 months.

4.1.4 Strabismic amblyopia

The cells in the ascending pathway are labeled lines. Labels relate to position on the retina and therefore position in the proximal stimulus. Labels also relate to spatial frequency and orientation. Labeled lines are important because the brain only knows what the ascending pathway tells it. If the labels are abnormal, vision is also abnormal. In strabismic amblyopia, the lines are mislabeled, which leads to distorted vision. In normal retinotopic organization, labels relate position in the distal stimulus to position upon the retina. Strabismic amblyopia is thought to be due to disordered (scrambled) retinotopic mapping between the LGN and V1 of the signals from one eye; therefore, leading to abnormal visual experience. The waves that happen after birth are not normal because the eye is not always pointing in the right direction. Recall that cells fire together after birth because of the wave of activity produced by the usual retinal stimulus. This postnatal wave may help guide the formation of synapses and determines which erroneous synapses are cut out for the normal mapping. This eye turn in early childhood produces an abnormal wave. The connection between the retina and the LGN remains normal because it is wired up prenatally, but the connection between the LGN and V1 is not. When cortical cells fire together abnormally they wire together abnormally. Clinical consequences of this disorder at the primary visual cortex are impaired visual recognition, crowding (nearby stimulus information obscures attended item), poor vernier acuity, poor stereo acuity, poor grating orientation identification acuity, and often near normal grating resolution acuity. The high spatial frequency gratings do not look like uniform gray, so they can be detected, but they are badly distorted, so the amblyope cannot discriminate between vertical and horizontal.

5. fMRI vision science studies

With a basic understading of the visual pathway and its development we can now review fMRI literature. As a result of the increase in general fMRI studies, there has also been an increase of studies investigating many aspects of the vision science. These studies include normal eye movements such as optokinetic nystagmus (OKN) (Bense et al., 2006a;b; Bucher et al., 1997; Dieterich et al., 1998; 2000; 2003; Kashou et al., 2006; Kashou, 2008; Kashou et al., 2010; Konen et al., 2005; Petit & Haxby, 1999; Schraa-Tam et al., 2008), saccades (Berman et al., 1999; Bodis-Wollner et al., 1997; Connolly et al., 2005; Cornelissen et al., 2002; Darby et al., 1996; Ettinger et al., 2008; Haller et al., 2008; Hayakawa et al., 2002; Kimmig et al., 2001; Konen et al., 2004; Luna et al., 1998; Merriam et al., 2001; Miller et al., 2005; Mort et al., 2003; Müri et al., 1996; 1998; Petit et al., 1997; Rosano et al., 2002), smooth pursuit (Barton et al., 1996; Berman et al., 1999; Freitag et al., 1998; Ohlendorf et al., 2010; Petit et al., 1997; Petit & Haxby, 1999; Rosano et al., 2002; Tanabe et al., 2002), and gaze (Andersson et al., 2007; Deutschländer et al., 2005). There have also been studies that look at varying aspects of visual perception such as: effect of age (Lewis et al., 2003; 2004), retinotopic mapping (Conner et al., 2004; Engel & Furmanski, 1997; Hadjikhani et al., 1998; Morland et al., 2001; Murray et al., 2006; Tootell et al., 1997; Warnking et al., 2002), magnocellular (M) and parvocellular (P) pathways (Kleinschmidt et al., 1996; Liu et al., 2006), ocular dominance (Cheng et al., 2001; Goodyear & Menon, 2001; Miki et al., 2001a), binocular rivalry (Lee et al., 2005), illusory contours (Mendola et al., 1999; Seghier et al., 2000), contrast detection (Leguire et al., 2011a; Ress & Heeger, 2003), visual attention (Büchel et al., 1998; Ress et al., 2000), perceptual filling-in (Mendola et al., 2006), lateral geniculate nucleus (LGN) (Büchel et al., 1997; Chen et al., 1998a;b; Chen & Zhu, 2001; Chen et al., 1999; Engel & Furmanski, 1997; Kleinschmidt et al., 1994; Miki et al., 2000; 2001b;c; Morita et al., 2000; Mullen et al., 2010), superior colliculus (SC) (Schneider & Kastner, 2005), motion perception (Paradis et al., 2000; Pelphrey et al., 2005), and illusory perception of real motion (Sterzer et al., 2006). There have also been fMRI studies undertaken for abnormal visual functions such as: amblyopia (Algaze et al., 2002; 2005; Choi et al., 2001; Goodyear et al., 2000; Lee et al., 2001; Leguire et al., 2004a;b; 2011a; Lerner et al., 2006; Lewis et al., 2003; 2004; Muckli et al., 2006; Rogers, 2003; Yang et al., 2003), albinism (Schmitz et al., 2004), infantile nystagmus syndrome (INS) (Leguire et al., 2011b), downbeat nystagmus (DBN) (Hüfner et al., 2007; Kalla et al., 2006), opsoclonus (Helmchen et al., 2003a;b), unilateral vestibular failure (UVF) (Deutschländer et al., 2008), convergence insufficiency (CI) (Alvarez et al., 2010), optic neuritis (ON) (Gareau et al., 1999; Langkilde et al., 2002; Levin et al., 2006; Rombouts et al., 1998; Toosy et al., 2002; 2005; Werring et al., 2000), Autism (Baron-Cohen et al., 2006; Hadjikhani et al., 2004a;b), and macular degeneration (Little et al., 2008; Sunness et al., 2004). Other studies include looking at callosal agenesis and colpocephaly (Bittar et al., 2000), vascular lesions and therapeutic intervention (Schlosser et al., 1997), ischemic lesions (Nyffeler et al., 2011), migrane aura (Hadjikhani et al., 2001), idiopathic Parkinsons disease (Holroyd & Wooten, 2006), Tourette syndrome (Mazzone et al., 2010), bipolar disorder (Martin et al., 2011), and schizophrenia (Nagel et al., 2007; Tregellas et al., 2004; 2005). This is not not an exhaustive but a brief list of fMRI studies related to vision science. We will now discuss some of the results of these studies in normal vision then in pathologies.

6. fMRI and oculomotor function

FMRI studies of the oculomotor function have been mostly limited to normal subjects and have concentrated on voluntary pursuit, saccadic eye movements and optokinetic nystagmus (OKN). Table 1 summarizes the details of these studies, imaging parameters and visual stimuli. Tanabe et al. (2002) have noted that fMRI studies of oculomotor function have employed few subjects and the reliability of mapping-out brain sites involved in oculomotor control have not been established. This statement was made almost 10 years ago and a lot has been accomplished since then. Overall, there appears to be two parallel cortical oculomotor systems for pursuit and saccadic eye movements. Both pursuit and saccadic eye movements appear to activate the same cortical areas including the frontal eye fields (FEF, precentral cortex), supplementary eye fields (SEF, superior frontal cortex), parietal eye fields (PEF, intraparietal cortex), precuneus, and MT/V5. However, pursuit or saccadic eye movements may selectively activate subregions of these cortical areas. Petit & Haxby (1999) found that the pursuit related activation areas were usually smaller than and consistently inferior to and/or posterior to the saccadic related activation areas. Dieterich et al. (2000) have shown that small field horizontal OKN as well as voluntary saccadic eye movements activate areas of both cerebellar hemispheres including the superior semilunar lobule, simple lobule, quadrangular lobule and inferior semilunar lobule. In addition, activation was found in the middle cerebellar peduncle, dentate nucleus, culmen (medially), and uvula of the cerebellar nuclei. Fixation during OKN suppressed activation in the uvula and culmen. Dieterich et al. (1998) also found OKN to activate subcortical areas including the caudate nucleus, putamen, globus pallidus and paramedium thalamus. Fixation increased activity in the FEF and anterior cingulate gyrus. (Dieterich et al., 2000) used a rotating drum that contained "colored figures" to stimulate OKN amplitude that ranged from $2 - 13^o$ visual angle, suggesting a mixture of voluntary and involuntary OKN or only voluntary OKN. Most recently it has been shown that voluntary OKN generates more cortical activation than does involuntary OKN (Kashou et al., 2006; 2010; Konen et al., 2005). Specifically, Kashou et al. (2010) showed that activation sites for OKN studies are dependent on subject instruction which influence the type of OKN generated. Bense et al. (2006a) found that there was no direction dependent activation in cortical eye fields, but there was asymmetry in the paramedian visual cortex areas. Also they found stronger activation in the hemisphere contralateral to slow OKN phase (pursuit). Bense et al. (2006b) found cerebellar activation was localized in the oculomotor vermis. In a comparison of gratings versus dots to stimulate an optokinetic response, the gratings evoked more activation in FEF, PEF, MT/V5 and the cerebellar area VI (Schraa-Tam et al., 2008).

Saccades in humans have been found to activate the precentral sulcus in FEF and in the precuneus along the intraparietal sulcus (IPS), extending in both superior and inferior parietal lobules (Luna et al., 1998). Saccades are traditionally divided into "reflexive" and "voluntary" saccade. Mort et al. (2003), demonstrated that voluntary saccades produced greater activation within FEF and the saccade related area of IPS. In an oculomotor study on oscillatory, predictable and unpredictable saccade, Konen et al. (2004) showed that predictable saccades with the shortest saccadic latency led to the most pronounced cerebral activity both in terms of cortical areas involved and signal intensity. The activation of FEF has also been found to be correlated with saccade reaction time (Connolly et al., 2005). Saccades are also distinguished as either pro or anti if they are made toward or away a stimulus respectively. Cornelissen et al. (2002) found similar BOLD activation in FEF during both pro- and antisaccades. It was suggested in a study looking at functional interactions between pro- and antisaccades that the presupplementary motor area (pre-SMA) coordinates with the FEF to maintain a controlled, preparatory set for task appropriate oculomotor execution (Miller et al., 2005). Saccade frequency and amplitude was varied (Kimmig et al., 2001) and high correlation between frequency and BOLD signal was found along with higher BOLD activation in antisaccades over prosaccades. Merriam et al. (2001) found that comparison of visually guided saccades with fixation revealed activation in all three cortical eye fields: SEF, FEF, and PEF. In

Reference	Type	Resolution	Slices	TR(s)	TE(ms)	Tesla	Stimuli	θ	Shot
Luna et al 1998	Saccade	3.125x3.125x5 gap=1	7	1.5	50	1.5	Circle	90°	1
Kimmig et al 2001	Saccade	2x2x4	16	4	66	1.5	Square	90°	1
Merriam et al 2001	Saccade	3.125x3.125x5 gap=1	7	1.5	50	1.5	Circle	90°	1
Hayakawa et al 2002	Saccade	2.5x2.5x5	25	10	56.05	1.5	Balloon-shaped	90°	1
Mort et al 2003	Saccade	3.75x3.75x4	24	3	50	1.5	Circle	90°	1
Konen et al 2004	Saccade	3x3x4.4	30	4	66	1.5	Square	90°	1
Cornelissen et al 2002	Pro-anti saccade	2x2x4	6	1.5	66	1.5	Spot	90°	1
Connolly et al 2005	Pro-anti saccade	3x3x6	6	0.5	28	4	Cross	30°	1
Miller et al 2005	Pro-anti saccade	3.5x3.5x5 gap=0.5	18	2	28	4	Circle	20°	2
Ettinger et al 2008	Pro-anti saccade	3.75x3.75x5 gap=0.5	–	2	40	1.5	Dot	80°	1
Haller et al 2008	Corrective saccade	3x3x4 gap=1	25	2.5	50	1.5	Dot	90°	1
Petit et al 1997	SPEM, saccade	3.75x3.75x5	26	3	40	1.5	Dot	90°	1
Petit & Haxby 1999	SPEM, saccade	3.75x3.75x5	26	3	40	1.5	Dot	90°	1
Rosano et al 20002	SPEM, saccade	0.8x1.3x3 gap=1	6	4.2	25	3	Spot	90°	2
Freitag et al 1998	SPEM	1.95x1.95x4	10/12/11	5	70	1.5	Dot (Random)	90°	1
Tanabe et al 2002	SPEM	3.75x3.75x6 gap=1	20	2.5	50	1.5	Dot	90°	1
Ohlendorf et al 2010	SPEM	3x3x3	36	2.5	30	3	Dot	90°	1
Konen et al 2005	OKN, SPEM	3x3x4.4	30	4	66	1.5	Gratings, dot	90°	1
Dieterich et al 2003	OKN	1.88x1.88x5	20	5	66	1.5	Rotating drum	90°	1
Bense et al 2006	OKN	3x3x4	40	4.2	60	1.5	Gratings	90°	1
Schraa-Tam et al 2008	OKN	–x–x5 gap=1	22	3	40	1.5	Gratings, dot	90°	1
Kashou et al 2010	OKN	3.75x3.75x5	23	1.5	35	3	Gratings	90°	1
Dieterich et al 1998	h/vOKN	1.95x1.95x5	17	5	40	1.5	Rotating drum	90°	1
Bense et al 2006a	h/vOKN	3x3x4	40	4.31	60	1.5	Gratings	90°	1
Andersson et al 1998	Fixation, gaze	3.75x3.75x5	21	3	60	1.5	Checkerboard	90°	1
Deutschlaender et al 2008	Fixation, gaze	3.75x3.75x3.75	32	4.5	60	1.5	LED	90°	1

Table 1. Specifications of fMRI studies performed on normal eye movements.

addition, the cerebellar vermis (declive and folium) and the bilateral cerebellar hemispheres (superior semilunar lobule) were associated with visually guided saccades (Hayakawa et al., 2002). In differentiating saccade inhibition from generation, the right supramarginal gyrus was responsible for inhibition and the right lateral FEF and bilateral intraparietal sulcus were responsible for antisaccade generation (Ettinger et al., 2008). Unlike pro- and anti-, corrective saccades may also occur, specifically during saccades, pursuit and fixation. This eye movement activated the anterior inferior cingulate, bilateral middle and inferior frontal gyri, bilateral insula and cerebellar areas (Haller et al., 2008).

FEF activation during smooth pursuit performance was found to be smaller than during saccades (Petit et al., 1997). The performance of pursuit eye movements induced activations in the cortical eye fields also activated during the execution of visually guided saccadic eye movements, namely in the precentral cortex [FEF], the medial superior frontal cortex [SEF], the intraparietal cortex [PEF], and the precuneus, and at the junction of occipital and temporal cortex (MT/MST) cortex (Petit & Haxby, 1999). Rosano et al. (2002) localized the saccade-related area to the upper portion of the anterior wall of the precentral sulcus and the pursuit-related area to a deeper region along the anterior wall, extending in some subjects to the fundus or deep posterior wall. It was suggested that the lateral occipitotemporal cortex has extraretinal signals during pursuit (Barton et al., 1996). Significant activation in V1 and V2 in both hemispheres as well as additional bilateral activation in the lateral extent of Brodmann's area 19 and 37 (BA 19/37) was evident during smooth pursuit (Freitag et al., 1998). Pursuit performance, relative to visual fixation, elicited activation in three areas known to contribute to eye movements in humans and in nonhuman primates: the frontal eye field, supplementary eye field, and intraparietal sulcus. It also activated three medial regions not previously identified in human neuroimaging studies of pursuit: the precuneus and the anterior and posterior cingulate cortices. All six areas were also activated during saccades (Berman et al., 1999). Tanabe et al. (2002) found activation consistently in dorsal cortical eye fields and cerebellum. Many studies are still being pursued on normal eye movements with hopes of mapping out or isolating specific anatomical areas responsible with the goal of future diagnostic and therapeutic interventions.

Before moving on to visual dysfunction we want to briefly mention a few visual perception studies. Goodyear & Menon (2001) were the first to demonstrate reproducible high resolution (0.55 mm x 0.55 mm) capabilities of fMRI in humans when using short duration (<6 sec) visual stimuli. Mullen et al. (2010) studied how the responses of the visual pathway to temporal frequency are modified as signals are transfered between the LGN and V1 to the dorsal and ventral streams (V2, V3, VP, V3A, VA, and MT). They concluded that the dorsal and ventral pathways develop characteristic differences in temporal processing that affect chromatic and achromatic stimuli. Differentiation between the magnocellular and parvocellular visual pathways has been recently demonstrated (Liu et al., 2006). Conner et al. (2004) compared retinotopic maps of children with adults in hopes that the study would be useful reference for studies of children with visual disorder, such as amblyopia. Retinotopic mapping is of importance in understanding visual field; a step by step study on this process has been summarized (Warnking et al., 2002). Studying the effects of age showed that the volume and degree of fMRI activation decreased with increasing age, particularly over the age of 40 years (Lewis et al., 2003; 2004).

7. fMRI and visual dysfunction

fMRI studies have been undertaken in normal subjects and in patients with amblyopia, commonly known as lazy-eye (Algaze et al., 2002; 2005; Goodyear et al., 2000; Leguire et al., 2004a;b; 2011a; Lewis et al., 2003; 2004; Rogers, 2003). Goodyear et al. (2000) showed that there were always fewer activated fMRI voxels during amblyopic stimulation than during normal eye stimulation. Algaze et al. (2002) also showed that the volume and level of occipital visual cortical activation was less from the amblyopic eye compared to the dominant eye of amblyopes or to normal eyes. Rogers (2003) and Algaze et al. (2005) have shown that L-dopa, a drug used in the treatment of Parkinson's disease, caused a reduction in volume of activation of occipital visual cortex while it improved visual acuity - a counterintuitive finding. (Yang et al., 2003) showed that the volume ratio between the amblyopic and sound eye stimulation significantly increased after L-dopa treatment. More recently, the amblyopic eye showed marked reduction in activation in the fusiform gyrus, with normal activation in the collateral sulcus (Lerner et al., 2006). Responses to grating stimuli showed reduced responses in higher areas on the central visual pathway (Muckli et al., 2006).

In albinism, there is an abnormal chiasmic projection system which favors the contralateral hemisphere (Schmitz et al., 2004). For example, in oculocutaneous albinism and in ocular albinism, monocular stimulation yields a greater fMRI reponse in the contralateral hemisphere than the ipsilateral hemisphere because of misrouting of the eye's afferents favoring the contralateral hemisphere. After using standard fMRI statistical analysis tools, the number of voxels activated in each hemisphere were counted for each subject. A crossing ratio was then computed by subtracting the voxels activated contralaterally from the ipsilateral ones and dividing by the total number activated. The mean of these ratios for left and right eyes were then calculated for correlations.

Reduced signal and greater asymmetry in the visual cortex has been shown in optic neuritis (ON) patients, compared with controls (Langkilde et al., 2002). They also showed that the volume of visual cortical activation was significantly correlated to the result of the contrast sensitivity test. They used an asymmetry index I_a to calculate the relative difference between size of activated area in the left and right hemisphere, in a similar fashion to the above study. This was done by simply counting the number of voxels in each hemisphere and taking the absolute value of the difference and dividing by the total number of voxels in both hemispheres. A value of $I_a = 1$ meant 100% asymmetry while a value of $I_a = 0$ meant no asymmetry. Toosy et al. (2002) showed that visual cortex activation is reduced during photic stimulation, whilst extra-occipital areas are extensively activated with a peak blood oxygen level dependent response during the OFF phase of the stimulus paradigm. More recently they suggested a genuine adaptive role for cortical reorganization within extrastriate visual areas early after optic neuritis (Toosy et al., 2005). Reduced activation was seen in V1 during stimulation of the affected eye, compared to the normal eye (Levin et al., 2006).

Parents of children with autism or Asperger Syndrome (AS) showed atypical brain function during both visual search and emotion recognition (Baron-Cohen et al., 2006). Hadjikhani et al. (2004a) found that retinotopic maps of individuals with autism were similar to normal subjects, indicating that low level visual processing is normal. A case study by Sunness et al. (2004) illustrated that retinotopic mapping can be performed successfully in patients with central scotomas from macular disease. An increase in the activation of the prefrontal cortex and intraparietal sucli and decrease in the visual cortex was reported in patients with macular degeneration (Little et al., 2008). The ability to look at anatomical reorganization of the visual cortex was demonstrated in a case of callosal agenesis and colpocephaly (Bittar et al., 2000), and in alteration by vascular lesions (Schlosser et al., 1997). Analyzing oculomotor recovery from ischemic lesions in frontal and parietal eye fields using visually triggered saccades has been recently implemented (Nyffeler et al., 2011).

In an eye blink inhibition study, patients with Tourette syndrome showed higher activation in the middle frontal gyrus, dorsal anterior cingulate and temporal cortices compared to controls (Mazzone et al., 2010). Most recently the declive of the cerebellum has been shown to be associated with INS (Leguire et al., 2011b). Similarly the cerbellar vermis, also has been found to be active in patients with bipolar disorder while performing SPEM (Martin et al., 2011). fMRI activation during downward smooth pursuit was less in both flocculi of the cerebellum for patients with DBN than controls (Kalla et al., 2006). Reduced activation in the paraflocular lobule and in the ponto-medullary brainstem of the patients was also seen (Hüfner et al., 2007). Saccadic oscillations in patients with opsoclonus may be a result of disinhibition of the cerebellar fastigial nuclei (Helmchen et al., 2003a;b). Monitoring vision therapy using fMRI for patients with CI revealed increase in activity in the frontal areas, cerebellum and brainstem (Alvarez et al., 2010). Understanding SPEM is also of interest in schizophrenia where greater activity in both posterior hippocampi and the right fusiform gyrus have been reported (Tregellas et al., 2004). The same investigators also found that nicotine was associated with greater activity in the anterior and posterior cingulate gyri, precuneus and area MT/MST and less activity in the hippocampus and parietal eye fields in patients with schizophrenia (Tregellas et al., 2005).

Data from Hadjikhani et al. (2001) suggested that an electrophysiological event such as cortical spreading depression (CSD) generates migraine aura in the visual cortex. This was determined using a standard t statistic computing the difference between activation amplitude during off period preceding aura. The time courses for independent voxels were then extracted from specific visual areas. A reference baseline (mean) and standard deviation was computed on the first 6 cycles and the pixels that exhibited a higher mean plus standard deviation and a standard deviation less than the reference standard deviation for at least 2 cycles were considered as activated. The visual cortex of patients with idiopathic Parkinsons disease with and without visual hallucinations were examined by Holroyd & Wooten (2006). They found that patients with visual hallucinations had increased activation in the visual association cortex and deficits in the primary visual cortex. Again these are samples of the fMRI studies published in literature. Table 2 lists a few pathologies related to vision investigated using fMRI.

Pathology
Albinism
Amblyopia
Autism
Bipolar Disorder
Callosal Agenesis & Colpocephaly
Convergence Insufficiency
Downbeat Nystagmus
Glaucoma
Infantile Nystagmus Syndrome
Ischemic Lesions
Macular Degeneration
Migrane Aura
Opsoclonus
Optic Neuritis
Parkinsons Disease
Schizophrenia
Tourette Syndrome
Vascular Lesions

Table 2. Pathologies investigated using fMRI.

8. Discussion

In this chapter we aimed to discuss the basics of visual development and then review fMRI vision science research. To recap, there are three main principles in visual development: labeled lines, cells firing together wire together, and synaptic competition. In summary, sensory cells send the same kind of signal, regardless of how, or how strongly, they are stimulates (labeled lines). The relations between the retina and the LGN, and between the LGN and the cortex, are crudely wired up at birth, by prenatal "visual" experience of the wave. That wire up is refined and related to the proximal stimulus by genuine postnatal visual experience and synaptic competition. This refinement includes creation of new synapses and culling of old ones.

Abnormalities early in life can cause disorders in the visual pathway. Rod monochromats do not have the normal photoreceptor connections from the retina and thus the rods take over the synaptic fields where the fovea usually falls in V1. Albinos seem to have a dysfunction in the chemical signposts that separate the nasal and temporal retina projections. In refractive amblyopia, there is a blur in the proximal stimuli of one eye and high frequency cells are not fully developed in V1 because they are cut out during the refinement process. Strabismic

amblyopes suffer from an eye turn early on that causes an abnormal wave which leads to miswiring between the LGN and V1.
The use of functional MRI has proved to be a successful imaging modality in understanding the visual development process and for basic research in vision science of controls and patients. Currently, neuroscientists, neurologists, ophthalmologists and others are using this imaging modality extensively to study vision science related problems. Further development of these studies will allow noninvasive diagnostic, pre-, and post- surgical techniques with the aim of improving the clinical sensitivity and specificity for visual cortex diagnosis.

9. Limitations of fMRI interpretation

The key to interpreting fMRI data is to understand the problem being studied. In this chapter some applications from vision science were discussed to show the extensiveness of the field. The more one knows about vision science in general the better they will be able to make an informed interpretation of the fMRI activation. However it is essential to have this knowledge before designing an fMRI study. It is also necessary to have firm knowledge of the MR technology and physics in order to appreciate the complexities and intricacies of the process. This in turn would help minimize errors and confounds in the results. The main limitations of interpretation lies in the knowledge of the user. Unfortunately, some believe that this is a pushbutton technology and whatever comes out is perfect. On the contrary, a good understanding of the field, in this case vision science, the technology, and the art of designing an fMRI experiment, will allow for respect and caution when interpreting and analyzing the data.

10. Future developments in fMRI

The advancement in technology will have the biggest influence on the future developments in fMRI. Most of the studies presented here were on 1.5 or 3 Tesla systems but ultra high field (UHF) 7 and 8 Tesla systems are now regulary being used for human research. The limiting factor for UHF MRI are the head coils, however continuous effort is being made for optimization and improvement. In the next few years 1.5 and even 3 Tesla systems will seem old in the field of research as the new UHF magnets have superior resolution (down to the μm). This will enhance the visualization of cortical areas and allow the parcellation of smaller anatomical regions such as the LGN and allow the functional localization of subregions that otherwise would be bulked into one region in the current scanners. Clinical imaging developments in the short term are focusing on enhancing the 3 Tesla technology by transition from 8 channel head coils to 32 channels so there will be a delay before the UHF systems make their way into hospitals.

11. References

Algaze, A., Roberts, C., Leguire, L., Schmalbrock, P. & Rogers, G. (2002). Functional magnetic resonance imaging as a tool for investigating amblyopia in the human visual cortex: a pilot study., *J AAPOS* 6(5): 300–308.

Algaze, A., Leguire, L. E., Roberts, C., Ibinson, J. W., Lewis, J. R. & Rogers, G. (2005). The effects of l-dopa on the functional magnetic resonance imaging response of patients with amblyopia: a pilot study., *J AAPOS* 9(3): 216–223. URL: *http://dx.doi.org/10.1016/j.jaapos.2005.01.014*

Alvarez, T. L., Vicci, V. R., Alkan, Y., Kim, E. H., Gohel, S., Barrett, A. M., Chiaravalloti, N. & Biswal, B. B. (2010). Vision therapy in adults with convergence insufficiency: clinical and functional magnetic resonance imaging measures., *Optom Vis Sci* 87(12): E985–1002.
URL: *http://dx.doi.org/10.1097/OPX.0b013e3181fef1aa*

Andersson, F., Joliot, M., Perchey, G. & Petit, L. (2007). Eye position-dependent activity in the primary visual area as revealed by fmri., *Hum Brain Mapp* 28(7): 673–680.
URL: *http://dx.doi.org/10.1002/hbm.20296*

Baron-Cohen, S., Ring, H., Chitnis, X., Wheelwright, S., Gregory, L., Williams, S., Brammer, M. & Bullmore, E. (2006). fmri of parents of children with asperger syndrome: a pilot study., *Brain Cogn* 61(1): 122–130.
URL: *http://dx.doi.org/10.1016/j.bandc.2005.12.011*

Barton, J. J., Simpson, T., Kiriakopoulos, E., Stewart, C., Crawley, A., Guthrie, B., Wood, M. & Mikulis, D. (1996). Functional mri of lateral occipitotemporal cortex during pursuit and motion perception., *Ann Neurol* 40(3): 387–398.
URL: *http://dx.doi.org/10.1002/ana.410400308*

Büchel, C., Josephs, O., Rees, G., Turner, R., Frith, C. D. & Friston, K. J. (1998). The functional anatomy of attention to visual motion. a functional mri study., *Brain* 121 (Pt 7): 1281–1294.

Büchel, C., Turner, R. & Friston, K. (1997). Lateral geniculate activations can be detected using intersubject averaging and fmri., *Magn Reson Med* 38(5): 691–694.

Bense, S., Janusch, B., Schlindwein, P., Bauermann, T., Vucurevic, G., Brandt, T., Stoeter, P. & Dieterich, M. (2006). Direction-dependent visual cortex activation during horizontal optokinetic stimulation (fmri study)., *Hum Brain Mapp* 27(4): 296–305.
URL: *http://dx.doi.org/10.1002/hbm.20185*

Bense, S., Janusch, B., Vucurevic, G., Bauermann, T., Schlindwein, P., Brandt, T., Stoeter, P. & Dieterich, M. (2006). Brainstem and cerebellar fmri-activation during horizontal and vertical optokinetic stimulation., *Exp Brain Res* 174(2): 312–323.
URL: *http://dx.doi.org/10.1007/s00221-006-0464-0*

Berman, R. A., Colby, C. L., Genovese, C. R., Voyvodic, J. T., Luna, B., Thulborn, K. R. & Sweeney, J. A. (1999). Cortical networks subserving pursuit and saccadic eye movements in humans: an fmri study., *Hum Brain Mapp* 8(4): 209–225.

Bittar, R. G., Ptito, A., Dumoulin, S. O., Andermann, F. & Reutens, D. C. (2000). Reorganisation of the visual cortex in callosal agenesis and colpocephaly., *J Clin Neurosci* 7(1): 13–15.
URL: *http://dx.doi.org/10.1054/jocn.1998.0105*

Blasdel, G. G., Lund, J. S. & Fitzpatrick, D. (1985). Intrinsic connections of macaque striate cortex: axonal projections of cells outside lamina 4c., *J Neurosci* 5(12): 3350–3369.

Bodis-Wollner, I., Bucher, S. F., Seelos, K. C., Paulus, W., Reiser, M. & Oertel, W. H. (1997). Functional mri mapping of occipital and frontal cortical activity during voluntary and imagined saccades., *Neurology* 49(2): 416–420.

Bucher, S. F., Dieterich, M., Seelos, K. C. & Brandt, T. (1997). Sensorimotor cerebral activation during optokinetic nystagmus. a functional mri study., *Neurology* 49(5): 1370–1377.

Calkins, D. & Hendry, S. (1996). A retinogeniculate pathway expresses the alpha subunit of cam ii kinase in the primate, *Soc. Neurosci. Abstr.* 22: 1447.

Callaway, E. M. & Wiser, A. K. (1996). Contributions of individual layer 2-5 spiny neurons to local circuits in macaque primary visual cortex., *Vis Neurosci* 13(5): 907–922.

Campbell, G. & Shatz, C. J. (1992). Synapses formed by identified retinogeniculate axons during the segregation of eye input., *J Neurosci* 12(5): 1847–1858.

Chen, W., Kato, T., Zhu, X. H., Ogawa, S., Tank, D. W. & Ugurbil, K. (1998). Human primary visual cortex and lateral geniculate nucleus activation during visual imagery., *Neuroreport* 9(16): 3669–3674.

Chen, W., Kato, T., Zhu, X. H., Strupp, J., Ogawa, S. & Ugurbil, K. (1998). Mapping of lateral geniculate nucleus activation during visual stimulation in human brain using fmri., *Magn Reson Med* 39(1): 89–96.

Chen, W. & Zhu, X. H. (2001). Correlation of activation sizes between lateral geniculate nucleus and primary visual cortex in humans., *Magn Reson Med* 45(2): 202–205.

Chen, W., Zhu, X. H., Thulborn, K. R. & Ugurbil, K. (1999). Retinotopic mapping of lateral geniculate nucleus in humans using functional magnetic resonance imaging., *Proc Natl Acad Sci U S A* 96(5): 2430–2434.

Cheng, K., Waggoner, R. A. & Tanaka, K. (2001). Human ocular dominance columns as revealed by high-field functional magnetic resonance imaging., *Neuron* 32(2): 359–374.

Choi, M. Y., Lee, K. M., Hwang, J. M., Choi, D. G., Lee, D. S., Park, K. H. & Yu, Y. S. (2001). Comparison between anisometropic and strabismic amblyopia using functional magnetic resonance imaging., *Br J Ophthalmol* 85(9): 1052–1056.

Conner, I. P., Sharma, S., Lemieux, S. K. & Mendola, J. D. (2004). Retinotopic organization in children measured with fmri., *J Vis* 4(6): 509–523.
URL: *http://dx.doi.org/10:1167/4.6.10*

Connolly, J. D., Goodale, M. A., Goltz, H. C. & Munoz, D. P. (2005). fmri activation in the human frontal eye field is correlated with saccadic reaction time., *J Neurophysiol* 94(1): 605–611.
URL: *http://dx.doi.org/10.1152/jn.00830.2004*

Cornelissen, F. W., Kimmig, H., Schira, M., Rutschmann, R. M., Maguire, R. P., Broerse, A., Boer, J. A. D. & Greenlee, M. W. (2002). Event-related fmri responses in the human frontal eye fields in a randomized pro- and antisaccade task., *Exp Brain Res* 145(2): 270–274.
URL: *http://dx.doi.org/10.1007/s00221-002-1136-3*

Cowan, W. M., Fawcett, J. W., O'Leary, D. D. & Stanfield, B. B. (1984). Regressive events in neurogenesis., *Science* 225(4668): 1258–1265.

Curcio, C. A. & Allen, K. A. (1990). Topography of ganglion cells in human retina., *J Comp Neurol* 300(1): 5–25.
URL: *http://dx.doi.org/10.1002/cne.903000103*

Darby, D. G., Nobre, A. C., Thangaraj, V., Edelman, R., Mesulam, M. M. & Warach, S. (1996). Cortical activation in the human brain during lateral saccades using epistar functional magnetic resonance imaging., *Neuroimage* 3(1): 53–62.
URL: *http://dx.doi.org/10.1006/nimg.1996.0006*

Derrington, A. M. & Lennie, P. (1984). Spatial and temporal contrast sensitivities of neurones in lateral geniculate nucleus of macaque., *J Physiol* 357: 219–240.

Deutschländer, A., Hüfner, K., Kalla, R., Stephan, T., Dera, T., Glasauer, S., Wiesmann, M., Strupp, M. & Brandt, T. (2008). Unilateral vestibular failure suppresses cortical visual motion processing., *Brain* 131(Pt 4): 1025–1034.
URL: *http://dx.doi.org/10.1093/brain/awn035*

Deutschländer, A., Marx, E., Stephan, T., Riedel, E., Wiesmann, M., Dieterich, M. & Brandt, T. (2005). Asymmetric modulation of human visual cortex activity during 10 degrees lateral gaze (fmri study)., *Neuroimage* 28(1): 4–13.
URL: *http://dx.doi.org/10.1016/j.neuroimage.2005.06.001*

Dieterich, M., Bucher, S. F., Seelos, K. C. & Brandt, T. (1998). Horizontal or vertical optokinetic stimulation activates visual motion-sensitive, ocular motor and vestibular cortex areas with right hemispheric dominance. an fmri study., *Brain* 121 (Pt 8): 1479–1495.

Dieterich, M., Bucher, S. F., Seelos, K. C. & Brandt, T. (2000). Cerebellar activation during optokinetic stimulation and saccades., *Neurology* 54(1): 148–155.

Dieterich, M., Bense, S., Stephan, T., Yousry, T. A. & Brandt, T. (2003). fmri signal increases and decreases in cortical areas during small-field optokinetic stimulation and central fixation., *Exp Brain Res* 148(1): 117–127.
URL: *http://dx.doi.org/10.1007/s00221-002-1267-6*

Engel, S. & Furmanski, C. (1997). Neural activity in human lateral geniculate nucleus measured with functional mri., *Invest Ophthalmol Vis Sci* 38(Suppl): 1689.

Ettinger, U., Ffytche, D. H., Kumari, V., Kathmann, N., Reuter, B., Zelaya, F. & Williams, S. C. R. (2008). Decomposing the neural correlates of antisaccade eye movements using event-related fmri., *Cereb Cortex* 18(5): 1148–1159.
URL: *http://dx.doi.org/10.1093/cercor/bhm147*

Fitzpatrick, D., Lund, J. S. & Blasdel, G. G. (1985). Intrinsic connections of macaque striate cortex: afferent and efferent connections of lamina 4c., *J Neurosci* 5(12): 3329–3349.

Fitzpatrick, D., Usrey, W. M., Schofield, B. R. & Einstein, G. (1994). The sublaminar organization of corticogeniculate neurons in layer 6 of macaque striate cortex., *Vis Neurosci* 11(2): 307–315.

Freitag, P., Greenlee, M. W., Lacina, T., Scheffler, K. & Radü, E. W. (1998). Effect of eye movements on the magnitude of functional magnetic resonance imaging responses in extrastriate cortex during visual motion perception., *Exp Brain Res* 119(4): 409–414.

Galli, L. & Maffei, L. (1988). Spontaneous impulse activity of rat retinal ganglion cells in prenatal life., *Science* 242(4875): 90–91.

Gareau, P. J., Gati, J. S., Menon, R. S., Lee, D., Rice, G., Mitchell, J. R., Mandelfino, P. & Karlik, S. J. (1999). Reduced visual evoked responses in multiple sclerosis patients with optic neuritis: comparison of functional magnetic resonance imaging and visual evoked potentials., *Mult Scler* 5(3): 161–164.

Goodman, C. S. & Shatz, C. J. (1993). Developmental mechanisms that generate precise patterns of neuronal connectivity., *Cell* 72 Suppl: 77–98.

Goodyear, B. G. & Menon, R. S. (2001). Brief visual stimulation allows mapping of ocular dominance in visual cortex using fmri., *Hum Brain Mapp* 14(4): 210–217.

Goodyear, B. G., Nicolle, D. A., Humphrey, G. K. & Menon, R. S. (2000). Bold fmri response of early visual areas to perceived contrast in human amblyopia., *J Neurophysiol* 84(4): 1907–1913.

Guillery (1970). The laminar distribution of retinal fibers in the dorsal lateral geniculate nucleus of the cat: a new interpretation, *J. Comp. Neurol.* 138: 339–68.

Hadjikhani, N., Liu, A. K., Dale, A. M., Cavanagh, P. & Tootell, R. B. (1998). Retinotopy and color sensitivity in human visual cortical area v8., *Nat Neurosci* 1(3): 235–241.
URL: *http://dx.doi.org/10.1038/681*

Hadjikhani, N., Rio, M. S. D., Wu, O., Schwartz, D., Bakker, D., Fischl, B., Kwong, K. K., Cutrer, F. M., Rosen, B. R., Tootell, R. B., Sorensen, A. G. & Moskowitz, M. A. (2001). Mechanisms of migraine aura revealed by functional mri in human visual cortex., *Proc Natl Acad Sci U S A* 98(8): 4687–4692.
URL: *http://dx.doi.org/10.1073/pnas.071582498*

Hadjikhani, N., Joseph, R. M., Snyder, J., Chabris, C. F., Clark, J., Steele, S., McGrath, L., Vangel, M., Aharon, I., Feczko, E., Harris, G. J. & Tager-Flusberg, H. (2004).

Activation of the fusiform gyrus when individuals with autism spectrum disorder view faces., *Neuroimage* 22(3): 1141–1150.
URL: *http://dx.doi.org/10.1016/j.neuroimage.2004.03.025*

Hadjikhani, N., Chabris, C. F., Joseph, R. M., Clark, J., McGrath, L., Aharon, I., Feczko, E., Tager-Flusberg, H. & Harris, G. J. (2004). Early visual cortex organization in autism: an fmri study., *Neuroreport* 15(2): 267–270.

Haller, S., Fasler, D., Ohlendorf, S., Radue, E. W. & Greenlee, M. W. (2008). Neural activation associated with corrective saccades during tasks with fixation, pursuit and saccades., *Exp Brain Res* 184(1): 83–94.
URL: *http://dx.doi.org/10.1007/s00221-007-1077-y*

Hayakawa, Y., Nakajima, T., Takagi, M., Fukuhara, N. & Abe, H. (2002). Human cerebellar activation in relation to saccadic eye movements: a functional magnetic resonance imaging study., *Ophthalmologica* 216(6): 399–405.
URL: *http://dx.doi.org/10.1159/000067551*

Helmchen, C., Rambold, H., Sprenger, A., Erdmann, C., & Binkofski, F. (2003). Cerebellar activation in opsoclonus: an fmri study., *Neurology* 61(3): 412–415.

Helmchen, C., Rambold, H., Erdmann, C., Mohr, C., Sprenger, A. & Binkofski, F. (2003). The role of the fastigial nucleus in saccadic eye oscillations., *Ann N Y Acad Sci* 1004: 229–240.

Hendry, S. H. & Reid, R. C. (2000). The koniocellular pathway in primate vision., *Annu Rev Neurosci* 23: 127–153.
URL: *http://dx.doi.org/10.1146/annurev.neuro.23.1.127*

Hendry, S. H. & Yoshioka, T. (1994). A neurochemically distinct third channel in the macaque dorsal lateral geniculate nucleus., *Science* 264(5158): 575–577.

Hüfner, K., Stephan, T., Kalla, R., Deutschländer, A., Wagner, J., Holtmannspötter, M., Schulte-Altedorneburg, G., Strupp, M., Brandt, T. & Glasauer, S. (2007). Structural and functional mris disclose cerebellar pathologies in idiopathic downbeat nystagmus., *Neurology* 69(11): 1128–1135.
URL: *http://dx.doi.org/10.1212/01.wnl.0000276953.00969.48*

Holmes, G. (1918). Disturbances of vision by cerebral lesions., *Br J Ophthalmol* 2(7): 353–384.

Holmes, G. (1944). The organization of the visual cortex in man., *Proc. R. Soc. London Ser. B* 132: 348–61.

Holroyd, S. & Wooten, G. F. (2006). Preliminary fmri evidence of visual system dysfunction in parkinson's disease patients with visual hallucinations., *J Neuropsychiatry Clin Neurosci* 18(3): 402–404.
URL: *http://dx.doi.org/10.1176/appi.neuropsych.18.3.402*

Horton, J. C. & Hoyt, W. F. (1991). The representation of the visual field in human striate cortex. a revision of the classic holmes map., *Arch Ophthalmol* 109(6): 816–824.

Horton, J. C. & Hubel, D. H. (1981). Regular patchy distribution of cytochrome oxidase staining in primary visual cortex of macaque monkey., *Nature* 292(5825): 762–764.

Hubel, D. H. & Wiesel, T. N. (1977). Ferrier lecture. functional architecture of macaque monkey visual cortex., *Proc R Soc Lond B Biol Sci* 198(1130): 1–59.

Humphrey, A. L. & Hendrickson, A. E. (1980). Radial zones of high metabolic activity in squirrel monkey striate cortex., *Soe.Neurosci. Abstr.* 6: 315.

Kaas, J. H., Guillery, R. W. & Allman, J. M. (1972). Some principles of organization in the dorsal lateral geniculate nucleus., *Brain Behav Evol* 6(1): 253–299.

Kaas, J. H., Huerta, M. F., Weber, J. T. & Harting, J. K. (1978). Patterns of retinal terminations and laminar organization of the lateral geniculate nucleus of primates., *J Comp Neurol*

182(3): 517–553.
URL: *http://dx.doi.org/10.1002/cne.901820308*

Kalla, R., Deutschlander, A., Hufner, K., Stephan, T., Jahn, K., Glasauer, S., Brandt, T. & Strupp, M. (2006). Detection of floccular hypometabolism in downbeat nystagmus by fmri., *Neurology* 66(2): 281–283.
URL: *http://dx.doi.org/10.1212/01.wnl.0000194242.28018.d9*

Kashou, N., Leguire, L. & Roberts, C. (2006). fmri on look vs stare optokinetic nystagmus (okn), *Invest Ophthal and Vis Sci* 47: 5873.

Kashou, N. H. (2008). *Development of Functional Studies and Methods to Better Understand Visual Function.*, PhD thesis, The Ohio State University.

Kashou, N. H., Leguire, L. E., Roberts, C. J., Fogt, N., Smith, M. A. & Rogers, G. L. (2010). Instruction dependent activation during optokinetic nystagmus (okn) stimulation: An fmri study at 3t., *Brain Res* 1336: 10–21.
URL: *http://dx.doi.org/10.1016/j.brainres.2010.04.017*

Kimmig, H., Greenlee, M. W., Gondan, M., Schira, M., Kassubek, J. & Mergner, T. (2001). Relationship between saccadic eye movements and cortical activity as measured by fmri: quantitative and qualitative aspects., *Exp Brain Res* 141(2): 184–194.
URL: *http://dx.doi.org/10.1007/s002210100844*

Kleinschmidt, A., Merboldt, K. D., Hänicke, W., Steinmetz, H. & Frahm, J. (1994). Correlational imaging of thalamocortical coupling in the primary visual pathway of the human brain., *J Cereb Blood Flow Metab* 14(6): 952–957.

Kleinschmidt, A., Obrig, H., Requardt, M., Merboldt, K. D., Dirnagl, U., Villringer, A. & Frahm, J. (1996). Simultaneous recording of cerebral blood oxygenation changes during human brain activation by magnetic resonance imaging and near-infrared spectroscopy., *J Cereb Blood Flow Metab* 16(5): 817–826.
URL: *http://dx.doi.org/10.1097/00004647-199609000-00006*

Konen, C. S., Kleiser, R., Seitz, R. J. & Bremmer, F. (2005). An fmri study of optokinetic nystagmus and smooth-pursuit eye movements in humans., *Exp Brain Res* 165(2): 203–216.
URL: *http://dx.doi.org/10.1007/s00221-005-2289-7*

Konen, C. S., Kleiser, R., Wittsack, H.-J., Bremmer, F. & Seitz, R. J. (2004). The encoding of saccadic eye movements within human posterior parietal cortex., *Neuroimage* 22(1): 304–314.
URL: *http://dx.doi.org/10.1016/j.neuroimage.2003.12.039*

Lachica, E. A., Beck, P. D. & Casagrande, V. A. (1992). Parallel pathways in macaque monkey striate cortex: anatomically defined columns in layer iii., *Proc Natl Acad Sci U S A* 89(8): 3566–3570.

Langkilde, A. R., Frederiksen, J. L., Rostrup, E. & Larsson, H. B. W. (2002). Functional mri of the visual cortex and visual testing in patients with previous optic neuritis., *Eur J Neurol* 9(3): 277–286.

Lee, K. M., Lee, S. H., Kim, N. Y., Kim, C. Y., Sohn, J. W., Choi, M. Y., Choi, D. G., Hwang, J. M., Park, K. H., Lee, D. S., Yu, Y. S. & Chang, K. H. (2001). Binocularity and spatial frequency dependence of calcarine activation in two types of amblyopia., *Neurosci Res* 40(2): 147–153.

Lee, S.-H., Blake, R. & Heeger, D. J. (2005). Traveling waves of activity in primary visual cortex during binocular rivalry., *Nat Neurosci* 8(1): 22–23.
URL: *http://dx.doi.org/10.1038/nn1365*

Leguire, L., Algaze, A., Murakami, J., Rogers, G. & Roberts, C. (2004). fmri more closely follows contrast sensitivity than visual acuity., *Invest Ophthal and Vis Sci.*

Leguire, L., Algaze, A., Murakami, J., Rogers, G., Lewis, J. & Roberts, C. (2004). Relation among fmri, visual acuity and csf., *American Association of Pediatric Ophthalmology and Strabismus.*

Leguire, L. E., Algaze, A., Kashou, N. H., Lewis, J., Rogers, G. L. & Roberts, C. (2011). Relationship among fmri, contrast sensitivity and visual acuity., *Brain Res* 1367: 162–169.
URL: *http://dx.doi.org/10.1016/j.brainres.2010.10.082*

Leguire, L. E., Kashou, N. H., Fogt, N., Smith, M. A., Lewis, J. R., Kulwin, R. & Rogers, G. L. (2011). Neural circuit involved in idiopathic infantile nystagmus syndrome based on fmri., *J Pediatr Ophthalmol Strabismus* pp. 1–10.
URL: *http://dx.doi.org/10.3928/01913913-20110118-03*

Lennie, P., Krauskopf, J. & Sclar, G. (1990). Chromatic mechanisms in striate cortex of macaque., *J Neurosci* 10(2): 649–669.

Lerner, Y., Hendler, T., Malach, R., Harel, M., Leiba, H., Stolovitch, C. & Pianka, P. (2006). Selective fovea-related deprived activation in retinotopic and high-order visual cortex of human amblyopes., *Neuroimage* 33(1): 169–179.
URL: *http://dx.doi.org/10.1016/j.neuroimage.2006.06.026*

Levin, N., Orlov, T., Dotan, S. & Zohary, E. (2006). Normal and abnormal fmri activation patterns in the visual cortex after recovery from optic neuritis., *Neuroimage* 33(4): 1161–1168.
URL: *http://dx.doi.org/10.1016/j.neuroimage.2006.07.030*

Lewis, J., Algaze, A., Leguire, L., Rogers, G., Murakami, J. & Roberts, C. (2003). Age effects on fmri using grating stimuli, *Association for Research in Vision and Ophthalmology.*

Lewis, J., Algaze, A., Leguire, L., Rogers, G., Murakami, J. & Roberts, C. (2004). Age effect on fmri using grating stimuli., *American Association of Pediatric Ophthalmology and Strabismus.*

Lichtman, J. W., Burden, S. J., Culican, S. M. & Wong, R. O. L. (1999). *Fundamental Neuroscience*, Acad. Press, chapter Synapse formation and elimination., pp. 547–580.

Linden, D. C., Guillery, R. W. & Cucchiaro, J. (1981). The dorsal lateral geniculate nucleus of the normal ferret and its postnatal development., *J Comp Neurol* 203(2): 189–211.
URL: *http://dx.doi.org/10.1002/cne.902030204*

Little, D. M., Thulborn, K. R. & Szlyk, J. P. (2008). An fmri study of saccadic and smooth-pursuit eye movement control in patients with age-related macular degeneration., *Invest Ophthalmol Vis Sci* 49(4): 1728–1735.
URL: *http://dx.doi.org/10.1167/iovs.07-0372*

Liu, C.-S. J., Bryan, R. N., Miki, A., Woo, J. H., Liu, G. T. & Elliott, M. A. (2006). Magnocellular and parvocellular visual pathways have different blood oxygen level-dependent signal time courses in human primary visual cortex., *AJNR Am J Neuroradiol* 27(8): 1628–1634.

Luna, B., Thulborn, K. R., Strojwas, M. H., McCurtain, B. J., Berman, R. A., Genovese, C. R. & Sweeney, J. A. (1998). Dorsal cortical regions subserving visually guided saccades in humans: an fmri study., *Cereb Cortex* 8(1): 40–47.

Lund, J. & Boothe, R. (1975). Interlaminar connections and pyramidal neuron organization in the visual cortex, area 17, of the macaque monkey., *J. Comp. Neurology* 159: 305–334.

Lund, J. S. (1988). Anatomical organization of macaque monkey striate visual cortex., *Annu Rev Neurosci* 11: 253–288.
URL: *http://dx.doi.org/10.1146/annurev.ne.11.030188.001345*

Lund, J. S., Henry, G. H., MacQueen, C. L. & Harvey, A. R. (1979). Anatomical organization of the primary visual cortex (area 17) of the cat. a comparison with area 17 of the macaque monkey., *J Comp Neurol* 184(4): 599–618.
URL: *http://dx.doi.org/10.1002/cne.901840402*

Martin, L. F., Olincy, A., Ross, R. G., Du, Y. P., Singel, D., Shatti, S. & Tregellas, J. R. (2011). Cerebellar hyperactivity during smooth pursuit eye movements in bipolar disorder., *J Psychiatr Res* 45(5): 670–677.
URL: *http://dx.doi.org/10.1016/j.jpsychires.2010.09.015*

Mazzone, L., Yu, S., Blair, C., Gunter, B. C., Wang, Z., Marsh, R. & Peterson, B. S. (2010). An fmri study of frontostriatal circuits during the inhibition of eye blinking in persons with tourette syndrome., *Am J Psychiatry* 167(3): 341–349.
URL: *http://dx.doi.org/10.1176/appi.ajp.2009.08121831*

Meissirel, C., Wikler, K. C., Chalupa, L. M. & Rakic, P. (1997). Early divergence of magnocellular and parvocellular functional subsystems in the embryonic primate visual system., *Proc Natl Acad Sci U S A* 94(11): 5900–5905.

Meister, M., Wong, R. O., Baylor, D. A. & Shatz, C. J. (1991). Synchronous bursts of action potentials in ganglion cells of the developing mammalian retina., *Science* 252(5008): 939–943.

Mendola, J. D., Conner, I. P., Sharma, S., Bahekar, A. & Lemieux, S. (2006). fmri measures of perceptual filling-in in the human visual cortex., *J Cogn Neurosci* 18(3): 363–375.
URL: *http://dx.doi.org/10.1162/089892906775990624*

Mendola, J. D., Dale, A. M., Fischl, B., Liu, A. K. & Tootell, R. B. (1999). The representation of illusory and real contours in human cortical visual areas revealed by functional magnetic resonance imaging., *J Neurosci* 19(19): 8560–8572.

Merigan, W. H. & Maunsell, J. H. (1993). How parallel are the primate visual pathways?, *Annu Rev Neurosci* 16: 369–402.
URL: *http://dx.doi.org/10.1146/annurev.ne.16.030193.002101*

Merriam, E. P., Colby, C. L., Thulborn, K. R., Luna, B., Olson, C. R. & Sweeney, J. A. (2001). Stimulus-response incompatibility activates cortex proximate to three eye fields., *Neuroimage* 13(5): 794–800.
URL: *http://dx.doi.org/10.1006/nimg.2000.0742*

Miki, A., Raz, J., Haselgrove, J. C., van Erp, T. G., Liu, C. S. & Liu, G. T. (2000). Functional magnetic resonance imaging of lateral geniculate nucleus at 1.5 tesla., *J Neuroophthalmol* 20(4): 285–287.

Miki, A., Liu, G. T., Fletcher, D. W., Hunter, J. V. & Haselgrove, J. C. (2001). Ocular dominance in anterior visual cortex in a child demonstrated by the use of fmri., *Pediatr Neurol* 24(3): 232–234.

Miki, A., Liu, G., Modestino, E., Liu, C. & Englander, S. (2001). Functional magnetic resonance imaging of lateral geniculate nucleus and visual cortex at 4 tesla in a patient with homonymous hemianopia., *Neuro-ophthalmology* 25: 109–14.

Miki, A., Liu, G. T., Raz, J., Englander, S. A., Bonhomme, G. R., Aleman, D. O., Modestino, E. J., Liu, C. S. & Haselgrove, J. C. (2001). Visual activation in functional magnetic resonance imaging at very high field (4 tesla)., *J Neuroophthalmol* 21(1): 8–11.

Miller, L. M., Sun, F. T., Curtis, C. E. & D'Esposito, M. (2005). Functional interactions between oculomotor regions during prosaccades and antisaccades., *Hum Brain Mapp*

26(2): 119–127.
URL: *http://dx.doi.org/10.1002/hbm.20146*

Morita, T., Kochiyama, T., Yamada, H., Konishi, Y., Yonekura, Y., Matsumura, M. & Sadato, N. (2000). Difference in the metabolic response to photic stimulation of the lateral geniculate nucleus and the primary visual cortex of infants: a fmri study., *Neurosci Res* 38(1): 63–70.

Morland, A. B., Baseler, H. A., Hoffmann, M. B., Sharpe, L. T. & Wandell, B. A. (2001). Abnormal retinotopic representations in human visual cortex revealed by fmri., *Acta Psychol (Amst)* 107(1-3): 229–247.

Mort, D. J., Perry, R. J., Mannan, S. K., Hodgson, T. L., Anderson, E., Quest, R., McRobbie, D., McBride, A., Husain, M. & Kennard, C. (2003). Differential cortical activation during voluntary and reflexive saccades in man., *Neuroimage* 18(2): 231–246.

Müri, R. M., Iba-Zizen, M. T., Derosier, C., Cabanis, E. A. & Pierrot-Deseilligny, C. (1996). Location of the human posterior eye field with functional magnetic resonance imaging., *J Neurol Neurosurg Psychiatry* 60(4): 445–448.

Müri, R. M., Heid, O., Nirkko, A. C., Ozdoba, C., Felblinger, J., Schroth, G. & Hess, C. W. (1998). Functional organisation of saccades and antisaccades in the frontal lobe in humans: a study with echo planar functional magnetic resonance imaging., *J Neurol Neurosurg Psychiatry* 65(3): 374–377.

Muckli, L., Kiess, S., Tonhausen, N., Singer, W., Goebel, R. & Sireteanu, R. (2006). Cerebral correlates of impaired grating perception in individual, psychophysically assessed human amblyopes., *Vision Res* 46(4): 506–526.
URL: *http://dx.doi.org/10.1016/j.visres.2005.10.014*

Mullen, K. T., Thompson, B. & Hess, R. F. (2010). Responses of the human visual cortex and lgn to achromatic and chromatic temporal modulations: an fmri study., *J Vis* 10(13): 13.
URL: *http://dx.doi.org/10.1167/10.13.13*

Murray, S. O., Olman, C. A. & Kersten, D. (2006). Spatially specific fmri repetition effects in human visual cortex., *J Neurophysiol* 95(4): 2439–2445.
URL: *http://dx.doi.org/10.1152/jn.01236.2005*

Nagel, M., Sprenger, A., Nitschke, M., Zapf, S., Heide, W., Binkofski, F. & Lencer, R. (2007). Different extraretinal neuronal mechanisms of smooth pursuit eye movements in schizophrenia: An fmri study., *Neuroimage* 34(1): 300–309.
URL: *http://dx.doi.org/10.1016/j.neuroimage.2006.08.025*

Nguyen, Q. T. & Lichtman, J. W. (1996). Mechanism of synapse disassembly at the developing neuromuscular junction., *Curr Opin Neurobiol* 6(1): 104–112.

Nyffeler, T., Hubl, D., Wurtz, P., Wiest, R., Hess, C. W. & Müri, R. M. (2011). Spontaneous recovery of visually-triggered saccades after focal lesions of the frontal and parietal eye fields: a combined longitudinal oculomotor and fmri study., *Clin Neurophysiol* 122(6): 1203–1210.
URL: *http://dx.doi.org/10.1016/j.clinph.2010.08.026*

Ohlendorf, S., Sprenger, A., Speck, O., Glauche, V., Haller, S. & Kimmig, H. (2010). Visual motion, eye motion, and relative motion: A parametric fmri study of functional specializations of smooth pursuit eye movement network areas., *J Vis* 10(14): 21.
URL: *http://dx.doi.org/10.1167/10.14.21*

Osterberg, G. (1935). Topography of the layer of rods and cones in the human retina, *Acta Ophthalmol Suppl* 6: 1–103.

Paradis, A. L., Cornilleau-Pérès, V., Droulez, J., Moortele, P. F. V. D., Lobel, E., Berthoz, A., Bihan, D. L. & Poline, J. B. (2000). Visual perception of motion and 3-d structure from motion: an fmri study., *Cereb Cortex* 10(8): 772–783.

Pelphrey, K. A., Morris, J. P., Michelich, C. R., Allison, T. & McCarthy, G. (2005). Functional anatomy of biological motion perception in posterior temporal cortex: an fmri study of eye, mouth and hand movements., *Cereb Cortex* 15(12): 1866–1876.
URL: *http://dx.doi.org/10.1093/cercor/bhi064*

Perry, V. H., Oehler, R. & Cowey, A. (1984). Retinal ganglion cells that project to the dorsal lateral geniculate nucleus in the macaque monkey., *Neuroscience* 12(4): 1101–1123.

Petit, L., Clark, V. P., Ingeholm, J. & Haxby, J. V. (1997). Dissociation of saccade-related and pursuit-related activation in human frontal eye fields as revealed by fmri., *J Neurophysiol* 77(6): 3386–3390.

Petit, L. & Haxby, J. V. (1999). Functional anatomy of pursuit eye movements in humans as revealed by fmri., *J Neurophysiol* 82(1): 463–471.

Purpura, K., Kaplan, E. & Shapley, R. M. (1988). Background light and the contrast gain of primate p and m retinal ganglion cells., *Proc Natl Acad Sci U S A* 85(12): 4534–4537.

Purpura, K., Tranchina, D., Kaplan, E. & Shapley, R. M. (1990). Light adaptation in the primate retina: analysis of changes in gain and dynamics of monkey retinal ganglion cells., *Vis Neurosci* 4(1): 75–93.

Purves, D. & Lichtman, J. (1985). *Principles of Neural Development*, Sinauer.

Rakic, P. (1976). Prenatal genesis of connections subserving ocular dominance in the rhesus monkey., *Nature* 261(5560): 467–471.

Rakic, P. (1977). Prenatal development of the visual system in rhesus monkey., *Philos Trans R Soc Lond B Biol Sci* 278(961): 245–260.

Ress, D., Backus, B. T. & Heeger, D. J. (2000). Activity in primary visual cortex predicts performance in a visual detection task., *Nat Neurosci* 3(9): 940–945.
URL: *http://dx.doi.org/10.1038/78856*

Ress, D. & Heeger, D. J. (2003). Neuronal correlates of perception in early visual cortex., *Nat Neurosci* 6(4): 414–420.
URL: *http://dx.doi.org/10.1038/nn1024*

Rogers, G. L. (2003). Functional magnetic resonance imaging (fmri) and effects of l-dopa on visual function in normal and amblyopic subjects., *Trans Am Ophthalmol Soc* 101: 401–415.

Rombouts, S. A., Lazeron, R. H., Scheltens, P., Uitdehaag, B. M., Sprenger, M., Valk, J. & Barkhof, F. (1998). Visual activation patterns in patients with optic neuritis: an fmri pilot study., *Neurology* 50(6): 1896–1899.

Rosano, C., Krisky, C. M., Welling, J. S., Eddy, W. F., Luna, B., Thulborn, K. R. & Sweeney, J. A. (2002). Pursuit and saccadic eye movement subregions in human frontal eye field: a high-resolution fmri investigation., *Cereb Cortex* 12(2): 107–115.

Sawatari, A. & Callaway, E. M. (2000). Diversity and cell type specificity of local excitatory connections to neurons in layer 3b of monkey primary visual cortex., *Neuron* 25(2): 459–471.

Schiller, P. H. & Malpeli, J. G. (1978). Functional specificity of lateral geniculate nucleus laminae of the rhesus monkey., *J Neurophysiol* 41(3): 788–797.

Schlosser, M. J., McCarthy, G., Fulbright, R. K., Gore, J. C. & Awad, I. A. (1997). Cerebral vascular malformations adjacent to sensorimotor and visual cortex. functional magnetic resonance imaging studies before and after therapeutic intervention., *Stroke* 28(6): 1130–1137.

Schmitz, B., Käsmann-Kellner, B., Schäfer, T., Krick, C. M., Grön, G., Backens, M. & Reith, W. (2004). Monocular visual activation patterns in albinism as revealed by functional magnetic resonance imaging., *Hum Brain Mapp* 23(1): 40–52.
URL: *http://dx.doi.org/10.1002/hbm.20046*

Schneider, K. A. & Kastner, S. (2005). Visual responses of the human superior colliculus: a high-resolution functional magnetic resonance imaging study., *J Neurophysiol* 94(4): 2491–2503.
URL: *http://dx.doi.org/10.1152/jn.00288.2005*

Schraa-Tam, C. K. L., van der Lugt, A., Smits, M., Frens, M. A., van Broekhoven, P. C. A. & van der Geest, J. N. (2008). fmri of optokinetic eye movements with and without a contribution of smooth pursuit., *J Neuroimaging* 18(2): 158–167.
URL: *http://dx.doi.org/10.1111/j.1552-6569.2007.00204.x*

Schwartz (2004). *Visual perception: a clinical orientation*, McGraw-Hill.

Sclar, G., Maunsell, J. H. & Lennie, P. (1990). Coding of image contrast in central visual pathways of the macaque monkey., *Vision Res* 30(1): 1–10.

Seghier, M., Dojat, M., Delon-Martin, C., Rubin, C., Warnking, J., Segebarth, C. & Bullier, J. (2000). Moving illusory contours activate primary visual cortex: an fmri study., *Cereb Cortex* 10(7): 663–670.

Shapley, R., Kaplan, E. & Soodak, R. (1981). Spatial summation and contrast sensitivity of x and y cells in the lateral geniculate nucleus of the macaque., *Nature* 292(5823): 543–545.

Shapley, R. & Perry, V. (1986). Cat and monkey ganglion cells and their visual functional roles.., *Trends Neuroscience* 9: 229–235.

Shatz, C. J. & Kirkwood, P. A. (1984). Prenatal development of functional connections in the cat's retinogeniculate pathway., *J Neurosci* 4(5): 1378–1397.

Sincich, L. C. & Horton, J. C. (2005). The circuitry of v1 and v2: integration of color, form, and motion., *Annu Rev Neurosci* 28: 303–326.
URL: *http://dx.doi.org/10.1146/annurev.neuro.28.061604.135731*

Sterzer, P., Haynes, J.-D. & Rees, G. (2006). Primary visual cortex activation on the path of apparent motion is mediated by feedback from hmt+/v5., *Neuroimage* 32(3): 1308–1316.
URL: *http://dx.doi.org/10.1016/j.neuroimage.2006.05.029*

Sunness, J. S., Liu, T. & Yantis, S. (2004). Retinotopic mapping of the visual cortex using functional magnetic resonance imaging in a patient with central scotomas from atrophic macular degeneration., *Ophthalmology* 111(8): 1595–1598.
URL: *http://dx.doi.org/10.1016/j.ophtha.2003.12.050*

Tanabe, J., Tregellas, J., Miller, D., Ross, R. G. & Freedman, R. (2002). Brain activation during smooth-pursuit eye movements., *Neuroimage* 17(3): 1315–1324.

Toosy, A. T., Werring, D. J., Bullmore, E. T., Plant, G. T., Barker, G. J., Miller, D. H. & Thompson, A. J. (2002). Functional magnetic resonance imaging of the cortical response to photic stimulation in humans following optic neuritis recovery., *Neurosci Lett* 330(3): 255–259.

Toosy, A. T., Hickman, S. J., Miszkiel, K. A., Jones, S. J., Plant, G. T., Altmann, D. R., Barker, G. J., Miller, D. H. & Thompson, A. J. (2005). Adaptive cortical plasticity in higher visual areas after acute optic neuritis., *Ann Neurol* 57(5): 622–633.
URL: *http://dx.doi.org/10.1002/ana.20448*

Tootell, R. B., Mendola, J. D., Hadjikhani, N. K., Ledden, P. J., Liu, A. K., Reppas, J. B., Sereno, M. I. & Dale, A. M. (1997). Functional analysis of v3a and related areas in human visual cortex., *J Neurosci* 17(18): 7060–7078.

Tregellas, J. R., Tanabe, J. L., Miller, D. E., Ross, R. G., Olincy, A. & Freedman, R. (2004). Neurobiology of smooth pursuit eye movement deficits in schizophrenia: an fmri study., *Am J Psychiatry* 161(2): 315–321.

Tregellas, J. R., Tanabe, J. L., Martin, L. F. & Freedman, R. (2005). Fmri of response to nicotine during a smooth pursuit eye movement task in schizophrenia., *Am J Psychiatry* 162(2): 391–393.
URL: *http://dx.doi.org/10.1176/appi.ajp.162.2.391*

Warnking, J., Dojat, M., Guérin-Dugué, A., Delon-Martin, C., Olympieff, S., Richard, N., Chéhikian, A. & Segebarth, C. (2002). fmri retinotopic mapping–step by step., *Neuroimage* 17(4): 1665–1683.

Werring, D., Bullmore, E., Toosy, A., Miller, D., Barker, G., MacManus, D., Brammer, M., Giampietro, V., Brusa, A., Brex, P., Moseley, I., Plant, G., McDonald, W. & Thompson, A. (2000). Recovery from optic neuritis is associated with a change in the distribution of cerebral response to visual stimulation: a functional magnetic resonance imaging study., *J Neurol Neurosurg Psychiatry* 68: 441–9.

Wiesel, T. N. (1982). Postnatal development of the visual cortex and the influence of environment., *Nature* 299(5884): 583–591.

Wong, R. (1999.). Retinal waves and visual system development., *Annu. Rev. Neurosci.* 22: 29–47.

Yang, C.-I., Yang, M.-L., Huang, J.-C., Wan, Y.-L., Tsai, R. J.-F., Wai, Y.-Y. & Liu, H.-L. (2003). Functional mri of amblyopia before and after levodopa., *Neurosci Lett* 339(1): 49–52.

Yazar, F., Mavity-Hudson, J., Ding, Y., Oztas, E. & Casagrande, V. (2004). Layer iiib-beta of primary visual cortex (v1) and its relationship to the koniocellular (k) pathway in macaque., *Soc.Neurosci. Abstr.* 34: 300.

2

Physiological Basis and Image Processing in Functional Magnetic Resonance Imaging: Neuronal and Motor Activity in Brain

Rakesh Sharma[1] and Avdhesh Sharma[2,3]
[1]*Amity Institute of Nanotechnology, Amity University, Uttar Pradesh, NOIDA*
[2]*Department of Electrical Engineering, Indian Institute of Technology Rajasthan, Jodhpur,*
[3]*Department of Electrical Engineering, Jai Narain Vyas University, Jodhpur Rajasthan, India*

1. Introduction

Functional magnetic resonance imaging or functional MRI (fMRI) is a type of specialized MRI scan used to measure the hemodynamic response (change in blood flow) related to neural activity in the brain or spinal cord of humans. Blood-oxygen-level dependence (BOLD) is the MRI contrast of blood deoxyhemoglobin, first discovered in 1990 by Seiji Ogawa at AT&T Bell labs and Functional Magnetic Resonance Imaging (fMRI) was soon introduced to map the changes in brain local blood flow, oxygenation or hemodynamics that correspond to regional neuronal activity of brain accompanying metabolic events [Ogawa et al. 1990]. Recent investigations focused on specific brain regional and functional specificity to delineate the specific distribution of neural activities at a given moment in the brain as a whole. It extended for brain anatomical imaging to map different structures and specific function of human brain. Present time, high resolution, noninvasive neural activity by a blood oxygen level dependent signal by fMRI has tremendous potentials for assessing the neurological status and neurosurgical risk [Tegeler et al. 1999; Lee et al. 1999; Singh et al. 2003; Bandettini et al. 2001]. Now fMRI applications have extended the understanding of neuronal and motor activities associated with different brain regional functions with additional information down to perfusion/diffusion of neurochemicals to cause neuroactivation. Presently, fMRI serves as non-invasive imaging and evaluation of neurophysiological/neuropsychological activities of brain that depend more on uncontrolled physiological motion in brain and functional characteristics of different locations such as cognition, sensory and motor active areas.

Present chapter serves a handful guide to practicing physician experts in fMRI. Functional magnetic resonance imaging (fMRI) is recently developing as imaging modality used for mapping hemodynamics of neuronal and motor event related tissue blood oxygen level dependence (BOLD) in terms of brain activation. In first section, we describe functional MR signal origin, physical basis of fMRI data generation, its physiological dependence on oxygen state in flowing blood and neuroactivation mechanism. In next section, image processing is described as performed by segmentation and registration methods. In next section, segmentation algorithms are illustrated to provide brain surface-based analysis, automated anatomical labeling of cortical fields in magnetic resonance data sets based on oxygen metabolic state. In next section, registration algorithms are illustrated to provide geometric features using two or more imaging modalities to assure clinically useful neuronal and motor information of brain activation. In nutshell, present chapter introduces basic concepts of fMRI and reviews the physiological basis of fMRI signal origin and contrast mechanisms with state-of-art fMRI segmentation and registration algorithms to identify cortical visual response and event related cortical areas associated with neurophysiological measurements and potential image post-processing directions in future. In the end, the chapter summarizes the current developments in physiological basis of fMRI signal, its origin, contrast enhancement, physical factors, anatomical labeling by segmentation, registration approaches of visual and motor activity in brain with a review of clinical applications of fMRI in motor sensory functions, multiple sclerosis and Alzheimer's Disease to explore the other different neurophysiological and imaging modalities.

2. The physiological basis of fMRI

2.1 Basics

It became clear in last decade that fMRI signal is coupled or 'blood linked' with neuroactivation due to regional changes of blood flow and its redox oxygen state or ferric-ferrous ionic state in hemoglobin. Idea was roped up as 'neurophysiological' effect sensitive to fMRI signal is generated due to 'neuropsychological' activity in specific regions in brain. As a result, neurovascular and neurometabolic coupling (neurophysiological effects) establishes the critical link between a focal change in neuronal activity and MRI-detectable observations. In fact, all neuroactivation task performances such as arousal, attention, alertness, adaptation, sleep, or consciousness that affect the blood perfusion or vascular hemodynamics do interfere with oxygenation-sensitive mapping by fMRI techniques. Increased neuronal activity needs the metabolic oxygen support. For that, blood flow provides the metabolic substrates or energy rich neurochemicals. Still there is paucity of information of metabolic requirements and hemodynamic response in different brain cognitive functions. Historically, these cognitive observations initially were supported by reports on local reduction in deoxyhemoglobin due to increased blood flow without change in oxygen extraction [Zaini et al. 1996]. Conceptually, weak susceptibility effect induced by deoxyhemoglobin acts as paramagnetic endogenous contrast agent to represent neuroactivation (active perfusion) or label of oxygen oversupply and alters the T_2* weighted pixel intensity (functional magnetic resonance image signal) [Reber et al.2002; Preibisch et al. 1999; Nakai et al. 2001; Bandettini et al.2000] and serves as the source of the neuroactivation signal (fluctuation of SNR) for fMRI. Such fluctuations originate in fMRI as a result of 3D variations in spatial frequencies and line width (B) in x, y, z directions (gradients define location of neuroactivation and slice position). Other physiological factors such as physiological drifts (fluctuations of SNR, frequency distribution, signal intensities, BOLD signals) also participate. It is based on the fact that spatial distribution of low-frequency drifts in human brain follows a tissue-specific pattern, with greater drift magnitude in the gray matter than in white matter. In gray matter, the dependence of drift magnitudes on TE remains similar to that of task-induced BOLD signal changes. For example, absolute drift magnitude reaches the maximum when TE approaches equal to T_2* whereas relative drift magnitude increases linearly with TE. By systematically varying the flip angle, drift magnitudes show a positive dependence on image intensity. Last decade was an excitement for clinical application of 3T-7T clinical scanners to observe functional activity of visual cortex using magnetic field susceptibility insensitive fast spin echo method [Turner et al.1993; Kwng et al. 1995; Russ et al. 2002; Miki et. al. 2001; Shibata et al. 2000; Fransson et al. 1997], the motor cortex [Kim et al. 1999; Mandeville et al. 1999; Toma et al. 2002; Kim et al. 1995; Nakada et al.2001] and Broca's area of speech and language-related activities [Kim et al. 1995; Nakada et al.2001]. fMRI and conventional neurophysiological techniques have been in use to localize the specific functions of the human brain [Logothetis et al.2001; Mayville et al.1999; Haslinger et al.2001; Kim et al. 2000; Ogawa et al. 1998; Jueptner et al. 1995]. Recent trend was focused on identification of brain regions involved with characteristic oxygenation-sensitive MRI response function. The art of other imaging techniques such as the neurochemical changes, chemical shift imaging, diffusion/perfusion dynamic imaging integrated with fMRI technique is in infancy. In next section, we describe the oxygen dependent nature of fMRI sensitive to neuroactivation and cerebrovascular blood flow.

2.2 Tissue oxygen content and framework for BOLD Signal

fMRI images can be made sensitive to local oxygen concentrations in tissue by choosing right MRI protocol. BOLD signal derives from the local concentration of deoxygenated hemoglobin that is modulated by several factors. The generator of this paramagnetic contrast agent is oxygen metabolism ($CMRO_2$). Blood oxygenation and blood magnetization both depend upon the balance of oxygen flow into and out of a region. The rate of oxygen inflow is proportional to cerebrovascular blood rate (CBR). During functional brain activation, increased CBF produces a washout of Hb_r as contrast agent by counteracting the effect of increased $CMRO_2$. Local blood volume fraction determines the deoxyhemoglobin content of a voxel at any level of blood oxygenation. As blood vessels swell, magnetic fields extend further into the brain tissue, causing a signal loss in the extravascular space. BOLD contrast can be approximated as changes in the BOLD relaxation rate scale with changes in the deoxy hemoglobin concentrations i.e. BOLD contrast (X) = K.A [Hb_r], where 'x' depends upon the magnetic field strength and the sample volume.

A BOLD framework is based upon conservation of oxygen mass (Fick's Law) i.e. at the steady-state, unidirectional extraction of oxygen from the blood is the difference between the 'flow' of oxygen 'into' and oxygen 'out' of the volume, FO_2^{IN} -, FO_2^{OUT} = dV/dt. The resulting expression takes a form like the following:

$$\Delta R_2 = -K\,[Hb_r]_o\{\Delta F/F_o - \Delta V/V_o - \Delta M/Mo\} \quad (1)$$

F, V, and M refer to CBF, CBV, and $CMR0_2$ respectively. Subscript "o" indicates baseline values prior to stimulation. BOLD signal changes are positive when the quantity in brackets is positive.

Positive stimulus-induced BOLD represent the relative changes in CBF that exceed over combined effect of changes in CBV and $CMR0_2$. $[Hb_r]_o$ is proportional to V and M_o and inversely proportional to F as shown in Figure 1 that combine to generate BOLD signal. Equation (1) stands good for small functional changes while intravascular signal contributions affect the linear relationship between ΔR_2, and $\Delta[Hb_r]$ dependence on blood oxygen and blood volume. The term $\Delta V/V_o$ is relative change in total venous hemoglobin.

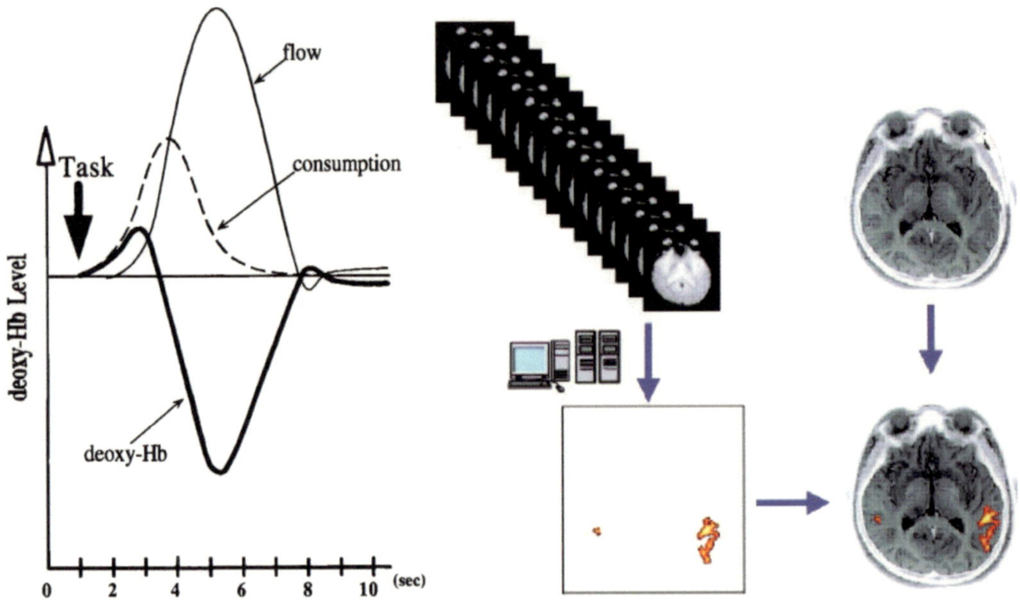

Fig. 1. Figure represents the "Oxygen oversupply" hypothesis. Regional deoxy-Hb (thick solid lines) decline is associated with increase in regional blood flow (thin solid line) and oxygen consumption (broken lines). In fMRI, T2* is described as blood flow based functional imaging of brain activation as sum of all activation pixels (yellow color) from all serial images shown in the figure (on right).

A rapid change in CBF produces an effect on BOLD signal that is both delayed and dispersed by transit through the vascular bed. The framework of Equation (1) of BOLD signal does not specify how oxygen is allocated, as long as the total amount is conserved. However, the quantities $\{\Delta F/F_o - \Delta V/V_o - \Delta M/M_o\}$ do not change arbitrarily during brain activation. The reproducibility of BOLD results across systems and BOLD stimuli poorly represent the coupling [Villringer et al.1999].

2.3 CBF and $CMRO_2$

Regional basal cerebral oxygen and glucose utilization show a molar ratio consistently less than 6($CMRO_2$/ CMR_{glu} - 5.5), suggesting that the oxidative glucose metabolism ($C_6H_{12}O_6$ + 6 O_2 + $6H_2O$ + $6CO_2$) is the primary source of energy. Tight linear couplings have been shown for regional basal measurements of CBF versus CMR_{glu} and CBF versus $CMR0_2$ [Buxton et al.1997].

2.4 BOLD stimulus-induced neuroactivation and physiological changes

Blood oxygen is delivered to the brain by gaseous-fluid diffusion along an oxygen concentration gradient that falls in the neuroactivated brain tissue. As a result, specific brain region gets low oxygen reserves. So blood flow in that region experiences the increases of oxygen delivery or MR sensitive changes (temporal resolution) resulting with following effects: reduced blood transit time through the capillaries; decreased oxygen; extraction fraction; restricted capillary area; and vascular resistance at the local level. So, the regional trajectories represent the temporal physiological quantities determined from the baseline or average state i.e. the diffusion and regional coupling of CBF and $CMRO_2$ match during the brain activation. The current viewpoint of CBF-$CMRO_2$ coupling and regional relationship with rate of oxygen delivery explained the events during brain activation by Buxton-Frank diffusion-limited model of oxygen delivery [Zaharchuk et al.1999]. The exact scaling between relative changes in blood flow (f) = F/F_d and relative changes in oxygen delivery (M) depend upon the baseline value of the extraction fraction (E_o) and extent of capillary dilation as:

$$(v) = V / V_o \tag{2}$$

$$M = f\,(1 - (1 - E_o)^{v/f}) / E_o \tag{3}$$

Empirically, the influence of $CMR0_2$ on BOLD signal can be deduced by comparing the responses of CBF and BOLD signal using stimuli that affect CBF and $CMRO_2$ i.e. hypercapnia modulates CBF without changing oxygen-utilization. Focal activation of the human visual cortex increases $CMRO_2$ [31]. By using graded levels of visual stimulus and hypercapnia, a linear coupling was measured between relative changes in CBF and $CMRO_2$ for flow [Disbrow et al.2000].

2.5 CBF and CBV

Cerebral vascular resistance is defined as the 'total pressure drop' across a vascular bed. In the brain, intravascular pressure drops from mean arterial blood pressure in large arteries to venous pressure in the large veins. The brain activation increases CBF by reducing cerebral vascular resistance corresponding to an increase in CBV. Blood flow and blood volume both exhibit different temporal responses [Cheng et al.2001]. However, the basal blood level of deoxygenated hemoglobin is determined by the ratio of $CMRO_2$ to CBF. Neurophysiological changes in fMRI alter BOLD signal by resetting the ratio of basal $CMRO_2$ to CBF, and altering CBV [Cox et al. 1996].

2.6 Sensitivity of fMRI signal

Blood volume fraction, oxygen extraction fraction, distribution of vessels, arterial oxygenation neurophysiological factors and intravascular or extravascular signals depend upon the applied MR pulse sequence, field strength, degree of neuroactivation and the physiology of the functional variable etc. Sensitivity is the product of the relative change in brain 'activation' (flow, volume, oxygenation, etc.) and 'amplification' factor expressing the intrinsic sensitivity per unit change:

$$\text{Sensitivity} = (\text{activation}) \times (\text{amplification}) \quad (4)$$

The amplification factor applies spatial resolution to the pattern of brain activation but it is independent of the degree of activation [32]. For detecting changes in local brain functional activity, fMRI signal-to-noise ratio (fSNR) refers to the time-averaged value of signal divided by the temporal standard deviation of the signal: fSNR = S_t/σ_t.

Similarly, contrast for fMRI or functional CNR per unit time (fCNR) may be expressed as the ratio of time dependent signal changes (δS) to time-dependent noise:

$$\text{fCNR} = \delta S_t / \sigma_t, \text{fSNR} \times \delta S_t/S_t \quad (5)$$

3. Basic functional MRI sequences and physical factors of functional MRI contrast

In routine, fast Flow Attenuated Short Echo (FLASH) or single-shot EPI pulse sequences with prolonged echo times are employed depending on the desired spatial or temporal resolution. These pulse sequences are shown in Figure 2. Typically, EPI sequences acquire all differently phase-encoded gradient echoes required for image reconstruction after a single slice-selective RF excitation pulse. The individual echoes are generated by multiple sinusoidal or trapezoidal reversal of the read or frequency-encoding gradient. Phase encoding is performed by a 'blipped' gradient, whereas the EPI technique uses a 'weaker' constant gradient. Echoes cover a large range of different echo times. The effective TE is given by the Fourier line representing the lowest spatial frequency, i.e. for zero phase encoding, as it dominates the image contrast. Basic emphasis is on high speed yield and image acquisition times of the order of 100 ms and excellent maximum volume coverage by multi-slice fMRI imaging at the expense of limited in-plane resolution.

In contrast, FLASH sequences require multiple RF excitations with low flip angles < 90° that normally generate only a single gradient echo per repetition interval. As large TE values also prolong the repetition time, typical imaging times are in the range of several seconds. The ability to select an arbitrary compromise between temporal and spatial resolution is best exploited for gaining access to high-resolution maps at the expense of less volume coverage. However, EPI images also suffer from several unavoidable artifacts. In following section, we describe different brain areas to correlate distribution of fMRI pixel intensities with cognitive functions as guideline to neuropsychological geography of brain.

4. Neuropsychological geography of neuroactivation in brain

Recent trend in fMRI research was to understand the relationship of physiological mechanisms and selective activation of different brain locations using fMRI techniques. However, the knowledge of the independent brain functions and control by different parts is still in infancy. fMRI has long way to answer the physiological stimuli and mechanism of different fMRI BOLD signals. The success of it solely depends on power of fMRI image processing. Recent investigations highlight the fMRI visible different brain areas as shown in FIG 3, new understanding of fMRI sensitive physiological stimuli and use of high field scanners.

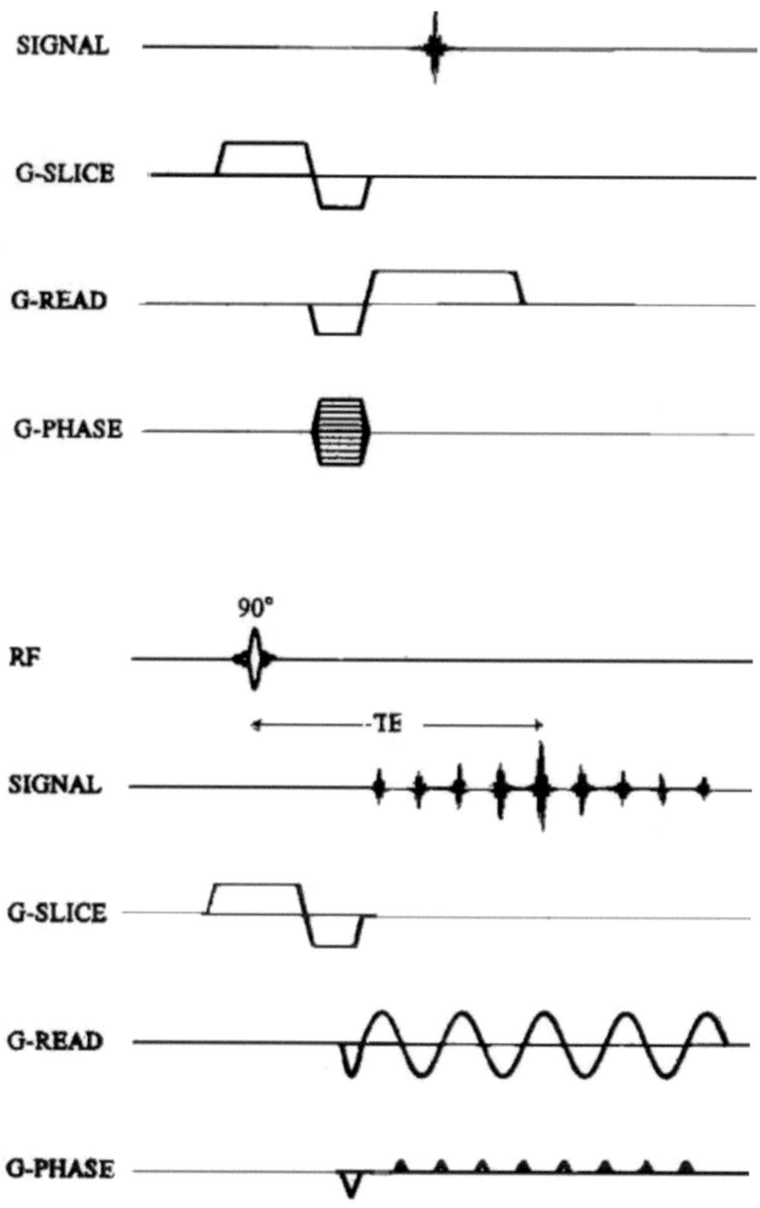

Fig. 2. A basic EPI sequence FLASH (top) and single-shot EPI Sequence (bottom) for functional Imaging is shown with reversible reading gradients and pulses to generate rapid images in less than a minute.

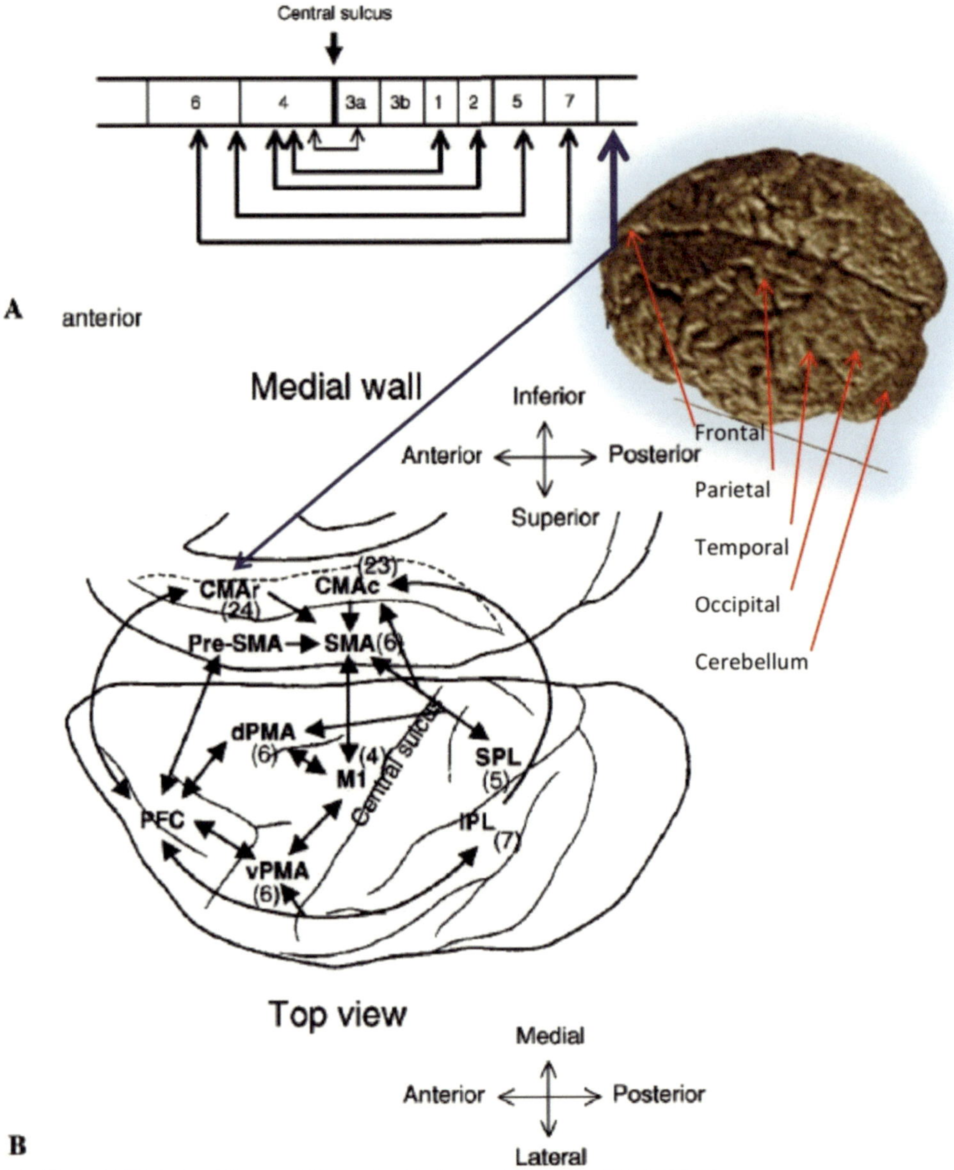

Fig. 3. An illustration of anatomical connections between motor areas are shown.
A: A sagittal section of gray matter shows reciprocal organization of frontal motor and parietal sensory cortices with respect to the central sulcus. Brodmann's area (BA), reciprocity between rimary areas (BA4 and BA3, 1 and 2 and reciprocity between nonprimary areas (BA6 and BA5 and 7) are shown by arrows. B. Interconnections between multiple motor-related cortices are represented with numbers in parentheses. These are: Brodmann's area M1: Primary motor cortex, SMA: Supplementary motor area, dPMA: Dorsal premotor area, vPMA: Ventral premotor area, CMAr: Rostral cingulated motor area, CMAc: Caudal cingulated motor area, PFC, Prefrontal cortex, SPL: Superior parietal lobe, IPL: Inferior parietal lobe.

5. Validation and physical factors in functional MRI

BOLD and fMRI characteristics are important determinants in validation process of ultrafast fMRI image acquisition of raw data and 'task to functional map' correlation by postprocessing and statistical analysis. We describe these concepts that validate brain activation, fMRI spatial resolution and BOLD events. Two assumptions support the validation of fMRI to pick up brain activation signal: 1. Any motor or sensory action of body generates specific motor or sensory response in neural circuit with a result in cerebrovascular blood flow change due to oxygen state in flowing blood; 2. 'Brain activation' is read as 'statistically significant pixel intensity changes' associated with a given set of tasks to denote the area of neuronal activation. It is a scalar number given by MRI system upon completion of image reconstruction including magnetic correction and other inherent factors. MRI spatial resolution is low in the range of 4 mm^3 on high field MR scanners. BOLD events are neuronal events. T2* contrast changes seen in fMRI are an empirically observed biological phenomenon. For fMRI, T2* contrast is 'weak' susceptibility effect of deoxy-hemoglobin (deoxy-Hb). In following sections we describe some known physical factors responsible of functional MRSI (task→oxygen change in blood Hb→change blood flow→brain activation→pixel intensity change→3D Talairach maps and changes in metabolites). Some known intrinsic and extrinsic factors are described to influence fMRI contrast in flowing section.

5.1 Susceptibility effects and T_2* contrast

In MRI, regional magnetic field inhomogeneity is common problem due to high paramagnetic susceptibility, ferromagnetic susceptibility and presence of air sinuses in brain, and B_o inhomogeneity. The susceptibility effect may affect a large area of the image matrix and can introduce image deformity. The smaller susceptibility effects introduce the pixel intensity changes in nearby pixels generating the T_2* contrast. This is the basis of fMRI that represents a 'statistical' method based on pixel intensity changes in the brain placed in high magnetic field B.

5.2 Magnet shimming

MRI is performed grossly by using high order gradient 1st and 2nd order shim coils to correct B_o inhomogeneity. Human brain undergoes the continuous motion and it makes hard to shim i.e. the line width of human brain is 200–400 Hz. Slice thickness and slab size over that focused shimming reduces the inhomogeneity. Fast spin echo (FSE) images are insensitive but echo planar images (EPI) are sensitive to inhomogeneity. In fMRI, selective RF excitation pulse applied through a gradient selects the appropriate slice thickness with appropriate inter slice gap between the slices.

5.3 Nyquist ghost

The unique k-space trajectory of the EPI sequence results in the appearance of a characteristic artifact termed 'Nyquist ghost'. However, in practice the most common cause of Nyquist ghost is minor field perturbation as shown in Figure 3. Nyquist ghost represents the fictitious activation encountered in fMRI. Direct adaptation of such paradigms to fMRI typically introduces task-correlated Nyquist ghost and fictitious activation.

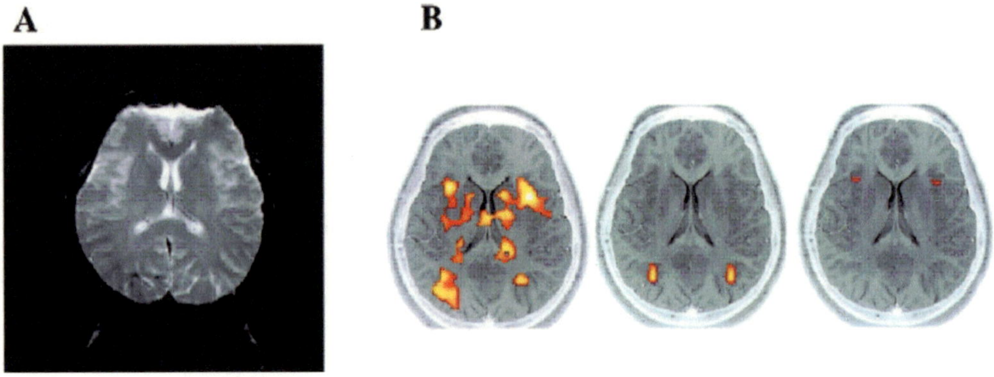

Fig. 4. The figure represents Nyquist ghost in panel A and representative fictitious activation in panel B. Notice the background bright signal as ghost (panel A) and activation areas (panels B) shown in yellow color spots which are not due to brain activation.

5.4 Pixel misalignment and limitation of spatial resolution

Pixel misalignment causes the fictitious activation due to subject motion as shown in Figure 4. Many "motion correction" post-processing algorithms have been developed based on the two-dimensional imaging and three-dimensional misalignments[Goodyear et al.2001; Kim et al. 2000; Kiebel et al. 2004]. The theoretical limit of the spatial resolution for fMRI is approximately 4 mm^3. fMRI image of the normal brain can be used to evaluate the relative intensity of cerebral cortex at various sites relative to CSF as shown in Figure 4. The substantial variation in the intensity of cortex is primarily due to the partial volume phenomenon as shown in Figure 5. The correction algorithms such as 're-slicing', 'standardization', or 'motion correction' image-processing methods as shown in Figure 6 have been reported [Meinzer et al.2011]. Basically, each raw image data is used for statistical analysis. In the following description, some representative examples of application of these physiological principles of fMRI are illustrated.

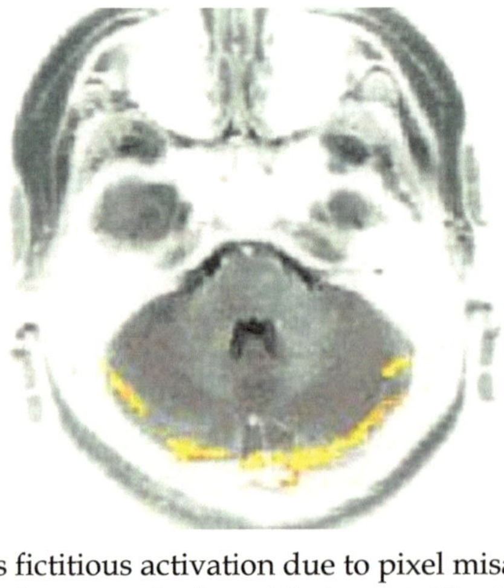

Fig. 5. The figure represents fictitious activation due to pixel misalignment. The bright spots around the bottom brain surface are misaligned that create illusion of active areas shown in yellow color.

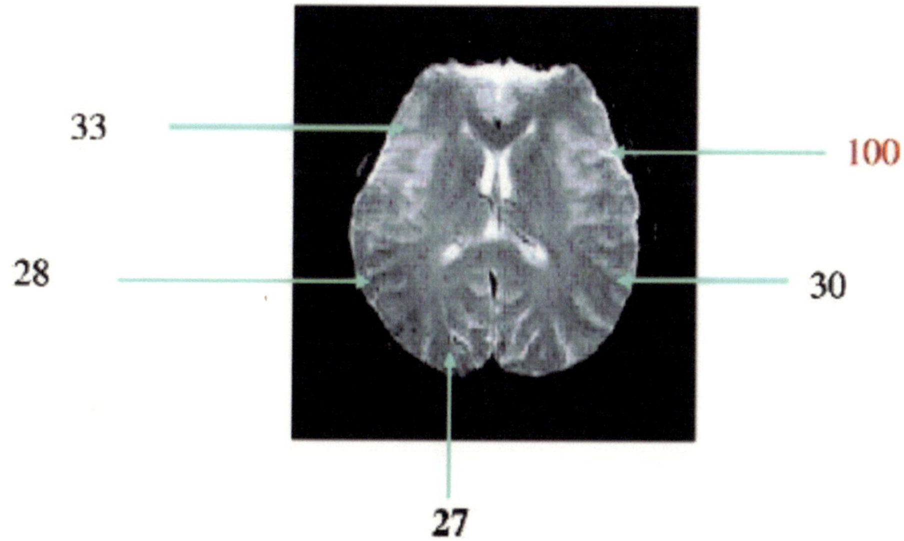

Fig. 6. An example of an fMRI image of the normal brain is shown. The numbers indicate the relative intensity of cerebral cortex at various sites relative to CSF which assigned a value of 100 (written in red). The substantial variation in the intensity of cortex is primarily due to the 'partial volume' phenomenon.

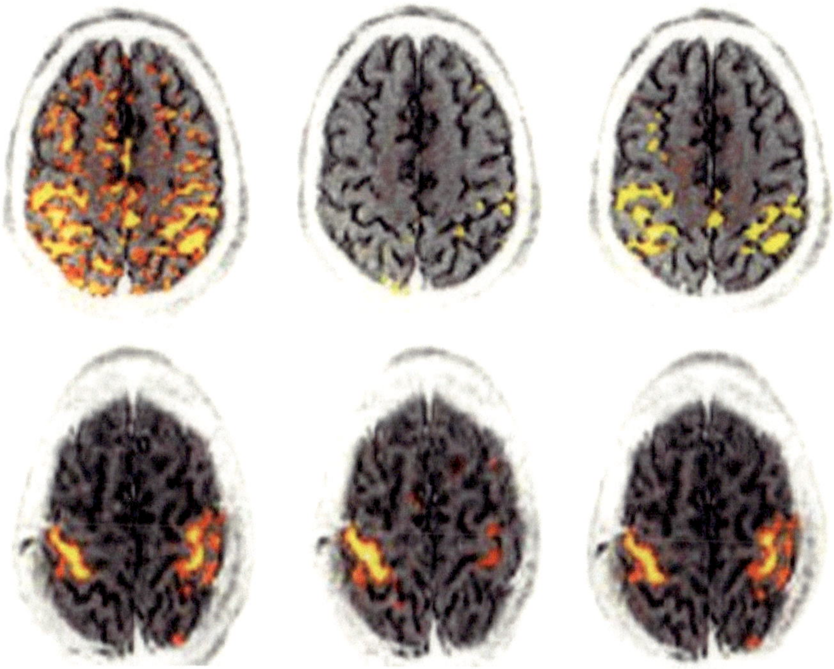

Fig. 7. The figure illustrates the effects of motion correction algorithm SPM 96. The activation maps were obtained for a bilateral hand motion paradigm using a horizontal 3 T MRI system with image voxel resolution of 3 mm × 3 mm × 5 mm. In this setting, acceptable pixel misalignment was determined to be 0.6 mm. Brain motion exceeding

0.6 mm (> 0.6 mm) produced significant pixel misalignment artifact. A motion correction algorithm wiped out these artifacts as well as actual activation. It also wiped out a small cluster of fictitious activation, while 'true' activation remained visible. In contrast, brain motion less than 0.6 mm provided activation maps of bilateral primary motor cortices. Application of motion correction algorithm artificially eliminated true activation areas.

Functional MRI is sensitive to some sensory and motor response functions. In following section, we illustrate visual response function in relation with fMRI.

5.5 The vision response function

The oxygen concentration in brain serves as a tool to map cortical regions responsible for performing various cognitive tasks because oxygenation level in active cortex changes between baseline and tasking conditions i.e. pattered lights protocols affect the spatiotemporal response and characteristics in the visual system. These visual stimulations generate the signal rise due to differences between tonic and phasic MRI hemodynamic responses after the onset of activation i.e. rapid rise in BOLD response due to rapid increase in the blood flow or enhanced oxygen delivery / oxygen consumption. Recently, the delayed upregulation of oxidative glucose consumption in brain and a slow venous blood volume (balloon model) suggested them as two processes. These were relevant for fMRI mapping studies with shorter protocol timings [Villringer et al. 1999]. The link between neuronal activity and blood flow characteristics forms the basis for functional mapping using fMRI. These characteristics such as cerebral blood flow (CBF), cerebral volume (CBV), metabolic regional oxygen ($CMRO_2$), and BOLD signal form an interconnected set of quantities that are coupled during normal brain activation. For details, readers are suggested to read chapter 9 in this book.

5.6 Neurophysiological factors in functional MRI contrast

In this section, we describe various measures currently used to identify the activated pixels in corresponding fMRI maps i.e. analysis of signal differences, variances, statistical parameters, temporal correlations or frequencies, principal components, clusters, phase information, and noise characteristics. In visual response, time-locked averaging of images and subsequent subtraction across the functional states i.e. summation of images was reported that was acquired during one condition (e.g. lights off) and subtraction of the result from that obtained for a different condition (e.g. lights on) [Cox et al.1996]. This robust and sensitive approach exploited the temporal structure of the known stimulation protocol and compared it to the oxygenation-sensitive MRI signal intensity time courses, on a pixel-by-pixel basis. This 'boxcar' function was employed to calculate the color-coded activation map for correlation coefficients identifying the activation centers and optimum area delineation i.e. retinotopic maps on brain V1, V2, V4 and MT (visual cortex) measured by fMRI for establishing the accuracy of visual maps as basis of hemodynamic responses in these two cortical areas [Cox et al.1996]. The stimuli used block-alternation design with relatively long intervals of stimulus vs rest state. However, fMRI has been widely used to image ocular dominance and orientation columns within a fraction of a millimeter [Goodyear et al.2001; Kim et al.2000; Kiebel et al. 2004].

5.7 Functional MRI signal of motor and visual stimulation

In following section, two common examples of fMRI experiments of motor and visual stimulation are described. Before details of fMRI experiments, a brief description is given on fMRI anatomical geography to correlate different language regions in brain with their functional neuropsychological activities. Readers are requested to read neuroanatomy for further details.

5.8 Neurostimulus in aphasia and fMRI

Functional MRI can map changes in brain functionality at different Brodmann and Broca areas following a treatment to assess its effectiveness as neuroimaging-guided rehabilitation neuroscience [Meinzer et al. 2011]. Broca's area "classical language area", supports various tasks related to memory, music [Maess et al. 2001; Patel 2003], calculation, object manipulation [Binkofski et al. 2004], motor imagery [Binkofski et al.2000], perception of meaningful but not meaningless sequences of hand and mouth actions [Fadiga et al.2006a; Fadiga et al.2006b], time perception, rhythmic perception, processing of complex geometric patterns [Fink et al.2006], prediction of sequential patterns, and so on. Major functions are: (a) selection of information from competing sources [Thompson-Schill 2005], (b) a broader cognitive control function [Novick et al.2010], (c) language specific linearization of hierarchical language dependencies [Greewe et al.2005], (d) processing of hierarchical dependencies like those found in language and musical syntax [Optiz et al. 2007] involving cognition, perception, and action. The syntactic subsystem, which too contributes to auditory comprehension, is supported by Broca's area (BA) [Fink et al. 2006; Thompson-Schill 2005], the angular gyrus (BA 39), the supramarginal gyrus (BA 40), the superior temporal gyrus (BA 22), involving also the white matter structures, such as the basal ganglia [Kutas et al. 2000; Caplan et al. 2000]. The dorsal stream in its posterior part involves a portion of the Sylvian fissure at the parietal-temporal boundary, supporting the sensory-motor interface. Its anterior portion in the frontal lobe includes Broca's area and its vicinity, while its more dorsal premotor component "corresponds to the portions of the articulatory network" [Hickok et al. 2007]. The ventral stream in its posterior portion (posterior middle and inferior portions of the temporal lobes) supports linking of phonological and semantic information (the lexical interface), while its more anterior areas support the combinatorial network. Phonological subsystem supporting auditory comprehension activates certain temporal areas as well as the dorsal region of Brodmann area (BA) 44. The semantic level of auditory comprehension is also distributed; e.g., passive listening activates temporal region BA 22/42 bilaterally, while other semantic tasks may activate left BA 47, BA 45/46 and BA 44 [Friederici 1998].

Together with structural and other functional neuroimaging methods as well as with new observer-independent methods of cytoarchitectonic analysis [Amunts et al.2003], fMRI has created a new picture of Brodmann area. Downing & Peelen (2011) have contradicted that the body areas in the occipitotemporal cortex (OTC) do not actually support processing of the body itself (as a category), but rather its shape and posture (that is, its features), forming a perceptual network that also supports processing in other cortical systems "overlapping and segregated system for object representation" (p. 9) in the ventral visual cortex for fronto-parietal activation [Peelen et al. 2011]. New fMRI evidences indicate activations of perilesional areas associated with small stroke lesions, while larger stroke lesions induce activation of the homologue areas in the opposite hemisphere [Cao et al. 1999]. A best example is Aphasia.

Much explored language disorder is Aphasia caused by brain damage due to a stroke, traumatic brain injury, tumour, atrophy and other neurological conditions. Neuroplasticity of brain can be associated with all aphasic types. Aphasia further can be divided into non-fluent (such as Broca's aphasia, transcortical motor or global aphasia) and fluent aphasias (e.g., Wernicke's aphasia, anomic and transcortical sensory aphasia). fMRI provides information on the remaining functionality of the injured brain after aphasia, involvement of other brain areas "taking over" the other brain functions, and the reorganization processes at work. To evaluate the "taking over" function, block design is used during blood oxygenation level-dependent (BOLD) fMRI based on "the temporal dynamics of the hemodynamic response delay" where increased blood flow remains 4 or 8 seconds after the response" to allow data collection after the task and "during the silent period of no speech, minimizing motion artifact from overt speech". Such neural activity involves Broca's area and the posterior perisylvian network (including Wernicke's area, the angular and supramarginal gyri), and RH homologues of these regions, plus the occipital area as a control area. Time to peak (TTP) data contain valuable information on patients' response to treatment, because changes in TTP reflect changes in the amount of time that a patient spends on a task from presentation of stimulus to verbal response. Brain cannot reorganize syntax after injury to left BA 45/47 and that the capacity of Right Hemisphere takes over function critically depends on the type of language function.

5.9 Visual stimulation and fMRI

The typical BOLD time course (shown in black) shows 4 'active' states and 4 'resting' states are shown in Figure 8. With prior knowledge of the activation timing (shown in red), a statistical test is performed on the data to determine active areas of the brain. In brief, MP-RAGE (magnetization prepared, rapid acquisition gradient echo) sequence generates a 3D anatomic image of the head and brain. fMRI is performed with T2*-weighted gradient recalled EPI. The visual stimuli are created on a visual stimulus generator graphics card. The stimuli are presented as dichoptic signals using polar filters and adjustable right-angle prisms for optical superimposition of the right and left image are shown in Figure 8. The stimuli appear as 'radial checkerboards', in which the high-luminance contrast checks exchanged position as a sinusoidal function of time. During rest (baseline) periods, subjects view a small black fixation mark superimposed onto a homogeneous field. The experimental paradigms contain five different epochs: Alternating monocular stimulation [A]; Simultaneous binocular stimulation [B]; left eye leading-right eye trailing [LR]; Right eye leading-left eye trailing [RL]; and baseline. Each rest epoch is followed by one of the described epochs of checkerboard stimulation. The complete sequence of one repetition is shown in Figures 8 and 9. In a recent report, BOLD contrast in visual cortex related to binocular interactions in primary visual cortex could be revealed by fMRI at high field 4 T MRI. Binocular and monocular stimulations were characteristic of high contrast radial checkerboard pattern-stimulated neurons tuned to high and low spatial frequencies. The different striate cells in ocular dominance columns interacted when they are simultaneously activated and reduced by binocular or monocular stimulation resulting with increased

BOLD response [Cao et al.1999]. However, binocular rivalry due to disparity appears as a source of error. Fixation of eye and maintaining it throughout scan period reduces the disparity which otherwise is commonly observed in area V3 by random-dot stereogram.

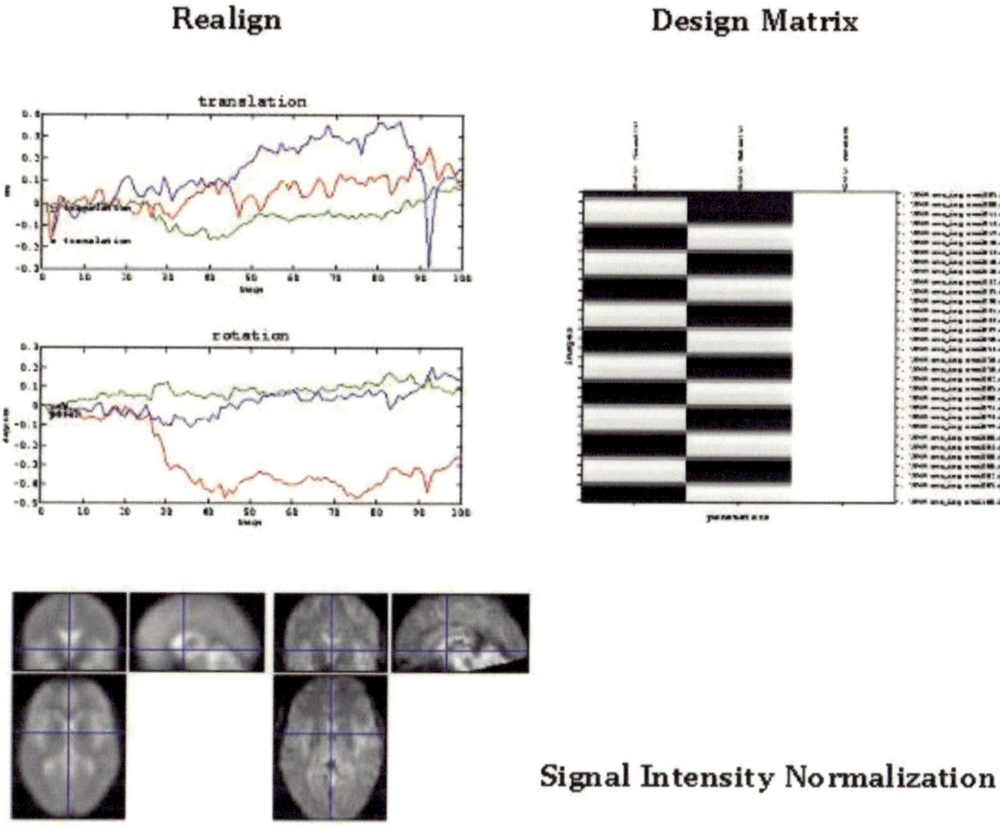

Fig. 8. Time course of activation for the four stimulus epochs (B binocular, M monocular RL right eye stimulated first, followed by left eye stimulation, LR left eye stimulation first, followed by right eye stimulation)(left panel). During stimulation period, the subjects perceived a single flickering radial checkerboard, whereas during the rest period they viewed a single black fixation mark at constant mean luminance (right panel). Typical time courses from region of interest (ROI) centered in one hemisphere in the primary visual cortex (VI) or in an extrastriate region. Statistical parametric maps of significant BOLD responses to alternating monocular stimulation compared to the binocular condition (right panel). Voxels in bright regions indicate strong response to alternating monocular stimulus. The cross hairs represent the most active voxel within the cluster used for normalization (bottom panels).

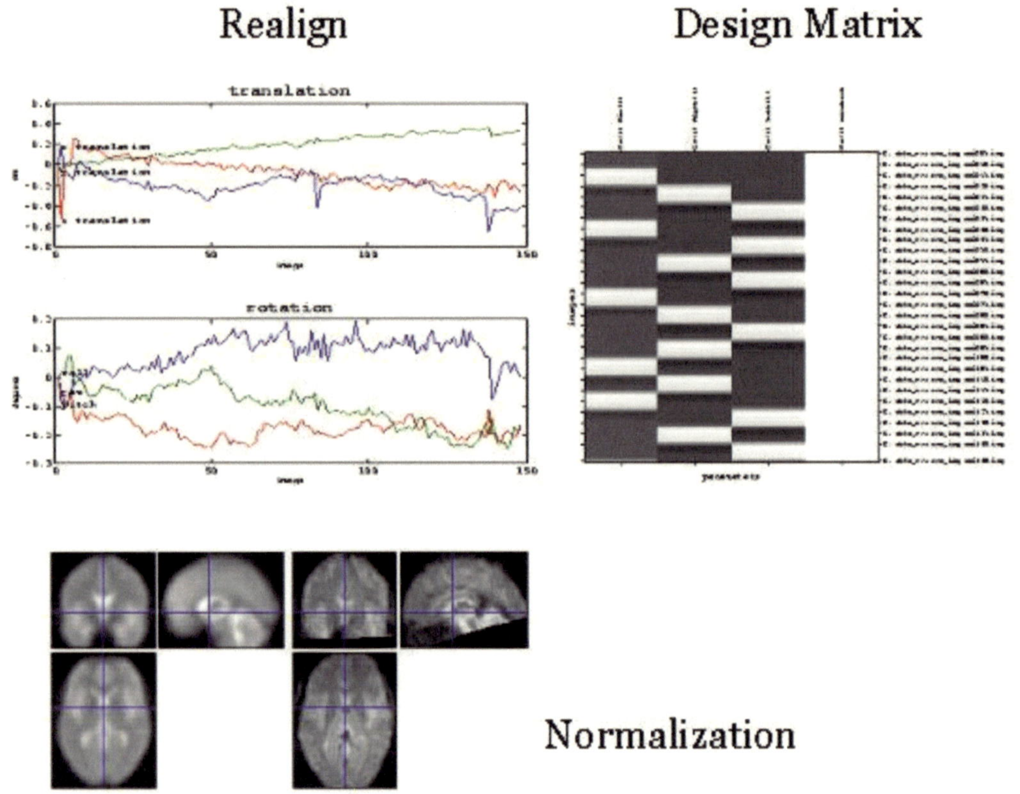

Fig. 9. Time course of activation for the four stimulus epochs (B binocular, M monocular RL right eye stimulated first, followed by left eye stimulation, LR left eye stimulation first, followed by right eye stimulation)(left panel). During stimulation period, the subjects perceived a single flickering radial checkerboard, whereas during the rest period they viewed a single black fixation mark at constant mean luminance (right panel). Typical time courses from region of interest (ROI) centered in one hemisphere in the primary visual cortex (VI) or in an extrastriate region. Statistical parametric maps of significant BOLD responses to alternating monocular stimulation compared to the binocular condition (right panel). Voxels in bright regions indicate strong response to alternating monocular stimulus. The cross hairs represent the most active voxel within the cluster used for normalization (bottom panels).

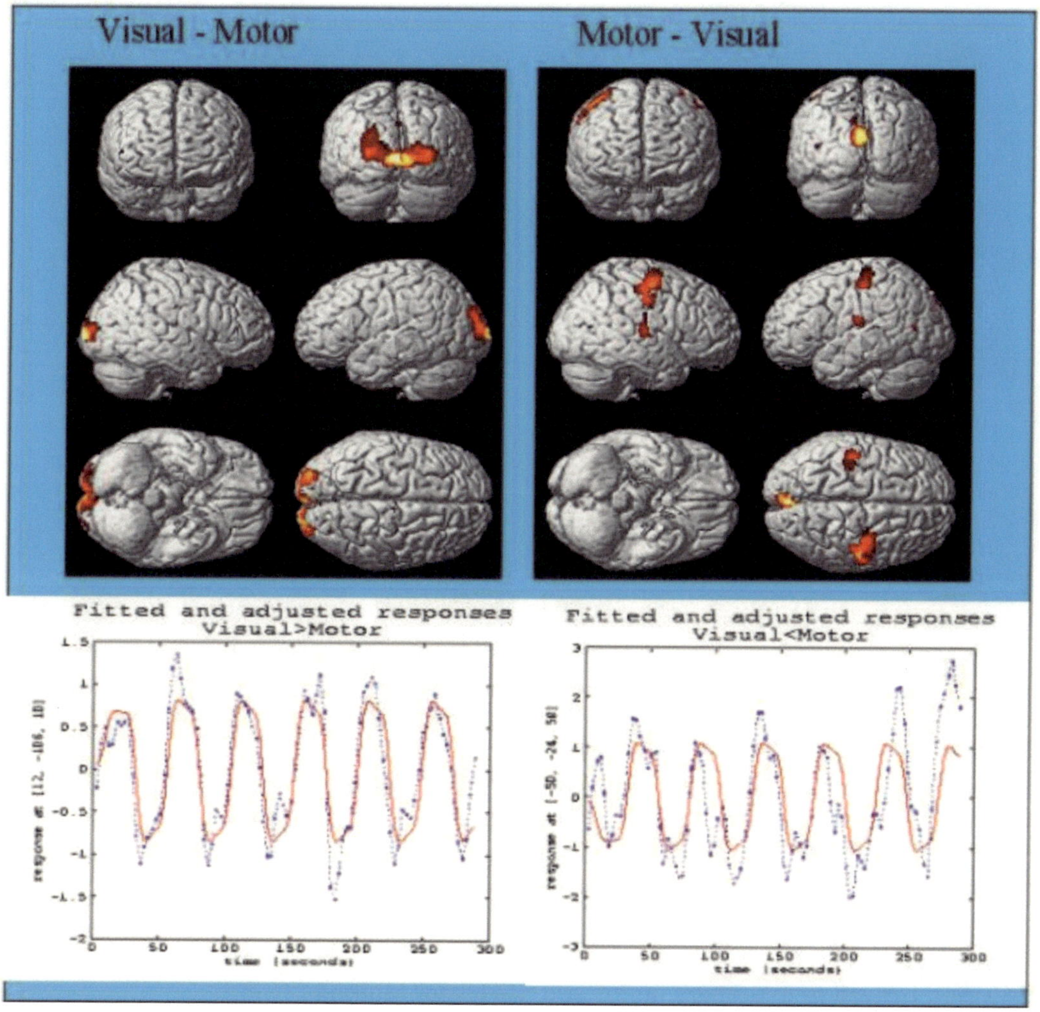

Fig. 10. Selected brain regions showing the activation areas observed by fMRI during finger movement. Regions with Z-score higher than threshold of 3.5 are displayed in red color. Stroke occurred in area colored as yellow. The time-course of on-off fMRI signal recorded in a typical voxel responding activation due to the stimulus paradigm (shown as red bold line).

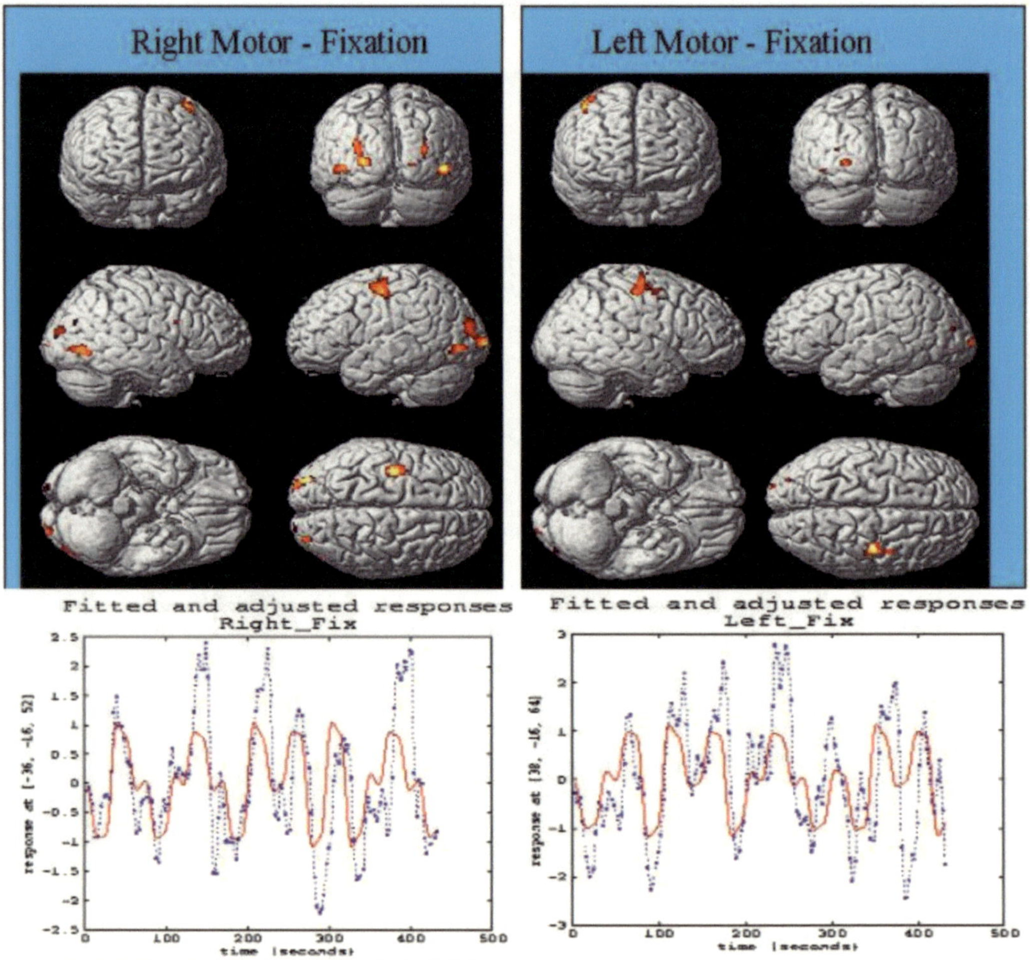

Fig. 11. Selected brain regions showing the activation areas observed by fMRI during finger movement. Regions with Z-score higher than threshold of 3.5 are displayed in red color. Stroke occurred in area colored as yellow. The time-course of on-off fMRI signal recorded in a typical voxel responding activation due to the stimulus paradigm (shown as red bold line).

5.10 fMRI activation in primary motor and pre-motor regions

Paralyzed patient retains the motor control. fMRI shows the activation in primary motor and premotor regions. An example is illustrated here for event-related finger tapping fMRI image acquisition and analysis. Right-handed subjects paralysed with eye blinking and restricted mouth movement with intact cognition were imaged by fMRI single-shot gradient recalled echo-planar imaging pulse sequence. Patients were simulated for the action of tapping fingers 'stimulus paradigm' as shown in Figure 10. Multiple regressions were applied to do statistical data analysis. Individual variables included 'box-car activation paradigm' and constants for activation signals. A ramp-regressor was used to remove linear-drift in the signal. Standard deviated Z-score map was superimposed on high-resolution anatomical image to display brain activation areas. Time course signal in each voxel was obtained to reveal hemodynamic response to the stimulus paradigm. The regions of activation were mainly in contralateral to the primary motor area (M1) and premotor regions (PM) in right motor cortex with little activation in supplementary motor area (SMA). However, ipsilateral activation in premotor (PM) area of left motor cortex was also observed. The time series of functional MRI signals from the voxel in labeled areas (see Figure 11). The time series corresponded with activation paradigm suggesting time-course on-off binary fMRI signal by simulated motor task due to neuronal or cognition activity. It suggested the association of motor cortex, somatosensory cortex and visual cortex with cerebellum through pontine nuclei during its motor activity and rCBF increases.

5.11 3D motion paradigm subtractive approach

It generates activation fMRI maps significant for evaluation of symmetry of activation in the frontal lobes. The cerebrum cortex is not motion physiology sensitive (see Figure 12) but cerebellum cortex is motion physiology sensitive so pixel intensity changes represent its true activation maps as shown in Figure 13. However, paradigm independent structures with high susceptibility effects, partial volume effect become apparent on simultaneously FSE and EPI images as shown in Figure 14. Common examples are air sinuses, air spaces, and ferromagnetic substrates. It is the reason coronal images are not acquired for fMRI imaging but axial images show specific task-related activation areas. The figure shows activation in the right intrapareital sulcus of cerebrum cortex lobes (as arrow). The raw image fMRI image did not show ghost or susceptibility effect to cause fictitious activation. After

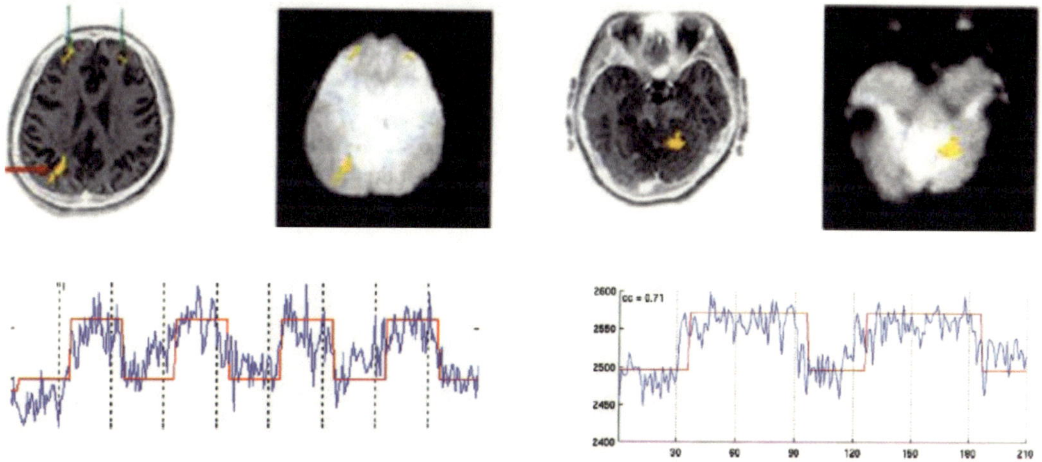

Fig. 12. The figure shows activation in the right intrapareital sulcus of cerebrum cortex lobes (as arrow). The raw image fMRI image did not show ghost or susceptibility effect to cause fictitious activation. After segmentation and processing, corresponding time series of activated pixels showed intensity changes. These intensity changes correlated with boxcar type paradigm. The frontal lobes showed fictitous activation while right intraparietal area showed valid activation map.

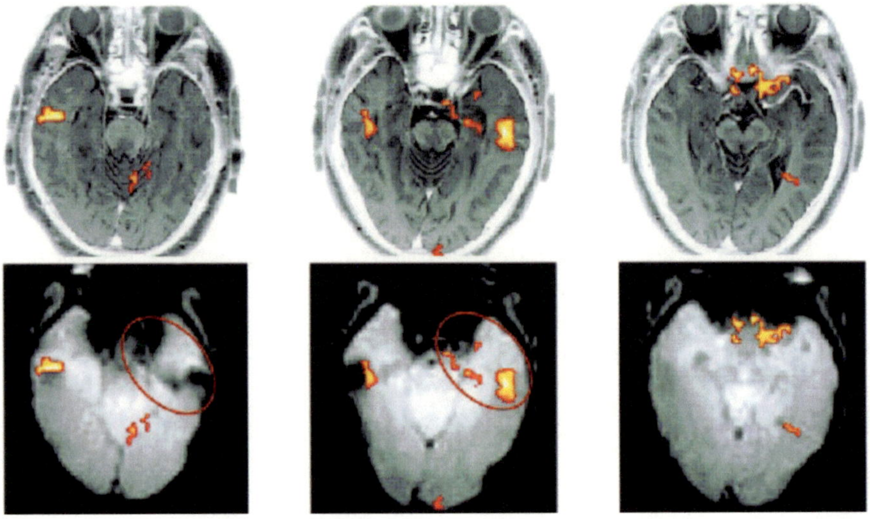

Fig. 13. The figure shows activation in the left cerebellum cortex lobes (as arrow). The raw image fMRI image did not show ghost or susceptibility effect to cause fictitious activation. After segmentation and processing, corresponding time series of activated pixels showed intensity changes. These intensity changes correlated with boxcar type paradigm. The left area showed fictitious activation map due to eye movement.

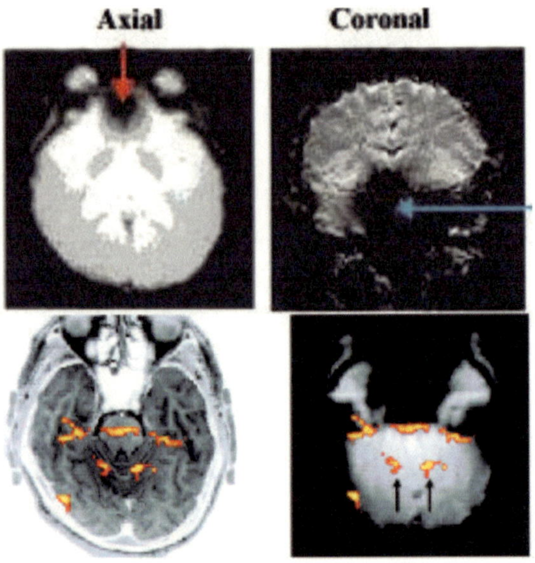

Fig. 14. (On left)The figure shows strong susceptibility effects in axial slice. Note the effect of partial presence of air sinus caused significant distortion in EPI image (arrow in left panel). In coronal slice, air sinus occupied larger image volume (arrow in right panel). (On right) A. activation map on structural (T2R) image. B. Activation EPI image. Emperical or fictitious activation occurred adjacent to structures with strong susceptibility (air sinuses and air cells) True activations sites caused by bilateral hand motion(see arrows in B) get affected by susceptibility on T_2* images.

segmentation and processing, corresponding time series of activated pixels showed intensity changes. These intensity changes correlated with boxcar type paradigm. The frontal lobes showed fictitous activation while right intraparietal area showed valid activation map.

6. Image processing principles

Image processing is the computation process to extract out or sort out important data from large set of image data. To perform extraction and analysis of brain activation locations or Talairach maps, we describe two basic segmentation and registration methods for fMRI image processing and their applications.

6.1 Segmentation

The segmentation task in fMRI is performed by recognition and distinguishing brain areas that respond to a given task or stimulus with high specificity and sensitivity. Two methods 'Bayesian approach' and 'General Linear Model' are common for computation of statistical parameter maps (SPM). The detection of brain activation due to an input stimulus is segmented by statistically comparing images acquired during stimulation (ON state) and those acquired when brain is at rest (OFF state). The results of comparison are expressed by test statistics for each brain voxel in terms of 'likelihood' or 'significant activation' of voxel by the stimulus. Whole brain voxels' likelihood generates SPM map. SPM is an image in which image intensity values represent statistics obtained under null hypothesis of no activation and conform to a certain probability distribution.

'Thresholding' technique using SPM at a significant value can detect brain activation and spatial correlation using 'Gaussian random fields' (GRF) for multivariate Gaussian distribution. This GRF performs the spatial filtering of functional images to minimize pseudo-active brain regions. Alternatively, binary 'Markov random fields' (MRF) models for activation patterns suggested the intensity distribution of SPMs and Bayesian modeling of fMRI time-series inferred the hidden psychological states in fMRI experiments using 'likelihoods' of activation probabilities from these SPMs as shown in Figure 15.

6.1.1 Bayesian approach

A functional brain image is a spatio-temporal signal from brain serial scans taken over time. The posterior probability (Gaussian conditional covariance $\eta_{\theta/y}$, where $(p(\theta/y)$ is proportional to the obtained data depending on times of prior probability of θ as: $p(\theta/y)\ \alpha\ p(y/\theta)\ p(\theta)$. The Guass-Markov estimator may be presented as:

$$\eta_{\theta/y} = (X^T C_\varepsilon^{-1} X)^{-1} (X^T C_\varepsilon - 1y) \quad (6)$$

First, preprocessing of images is done and then detection of brain activation analysis is performed [56]. For it, the set of brain voxels is identified from image domain, and the brain scans are corrected for baseline intensity variation and person's head motion. In next step, derivation of SPMs and their statistical analysis by GLM, detects regions of significant activation.

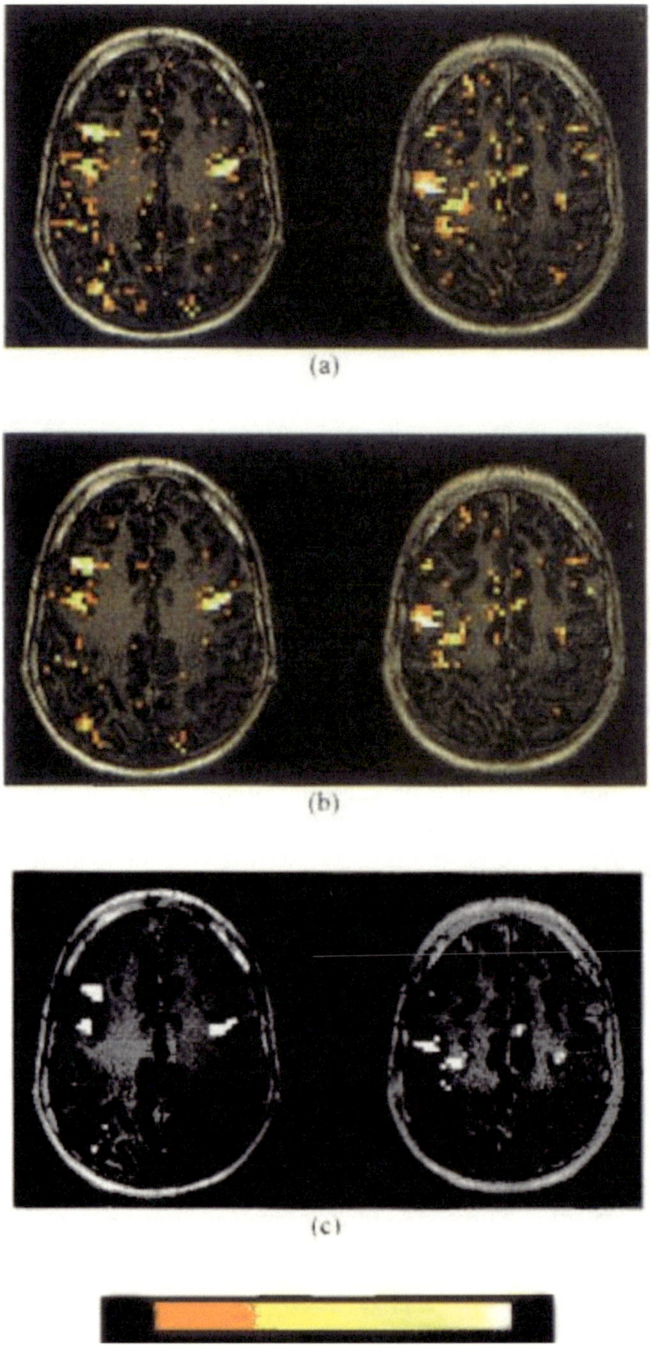

Fig. 15. Activation obtained on two axial brain slices of a representative volunteer in the memory retrieval task by (a) thresholding the SPM{z} at a significant P value = 0.01, (b) using the SPM approach on the SPM{z} with a minimum blob size of three voxels and a significance threshold z = 3.5, and (c) using the MRF approach on the SPM{z}. The significance values (z-values) of the activated voxels are shown color-coded.

6.1.2 F contrasts

Event-related conditions for motor responses are interpreted as hemodynamic response function (HRF) to generate SPM 't' maps as shown in Figure 9. Using design matrix X_o for 'right motor response' regressors look for variance of residuals. The 'F' test computes the sum of squares of "right hand regressors" as following:

$$Fdf_1, df_2 = \frac{[Y^T(1-P_{xo})Y - Y_T(I-P_x)Y]/v_1}{[Y^T(1-P_{xo})Y/v_2} \tag{7}$$

with $v_1 = tr[(R_o - R)\Sigma_i]$ and $v_2 = tr(R\ \Sigma_i)$; $df_1 = tr\ [R_o - R)\ \Sigma_i\ (R_o - R)\ \Sigma_i\ / tr(R_o - R)\ \Sigma_i]_2$ and $df_2 = tr\ [R\ \Sigma_i\ R\ \Sigma_i\ / tr(R\ \Sigma_i]_2$

where R_o is projector onto residual space of x_o, and P_x is orthogonal projector onto X. The 'F' contrasts are one-dimensional, in which case 'F' statistics is simply the square of the corresponding 't' statistics. In SPM interface, 'F' contrasts are displayed as images and 't' statistics is displayed as bars [Cao et al. 1999;Rajapakse et al. 2001].

6.1.3 General linear model

Consider an fMRI experiment involving multiple-input stimuli. Let y(t) and $x_o(t)$ denote the values of the fMRI time-series reponse and the input stimulus 'o' at time t, respectively. Let $X_o = (X_o(t);\ t \in \theta)^T$ and the design matrix of experiment by $[X_1X_2....X_n\ x_{n+1}....x_{n+m}]$ where X_1, $X_2....X_n$ represent n stimulus covariates and X_{n+m} represent 'm' dummy covariates such as age, gender etc. If $y = (y(t):\ t \in \theta)^T$ represents the fMRI time-series, the GLM can be written as $y = X_{\beta + \eta}$, $\beta = (\beta_1, \beta_2, ..\beta_{n+m})^T$ denotes the regression coefficients relating the input covariates to the fMRI response, the matrix $X = [H_1X_1\ H_2X_2 ....H_nX_n\ X_{n+1}.....X_{n+m}]$ represent the design matrix having covariates modified with the modulation matrices $H_o = \{h^k{}_{ij}\}_{n.m}$ and the components of noise factor η will correlate and distribute normally. The multiplication of 'input' stimulus with 'modulation matrix' both auto-correlate the dispersion in fMRI response. The 'F' statistics estimates the significance of stimulus to generate time-series 'y' and least square estimate of regression coefficients 'β'. Using time-series at voxel site and stimulus condition X_o, the F_o (statistical score) = $\{F_o(p):\ p \in \theta\}$ represents 'F' statistical maps for stimulus 'o' and denoted by SPM $[F_o]$. SPM obtained using one statistics can be converted to another statistics using their grand mean scaling, regressors by parametric modulation, high-resolution basic functions and serial covariance matrix to get cumulative distributions in each voxel. The applications of these smooth and filtered SPM intensity profiles indicate spatial extents of the activated blobs [Rajapakse et al. 2001].

6.1.4 Markov Random Field (MRF) model

This approach presumes that brain activation patterns form MRF to incorporate contextual information. Let us assume that set $a_o = \{a_o(p):p \in \theta\}$ denote a segmentation of an SPM or a configuration of brain activation, where $a_o(p)$ denotes the state of the brain voxel at site p and $a_o(p) = 0$ if the voxel is inactive and $a_o(p) = 1$ if the voxel is activated by the stimulus 'o'. Here a_o represents MRF or activation pattern [Rajapakse et al. 2001]. As the brain voxel is either activated or inactive, the MRF is assumed as binary logistic model. For this contextual information, preprocessed images find height threshold for smooth statistical map to detect and distinguish activated areas by using 'Euler Characteristics', Benferroni Correction and contextual clustering algorithm [Cao et al. 1999; Rajapakse et al. 2001]. The Euler characteristics E [EC] is:

$$E[EC] = R(4 \log_e 2)(2\pi)^{-3/2} Z_t e^{-1/2} Z_t^2 \quad (8)$$

Where Z-score thresholds between 0–5, R is number of resels. The later is based on the fact that SPM voxel is adjusted with neighborhood information, if differs from expected non-activation value more than a specified decision value. The 'contextual clustering algorithm' estimates cluster parameter, calculates probability distribution and estimates modulation function to classify the voxel as the 'activation' class, otherwise 'nonactivation' class. However, three algorithms viz. 'voxel-wise thresholding', 'cluster-size thresholding' and 'contextual-clustering' have been described earlier [Rajapakse et al. 2001]. Contextual clustering detects activations in small areas with high probability and voxel-wise specificity. 'Benferroni Correction' is based on probability rules and used for calculating family-wise error (FEW) rates P^{fwe} for fMRI as $P^{fwe} = 1 - (1 - \alpha)^n$ where α is single-voxel probability threshold.

6.1.5 Computation of a statistical parametric map

For the purpose of this segmentation, SPM in the voxel i is represented as:

$$SPM\{F_x\}=\{F_k(p): p \in \Omega_B\} \quad (9)$$

Where F statistical map of $F_k(p)$ for stimulus k represents F statistical score and indicates significance of predicting time-series of voxel site p. For image data, first spatial low-pass filtration increases signal-to-noise ratio and sensitivity then $SPM\{F_x\}$ is computed [Rajapakse et al. 2001].

6.1.6 Applied segmentation methods

Voxel-wise thresholding (VWTH) segmentation method of an SPM applies thresholding to each voxel separately. The voxel at location I is considered as active if and only if $z_i < T$ where T is threshold. Cluster-size thresholding (CSTH) explains the cluster 'c' as active if and only if for all voxels within the cluster $z_i < T$ and the size of cluster 'c' is at least 'T' size voxels. Other common use 'contextual clustering algorithm' (CC) was described in steps [Cao et al. 1999;Rajapakse et al. 2001] as:

1. Label the voxels with zi <T as active and other voxels as non-active. Voxels outside the image volume are considered as non-active.
2. Compute for all voxels I the number of active neighbor voxels u_i.
3. Relabel the voxels for which

$$Z_i + \beta/T\,(u_i - N/2) < T \quad (10)$$

Equation 10 represents voxels as active and other voxels as non-active. The number of neighbor voxels equals to 26-connectivity N = 26. The parameter determines the weighing of the contextual information and is usually positive.

4. If the current labeling is same as the labeling in the previous cycle before that, then stop iterations, otherwise return to step 2.

Probability of observing false activation voxels in a whole volume compares the sensitivity of methods by algorithm applied to different data parameter values. The decision parameter value is chosen that gives false activation in approximately 5 % images and 5 % measured false activation voxels.

6.1.7 Sensitivity, segmentation accuracy and robustness

Generally averaged 500 SPMs achieved by different segmentation methods give mean image probability at voxel-level. The less number of false classified voxels as 'active' in the neighborhood of activation represents segmentation accuracy. Noise evaluation by segmentation of different data determines the robustness against spatial autocorrelations. Low robustness is high probability of false activation detection more than the expected probability. To minimize the false detection of activation, registration algorithms are used to perform 3D geometric matching.

6.2 Registration

6.2.1 Basics

Image registration estimates the mapping between a pair of images. Registration performs for each 3D volume with display of movement parameters in continually updating graph to get matching criteria. Combination of 2D shearing operations and Fourier transform based shifting generate accurate high-speed 2D MR image rotation based on factorization of a general 2D planar rotation matrix. 3D arbitrary orthogonal matrix can be factored in to 3D rotations to accomplish 3D image rotation from nine 2D shears. Other approach of linear-in-frequency phase shift in frequency domain applied to 1D fast Fourier transforms (FFTs) generated the image rotation with polynomial interpolation methods [Cox et al.1999; Sarkissian et al. 2003; Ciulla et al.2002].

However, 3D real time image registration (rotation) algorithm chose the axes ordering that resulted in the least intermediate image distortion (minimum net rotation) at proper flip angle about x, y or z-axes i.e. generalized and windowed sinc interpolation. It applied real-time functional MRI acquisition and activation analysis modules within AFNI package. Functional MRI requires the rigid body transformations: small rotations, translations, zooms, rotating tensors and shears in 1-2 degrees or 1-2 voxel dimensions [Cox et al. 1999;Ciulla et al. 2002]. So, repeated linearization of weighted least squares penalty functions with respect to motion parameters accomplishes the registration of a base image to a target image. This method minimized the regional influences and intrinsic variability in functionally active voxels in the brain. However, fMRI registration suffers from motion-related artifacts: interpolation errors, spin excitation in slice, spatial distortion by Gy and Nyquist ghosts. Intensity based intermodal registration AIR use variance of intensity ratios (VIR) cost function. Real-time image reconstruction was reported using Vision 3.5 software in communication with AFNI or TCP/IP sockets for intra- or intercomputer communications. These registration and rotation algorithms are available as AFNI registration and Visualization program [Cox et al. 1999; Nichols et al.2004].

6.3 Post-processing methods for fMRI images

Several post-processing programs 'BrainVoyager', 'AFNI', 'LOFA', 'AIR' etc (read the directory of fMRI softwares in preface) are available as a highly optimized and user-friendly software systems for the analysis and visualization of functional magnetic resonance imaging data [Gokcay et al.1999; Gold et al.1998; Vemuri et al.2003; Friston et al.2002]. These combine surface-based and volume-based tools to study the structure and function of the brain to explore the secrets of the active brain by fast and highly optimized 2D and 3D image analysis and visualization routines, as shown in Figure 16. These are built-in-support for major standard and advanced data formats.

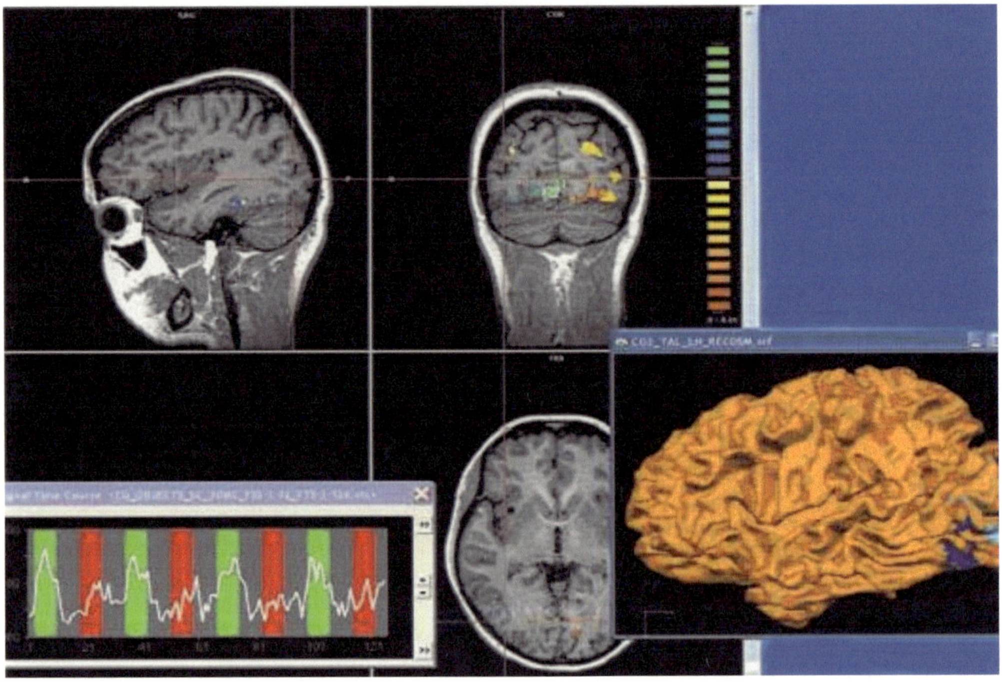

Fig. 16. BrainVoyager is a highly optimized and user-friendly software system for the analysis and visualization of functional and anatomical magnetic resonance imaging data. It combines surface-based and volume-based tools to study the structure and function of the primate brain.

In general, post-processing is completed in following steps:

6.4 Volume-based statistical analysis

Methods include conjunction and Random Effects Analysis (RFX) for single and group analysis via Summary Statistics as following:

1. Fit the model for each subject using different GLMs for each subject or by using a multiple subject GLM.
2. Define the effect of interest for each subject with the contrast factor. Each produces a contrast image containing the contrast of the parameter estimates at each voxel.

3. Feed the contrast images into a GLM that implements a one-sample t test.

The RFX analysis is good technique for making inference from representative subjects [Moutoussis et al.2004]. In fMRI, block analysis, event-related easy selection of regions-of-interest, display of time courses, integration of volume and surface rendering are powerful tools for creation of high-quality figures and movies.

6.5 Advanced methods for automatic brain image-processing

The post-processing offers a comprehensive set of analysis and visualization tools that start its operation on raw data (2D structural and functional matrices) and produces visualization of the obtained results. Now a day, all advanced software features are available via a 'intuitive Windows interface'. Several approaches were performed for surface reconstruction, cortex inflation and flattening; cortex-based statistical data analysis (cbGLM) and inter-subject alignment based on gyral / sulcal pattern; cortex based Independent Component Analysis (cbICA); creation and visualization of EEG / MEG multiple dipole models (fMRI "seeding"); multi-processor support, for ultimate performance; open architecture via COM interface, including scripting and automation [Hong et al. 1999; Kin et al. 2003; Schmitt et al. 2004; Henson et al. 2001].

6.6 Data analysis

It includes data analysis (motion correction, Gaussian spatial and temporal data smoothing, and linear-trend removal, filtering in the frequency domain), correlation analysis, and determination of Talairach coordinates, volume rendering, surface rendering and cortex flattening [Moutoussis et al.2004]. Statistical maps may be computed either in the 2D or 3D representation since structural as well as functional 4D data (space × time) is transformed into Talairach space (see Figures 10 and 11). Talairach transformation is performed in two steps. The first step consists of rotating the 3D data set for each subject to be aligned with the stereotaxic axes. For this step, the locations of the anterior commissure (AC) and the posterior commissure (PC) as well as two rotation parameters for midsagittal alignment have to be specified interactively. In the second step, the extreme points of the cerebrum are specified. These points together with the AC and PC coordinates are then used to scale the 3D data sets into the dimensions of the standard brain of the Talairach and Tournaux atlas [Moutoussis et al.2004]. Isolating the brain gray matter and white matter tissues using region-growing methods, filter operations and the application of 3D templates performs segmentation. Segmentation explores a 3D volume with superimposed pseudocolor-coded statistical maps in a four-window representation showing a sagittal, coronal, transversal and oblique section. Based on a (segmented) 3D data set, a 3D reconstruction of the subjects' head and brain can be calculated and displayed from any specified viewpoint using volume or surface rendering. Parametric and non-parametric statistical maps may be computed and superimposed both on the original functional scans as well as onto T1-weighted 2D or 3D anatomical reference scans. Nonparametric-permutatation approaches are alternate options at low degree of freedom (small sample size to determine intersubject variability) for noisy statistic images when random fields are conservative i.e. smooth variances [Moutoussis et al.2004].

6.7 Volume rendering

It is performed with a fast 'Ray-Casting algorithm'. Lightning calculations are based on 'Phong-shading'. Surface rendering of reconstructed surfaces was performed using OpenGL [Hong et al. 1999].

6.8 The surface reconstruction

The surface reconstruction starts with a sphere (recursively tessellated icosahedron) or a rectangle, which slowly wraps around a (segmented) volume data set. Blood oxygenation level-dependent (BOLD)-based fMRI was performed in the visual cortex, and the foci of fMRI activation utilized as seeding points for 3D fiber reconstruction algorithms, thus provided the map of the axonal circuitry underlying visual information processing [Kim et al. 2003]. A reconstructed cortical surface may be inflated; cut interactively and slowly unfolded minimizing area distortions. Statistical 3D maps may be superimposed on reconstructed, inflated or flattened cortex. Signal time courses may be invoked by simply pointing to any region of a visualized surface.

7. Present knowledge and advances in fMRI data analysis

In last two decades, fMRI technique was improved for fast data acquisition by motion and susceptibility insensitive T_2* weighted EPI, FSE sequences, new task paradigms, motor or sensory task related fMRI robust automated data analysis of brain activation in x, y, and z coordinates as function of time to map out Talairach spaces. SPM data analysis software was developed for matching Talairach coordinates with morphological MRI features. Recent advances in fMRI research in visual and motor events response are extensively reported mainly to identify localized cortical regions by robust image processing segmentation and registration methods, statistical analysis and better spatial resolution using multimodal approaches (fMRI combined with MR spectroscopy, diffusion-weighted imaging, MRI/PET as reviewed in following section. Conventionally, fMRI serves as surface topography patterns related with cognition brain functionality but now art is growing as multimodal fMRI with its adjuncts in characterizing focal or localized region analysis associated with neurological lesions to rule out if focal lesions can affect brain functionalities in various brain areas such as multiple sclerosis lesions, hippocampus size in Alzheimer's Disease, epilepsy as examples. In following sections, we describe advantages of growing imaging technology at high-magnetic field and new possibilities of multimodal imaging.

7.1 High-field MR scanner system is an advantage in fMRI

For high-field fMRI imaging at 3T-11.7T MRI scanners, paramagnetic susceptibility of spin may be related with gyromagnetic ratio (γ) and represented by the Brillouin equation as:

$$\text{Paramagnetic susceptibility} = \frac{h\gamma}{2B_o}\tanh[\frac{|h\gamma B_o|}{|2kT|}] \tag{11}$$

where k is the Boltzmann constant and T absolute temperature.

Susceptibility effect in fMRI increases exponentially as the hyperbolic tangent associated with an increase in the main field, B_o, of the system. T2* detectable activation (ΔI) is significantly increased as shown in Figure 17. Simultaneously, artifacts inducing perturbations also increase. High-field MRI imager system generates T2* contrast for analysis of complex behavioral tasks. It is performed by Independent component-component cross correlation sequence epoch (ICS) as shown in Figure 18. Single subject Ideographic analysis was reported at 3 T systems to locate face-exemplar by regional cortical flat-mapping [Schmitt et al. 2004]. For clinical purposes, 1.5 T systems work well. For advanced neuroimaging investigation, higher field MR systems are essential.

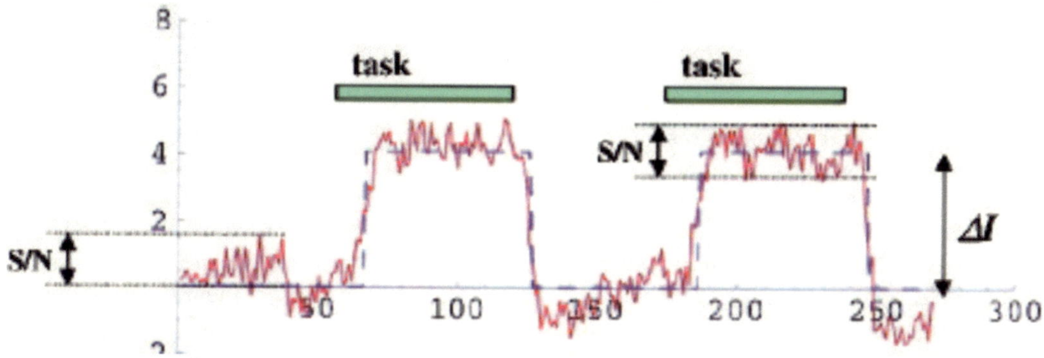

Fig. 17. A typical time series of an activated pixel in primary cortex is shown to represent the performance of horizontal 3T system optimized for fMRI. S/N indicated variation of EPI images, while ΔI, activation induced increase in signal intensity. This time series represents signals from a single voxel volume of 3 mm × 3 mm × 5 mm. The red curves represent raw data and boxcar type model functions shown in blue color.

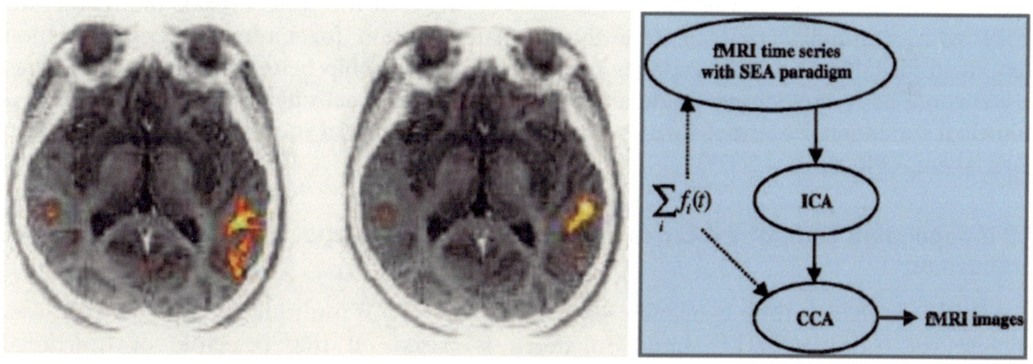

Fig. 18. (On left) Figure represents functional maps shown for comprehension tasks: for reading task (eft panel) and hearing task (right panel). Paradigms requiring tasks of different modalities (visual vs auditory) may provide almost identical activation maps based on the identical abstract concept of "comprehension". Using high field fMRI may provide high quality activation maps to distinguish these activation maps. (On right) Figure shows the Independent component-component cross correlation sequence epoch (ICS).

7.2 fMRI time series analysis

In fMRI, 'time series analysis' by SPM99 is recently used for autocorrection and smoothening. For it, generalized linear model can be expressed as a function of discrete time series, y(t) as:

$$Y(t) = x_c(t)\beta_c + \varepsilon(t) \quad (12)$$

where $x_c(t)$ and $\varepsilon(t)$ are function of time, β_c are time-invariant parameters. Linear time invariance distinguishes neural activity (event) and post-stimulation (epoch) onsets. In general, the resolution of delta function, dt = Tr/T sec and the number of columns = N_c = $N_iN_jN_kN_b$ represent invariance in design matrix. High pass filtering of 'time series' frequency components y(t) get Fourier transformed to remove noise and convolution. Temporal autocorrection in fMRI series is done by 'temporal smoothing' and 'intrinsic autocorrelation' and estimated by 'Auto-Regression' or '1/ f low-pass smoothing' methods to remove bias [Henson et al. 2001].

SPM99 offers 'finite impulse response' (FIR) sets for increased neural activity increases BOLD response 'amplitude' over few seconds based on BOLD from different brain regions such as V1, S1, A1 and higher cortical regions with different vasculature 'Temporal Basis Functions'. FIR sets consist of N_k contiguous box-car functions of peristimulus time, each of duration TH/N_k. TH is maximum duration of high-pass filter. The Fourier set consists of sine Ns and cosine functions of harmonic periods TH, TH/2...TH/N_s. Linear combination of FIR, Fourier sets captures any shape of response in timescale TH/N_k or N_s/TH respectively [Rugg et al. 2002]. 'Event-related Response' and 'Basis sets' were chosen based on stimulus variability and canonical 'Hemodynamic Response Function' and 'F' contrasts determine contribution of different basis sets. Single event- Multi-event type design minimizes the 'contrast error'. Deterministic, static and dynamic stochastic designs use minimum 'stimulus onset synchrony' (SOA_m) and probability of event (for single event design) or transition matrix (for multi-event design) to induce variance over a range of frequencies. Extended softwares are VoxBo, IBASPM, SPM2/5/8,MRIcro, and FSL for better data analysis.

Linear Transform model interprets fMRI signals, origin of the fMRI signals and compares fMRI with neuronal signals. Left and right lateralization for motor cortex stimulation generated visual flash motor response indicative of relationship between different measures of neuronal activity such as single-and multi-unit spiking activity, LFP etc. and reflected neuronal functions. Recently, fMRI signal measured the signal induced by the inputs to a cortical area [Meyer et al.2003].

7.3 Independent component-cross correlation-sequential epoch (ICS) analysis: Image processing

The fMRI acquisition time is usually less per paradigm. For multiple task-oriented studies, analysis of complex higher brain functions is based on the 'principle of functional independence' and functional distinct areas (chronoarchitecture). Independent component-cross correlation-sequential epoch (ICS) segregates distinct areas in cerebral and temporal chronoarchitectonic maps. The different exposures of the brain to natural conditions for different 'durations' segregate the different brain areas for their temporal differences. One subset of natural conditions, reflect free-viewing activity of visual, parietal, temporal areas. However, frontal, pre-frontal cortices functional subdivisions or multivariate paradigms were recently illustrated as shown in Figure 19. A sequential epoch paradigm is composed to embed the function which correlates to the target multiple behavioral hypothesis **(Σifi(t))**. The simplest function is a 'boxcar function' as employed in many fMRI studies. For it, fMRI time series are subjected to blind separation into independent components by independent component analysis. Subsequently, cross correlation analysis is performed utilizing each embedded function, **f(t)**, as model function to achieve multiple fMRI images as behavioral correlates given by the selected function as an activation map. For the hemodynamic reference function (HRF) following a single sensory stimulation, the time course function represents as model function and ICS becomes a reliable method for event-related fMRI. ICS is useful for event related high-field fMRI where T2* contrast enhances the magnitude of activation than that performed on conventional 1.5 T clinical systems [Kiviniemi et al.2004].

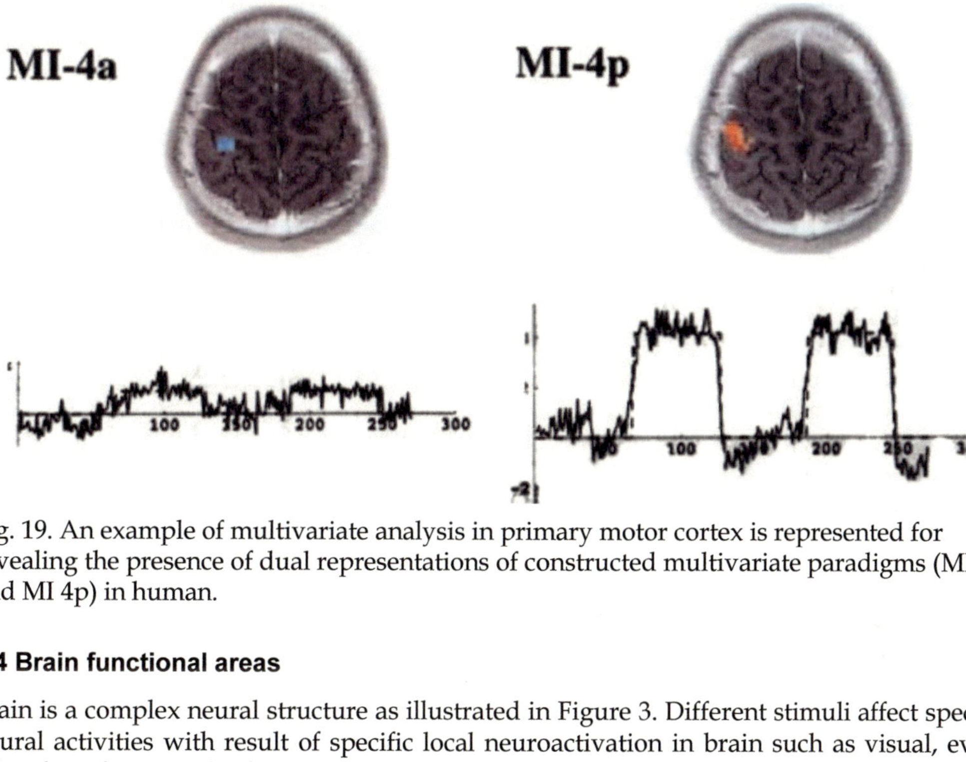

Fig. 19. An example of multivariate analysis in primary motor cortex is represented for revealing the presence of dual representations of constructed multivariate paradigms (MI 4a and MI 4p) in human.

7.4 Brain functional areas

Brain is a complex neural structure as illustrated in Figure 3. Different stimuli affect specific neural activities with result of specific local neuroactivation in brain such as visual, event related, auditory and other motor sensory stimuli cause fMRI visible activation of specific locations in frontal, parietal and temporal lobe regions. We review some of these well-established reports of stimuli in following description.

7.5 Visual stimuli and fMRI activation patterns

- Visual stimuli and event related neural activity by fMRI and image processing methods are reviewed significantly in recent years [18]. Visual areas are recently identified as the boundaries of visual areas V1, V2, V3, V3A, V4, MT/V5, and TEO/V4A in visual cortex and their distribution within the occipital lobe. Motor related areas are known as M1. These corresponding areas are: Broadmann's area (BA 4), SMA (BA 6) and premotor area (BA 6). These fMRI visible areas as shown in Figure 19, are important to interpret fMRI stimulation and its location [Mandeville et al. 1999; Brewer et al.2002]. Recently, new understanding of quantitative visual field eccentricity function measurements on visual field maps by fMRI were made in macaque visual cortex visual areas. fMRI estimated the average receptive field sizes of neurons in each of several striate and extrastriate visual areas of the human cerebral cortex. Retinotopic mapping procedures determined the boundaries of the visual areas and visualized on flattened occipital cortex, primary visual cortex V1, V2, V3/VP and V3A and V4. In all these areas, receptive fields increased in size with increasing stimulus eccentricity similar to macaque monkeys [Schoenfeld et al.2002]. fMRI maps and the visual area maps represent the distribution of cortical signals and computational homologies between human and monkey. Neural activity and the creation of a new memory trace were observed using functional magnetic resonance imaging (fMRI). Event-related fMRI demonstrated the activity in prefrontal and medial temporal lobe areas associated with successful memory storage. Contrast activity was associated with encoding success and encoding effort using a cue in the form of a letter (R or F). These recent studies suggested the prefrontal activation strongly associated with intentional verbal encoding and left medial temporal activation for successful memory on the subsequent test. Cortical regions sensitive to motion processing receive their inputs only via the primary visual cortex (striate cortex).

- Recently, fMRI evidenced higher-order motion-processing in primates and humans with damaged primary visual cortex (e.g., "blindsight" for motion in the blind visual hemifield) for the existence of a direct thalamic functional pathway exists to extrastriate visual cortical motion processing areas that bypasses primary visual cortex [Schoenfeld et al.2002]. Highfield fMRI retinotopic method was reported to map the neural substrate of retinal slip compensation during visual jitter in flattened cortical format. A novel illusion (visual jitter) suggested the compensation mechanism based on retinal motion. fMRI suggested the pathway from V1 to MT+ involved in the compensation stage in stabilizing the visual world [Sasaki et al.2002]. fMRI demonstrated the sensitivity changes controlled within the visual pathway for responses in human visual area V1 to a constant-amplitude, contrast reversing probe presented on a range of mean backgrounds. fMRI signals from probes initiated in the L and M or S cones. Psychophysical tests showed changes in V1 fMRI cortical BOLD signals by 'mean-field adaptation model' within cone photoreceptor classes [Wade et al.2002]. A new mechanism of hypercapnia and hypocapnia was described as alveolar oxygen and CO_2 gases flux and their effect on BOLD response to visual stimulation. At high magnetic field 7 T, the BOLD signal magnitude and dynamics of hemodynamic response represented the effect of CBF under conditions: hypocapnia, normocapnia, and hypercapnia [Cohen et al.2002].
- Binocular interactions present checkerboard stimuli occurring when subjects view dichoptically. A flickering radial checkerboard stimulation of eyes in binocular or monocular conditions, generate specific responses in striate and extrastriate visual cortex on T2*-weighted images of visual cortex acquired with gradient-echo, echoplanar imaging. The striate area, calcarine fissure BOLD response differed for these stimulation conditions [Buchert et al.2002]. Recently, a neuron location by color-selective mapping method has attracted to compare the relationships of ocular dominance and orientation with responses to high-contrast luminance stimulus and patchy distribution of color selectivity to locate different functional subdivisions of striate cortex in macaque. These color patches with the cytochrome-oxidase (CO) blobs speculated the ocular dominance (OD) column. For it, "Ice cube" model of color-selective regions predicted the organization of orientation and ocular dominance functional hypercolumns in V1

[Landisman et al.2002]. Dipole locations in cortical brain (regional visualization) is developed as a new art by fMRI activations. Neural generators of the visual evoked potential (VEP) generate isoluminant checkerboard stimuli. Using Multichannel scalp recordings, retinotopic mapping and dipole modeling techniques estimated the dipole locations of the cortical regions giving rise to C1, P1, and N1 components of VEP [Di Russo et al.2002]. These locations could be matched to both MRI-visible anatomical brain regions and fMRI activations. Several locations are broadly identified as C1 component (striate cortex; area 17), early phase of the P1 component (dorsal extrastriate cortex of the middle occipital gyrus), late phase of the P1 component (ventral extrastriate cortex of the fusiform gyrus), posterior N 150, anterior N 155 (parietal lobe) in relation to visual-perceptual processes. In other development for complex cognitive tasks, neuronal encoding and fMRI processing strategies segregate retention and retrieval phases of visual short-term memory for objects, places and conjunctions in humans. These tasks were associated with spatio-temporal activation of parietal and prefrontal areas during the retention phase and posterior-anterior and right-left dissociation for spatial versus non-spatial memory [Munk et al.2002].

- The 'perceptual switch' stimulus induces responses in areas calcarine to parieto-occipital and ventral and lateral temporo-occipital cortex to anterior insula. During vection, early motion-sensitive visual areas and vestibular parieto-insular cortex deactivate, whereas higher-order parieto- and temporo-occipital areas respond to optical flow retained identical activity levels. Recent fMRI study showed that these areas displayed transient activations as response to the type of visual motion stimulus and perceptual biostability [Kleinschmidt et al.2002]. fMRI distinguished different neural substrates as 'visual object recognition' sites i.e. lateral occipital and posterior inferior temporal cortex with lower activity for repetitions of both real and non-sense objects; fusiform and left inferior frontal regions with lower activity for repetitions of only real 3D objects; left inferior frontal cortex for different exemplars evidencing dissociable subsystems in ventral visual cortex with distinct view-dependent and view-invariant object representations. Repetition-priming method was proposed for visual stimuli recurring at unpredictable intervals, either with the same appearance or with changes in size, viewpoint or exemplar [Vuilleumier et al.2002].

7.6 Event related potentials and fMRI activation patterns

- Combining event-related potentials (ERP) and fMRI activation provide temporal and spatial resolution, functional connectivity of neural processes of same neural networks within the bilateral occipital gyrus, lingual gyrus; precuneus and middle frontal gyrus; and the left inferior and superior parietal lobe; middle and superior temporal gyrus; cingulate gyrus, superior frontal gyrus and precentral gyrus. It evidenced the correlation within the common activity and time-range in a complex visual language task [Jackson et al.2004]. These tasks comprise specific stimulus-response associations and activate a variety of non-specific cortical regions [Maclin et al.2001]. Dystonia, a movement disorder involves involuntary coordination of agonist and antagonist muscles, which cause abnormal posture or twisting. Event related fMRI technique revealed impairment of muscle contraction and relaxation. Comparison of activated volume in cortical motor areas in dystonia patients with volunteers showed different muscle relaxation and contraction activation volumes as shown in Figure 20. In these tasks, mainly SM1 and SMA activated areas were reduced contra- laterally in dystonia patients as evidenced by time course of fMRI signal in SMA activation area [Oga et al.2002].

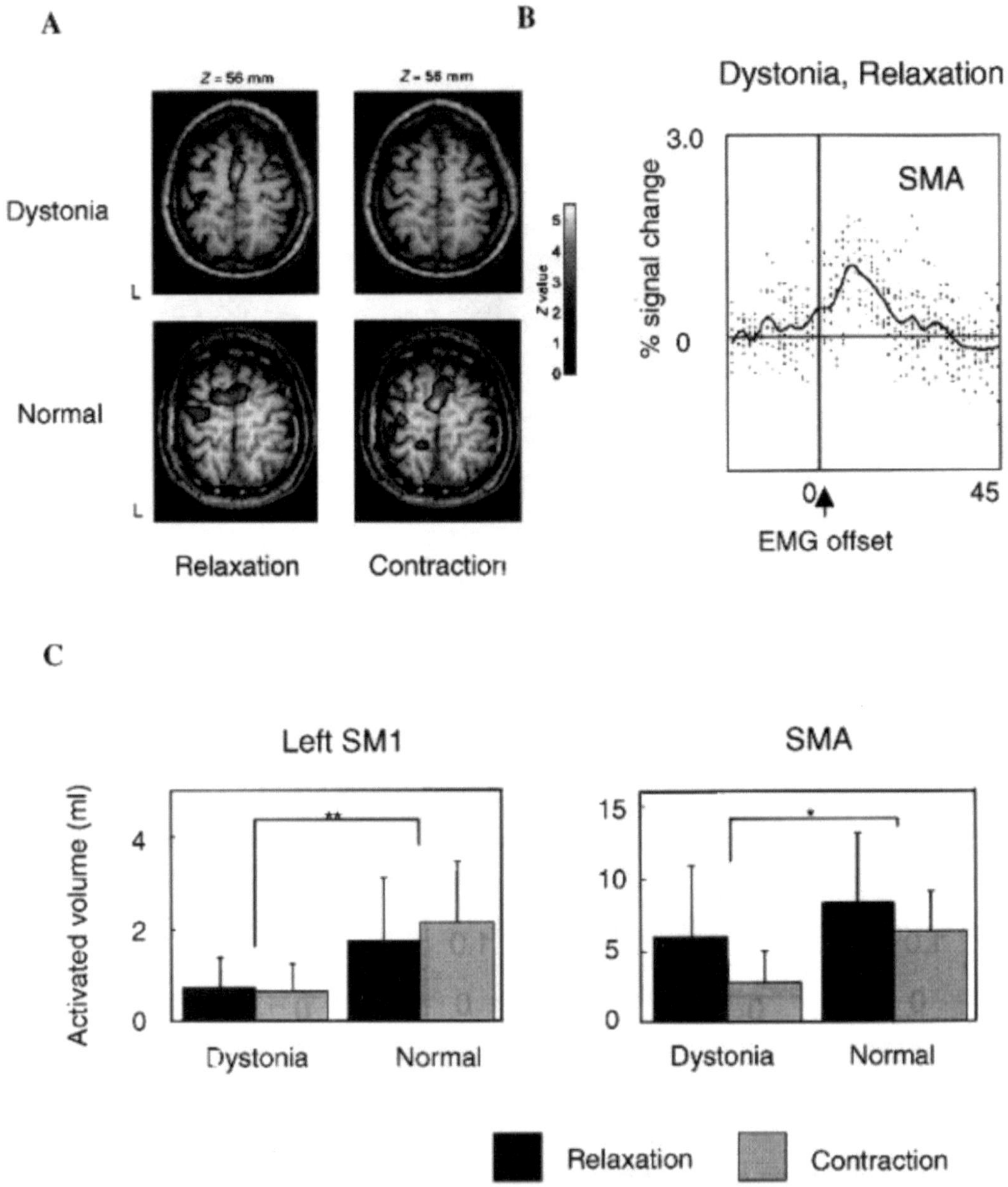

Fig. 20. Figure represents the application of event-related fMRI to dystonia. Comparison of activated volume in motor cortical areas in a patient with dystonia and a normal subject is represented in the muscle relaxation and contraction task. In both tasks, the activated areas in the M1 and SMA were smaller for dystonia while in normal these activated areas were larger (see top 4 panels shown as A). A solid line indicates a mean signal change across ten trials shown as dots. The transient signal change timelocked to EMG offset was observable even in single trial (see panel B). Group data from eight patients and twelve healthy volunteers; demonstrate that activated volumes in the contralateral SM1 and SMA are greater in the healthy volunteers than in the dystonic patients.

7.7 Sensory and motor systems

- Sensory and motor systems interact in complex ways. Voluntary movements with visual attention yield distinct fMRI hemodynamic signals and brain activations i.e. making repetitive finger movements, attending to the color of a visual stimulus or simultaneous finger movement and visual attention. In these processes, the primary motor cortex, supplementary motor area, cerebellum, sparse cerebral cortical and substantial bilateral cerebellar locations get active. Activation-related interactions in the left superior parietal lobule, the right fusiform gyrus, and left insula, recently were indicated their role in visual attention and movement [Indovina et al.2001].
- Different psychological tests have been developed to evaluate frontal tasks of macaque monkeys and humans. Wisconsin Card Sorting Test (WCST) characterized the frontal lobe lesions in macaque monkeys and humans based on behavioral flexibility in the form of cognitive set shifting. Equivalent visual stimuli and task sequence showed transient activation related to cognitive set shifting in focal regions of prefrontal cortex in both monkeys and humans. These functional homologs were located in cytoarchitectonically equivalent regions in the posterior part of ventrolateral prefrontal cortex. This comparative imaging provided insights into the evolution of cognition in primates [Nakahara et al.2002].
- Test-retest precision of functional magnetic resonance imaging (fMRI) by student 't' mapping (STM) is recently described for independent component analysis (ICA) using two or three iterations of visual and auditory stimuli for fMRI scans. Concurrence ratios of the activated voxels divided by the average number of voxels activated in each repetition showed similar test-retest precision of ICA as STM [Nybakken et al.2002].

7.8 High spatial resolution fMRI

High spatial resolution in fMRI showed as dependent on hyperoxic hemodynamic response to neural activity in short duration and it was used to investigate the columnar architecture of ocular dominance within the primary visual cortex [Yoo et al.2004]. For intensity-based non-rigid registration of medical images was developed for atlas based segmentation and intensity-based geometric correction of functional magnetic resonance imaging (fMRI) images by 'Adaptive bases algorithm' to register the smallest structures in the image [Rohde et al.2003].

8. Present developments and future perspectives on fMRI and adjunct imaging multimodal techniques

The goal of this chapter was to introduce the neurophysiological factors and image processing principles of fMRI to suggest potential future applications in neuroscience and physiology. These future directions include neurosurgical planning and improved assessment of risk for individual patients, improved assessment and strategies for the treatment of chronic pain, improved seizure localization, and improved understanding of the physiology of neurological disorders. We look ahead to newer algorithms, enhanced fMRI sensitivity and spatial resolution by use of high field systems, ASL and phase array coils or newer contrast agents [Ugurbil et al.2002]. Presently, other emerging applications of

EEG/MEG, PET and neuropsychological testing along with fMRI are coming up as the benefits of this fMRI technology incorporated into current neuroscience and future patient care. These adjunct methods are:

8.1 Diffusion based functional MRI

Neuronal activity produces some immediate physical changes in cell shape that can be detected because they affect the compartment shape and size for water diffusion. A much improved spatial and temporal resolution for fMRI data collection has now been achieved by using diffusion MRI methodology that can detect these changes in neurons. The abrupt onset of increased neuron cell size occurs before the metabolic response commences, is shorter in duration and does not extend significantly beyond the area of the actual cell population involved. This technique is a diffusion weighted technique (DWI). There is some evidence that similar changes in axonal volume in white matter may accompany activity and this has been observed using a DTI (diffusion tensor imaging) technique. The future importance of diffusion-based functional techniques relative to BOLD techniques is not yet clear.

8.2 Contrast MR

An injected contrast agent such as an iron oxide that has been coated by a sugar or starch (to hide from the body's defense system), causes a local disturbance in the magnetic field that is measurable by the MRI scanner. The signals associated with these kinds of contrast agents are proportional to the cerebral blood volume. While this semi-invasive method presents a considerable disadvantage in terms of studying brain function in normal subjects, it enables far greater detection sensitivity than BOLD signal, which may increase the viability of fMRI in clinical populations. Other methods of investigating blood volume that do not require an injection are a subject of current research, although no alternative technique in theory can match the high sensitivity provided by injection of contrast agent.

8.3 Arterial spin labeling

Arterial Spin Labelling (ASL), also known as arterial spin tagging, is an MRI technique capable of measuring cerebral blood flow (CBF) *in vivo*. ASL is capable of providing cerebral perfusion maps, without requiring the administration of a contrast agent or the use of ionising radiation, as it uses magnetically-labelled endogenous blood water as a freely-diffusible tracer. It was first proposed in 1992 and has since benefited from a number of modifications aimed at improving its robustness. ASL can monitor changes in CBF with activation and fMRI studies can therefore be conducted using ASL instead of relying on the BOLD effect. ASL fMRI is less popular than BOLD, as it suffers from a lower signal to noise ratio, can be less sensitive to weak stimuli and its temporal resolution is poorer than in BOLD studies. On the plus side, it can provide quantitative measures of a single well-defined parameter, CBF, whose baseline value can also be determined in the same experiment. It has also been found to outperform BOLD in terms of stability to slow signal drifts and localization of the activation area. The ASL activation signal is believed to be dominated by changes in the capillary bed of the activated area of the cortex, wheareas the BOLD signal is likely to be dominated by changes in the oxygenation of nearby veins.

8.4 Magnetic resonance spectroscopic imaging

Magnetic resonance spectroscopic imaging (MRS) is another, NMR-based process for assessing function within the living brain. MRS takes advantage of the fact that protons (hydrogen atoms) residing in differing chemical environments depending upon the molecule they inhabit (H_2O vs. protein, for example) possess slightly different resonant properties (chemical shift). For a given volume of brain (typically > 1 cubic cm), the distribution of these H resonances can be displayed as a spectrum.

The area under the peak for each resonance provides a quantitative measure of the relative abundance of that compound. The largest peak is composed of H_2O. However, there are also discernible peaks for choline, creatine, N-acetylaspartate (NAA) and lactate. Fortuitously, NAA is mostly inactive within the neuron, serving as a precursor to glutamate and as storage for acetyl groups (to be used in fatty acid synthesis) – but its relative levels are a reasonable approximation of neuronal integrity and functional status. Brain diseases (schizophrenia, stroke, certain tumors, multiple sclerosis) can be characterized by the regional alteration in NAA levels when compared to healthy subjects. Creatine is used as a relative control value since its levels remain fairly constant, while choline and lactate levels have been used to evaluate brain tumors.

8.5 Diffusion tensor imaging

Diffusion tensor imaging (DTI) is a related use of MR to measure anatomical connectivity between areas. Although it is not strictly a functional imaging technique because it does not measure dynamic changes in brain function, the measures of inter-area connectivity it provides are complementary to images of cortical function provided by BOLD fMRI. White matter bundles carry functional information between brain regions. The diffusion of water molecules is hindered across the axes of these bundles, such that measurements of water diffusion can reveal information about the location of large white matter pathways[Awojoyogbe et al. 2011]. Illnesses that disrupt the normal organization or integrity of cerebral white matter (such as multiple sclerosis) have a quantitative impact on DTI measures.

8.6 fMRI and EEG

Functional MRI has high spatial resolution but relatively poor temporal resolution (of the order of several seconds). Electroencephalography (EEG) directly measures the brain's electrical activity, giving high temporal resolution (~milliseconds) but low spatial resolution. The two techniques are therefore complementary and may be used simultaneously to record brain activity.

Recording an EEG signal inside an MRI system is technically challenging. The MRI system introduces artifacts into the EEG recording by inducing currents in the EEG leads via Faraday induction. This can happen through several different mechanisms. An imaging sequence applies a series of short radiofrequency pulses which induce a signal in the EEG system. The pulses are short and relatively infrequent, so interference may be avoided by blanking (switching off) the EEG system during their transmission. Magnetic field gradients used during imaging also induce a signal, which is harder to remove as it is in a similar frequency range to the EEG signal. Current is also induced when EEG leads move inside the magnet bore (i.e. when the patient moves during the exam). Finally, pulsed blood flow in the patient in the static magnetic field also induces a signal (called a ballistocardiographic artifact), which is also within the frequency range of interest. The EEG system also affects the MRI scan. Metal in the EEG leads and electrodes can introduce susceptibility artifacts into MR images. Care must also be taken to limit currents induced in the EEG leads via the MRI RF system, which could heat the leads sufficiently to burn the subject. Having simultaneously recorded EEG and fMRI data, the final hurdle is to co-register the two datasets, as each is reconstructed using a different algorithm, subject to different distortions in EEG-fMRI.

In recent years, lot of future excitement is evident in the following areas of brain information extraction by segmentation and registration methods applied to fMRI and above-mentioned multimodal adjunct methods. These include mainly automated nonlinear labeling; and automated surface reconstructions. Automated surface reconstruction appears to be possible by: i. cortical surface-based analysis by segmentation and surface reconstruction [Fischl et al.1999a]; ii. cortical surface-based analysis by inflation, flattening, and a surface-based coordinate system [Fischl et al.1999b]. Automated anatomical brain labeling may be performed by: i. whole brain segmentation: automated labeling of neuro-anatomical structures in the human brain [Fischl et al.2002]; ii. multipatient registration of brain fMRI using intensity and geometric features [Cachier et al.2001]; iii. automatic detection and labeling of the human cortical fields in magnetic resonance data sets [Lohmann et al.1998]. With advancement of neurophysiological principles, more and more facts are explored on physiological origin of neuroactivation and brain functional relationships. Recently a biophysical mechanism of low-frequency drift in blood-oxygen-level-dependent (BOLD) functional magnetic resonance imaging (fMRI) (0.00-0.01 Hz) was reported by exploring its spatial distribution, dependence on imaging parameters, and relationship with task-induced brain activation. Authors showed that the spatial distribution of low-frequency drifts in human brain followed a tissue-specific pattern, with greater drift magnitude in the gray matter than in white matter. In gray matter, the dependence of drift magnitudes on TE was similar to that of task-induced BOLD signal changes, i.e., the absolute drift magnitude reached the maximum when TE approached T(2)* whereas relative drift magnitude increased linearly with TE. By systematically varying the flip angle, it was found that drift magnitudes possessed a positive dependence on image intensity. In fMRI studies with visual stimulation, a strong positive correlation between drift effects at baseline and task-induced BOLD signal changes was observed both across subjects and across activated pixels within individual participants. Unique point was that intrinsic, physiological drift effects are a major component of the spontaneous fluctuations of BOLD fMRI signal within the frequency range of 0.0-0.1 Hz[Yan et al.2009]. A rare attempt was made to integrate complementary functional and structural MRI data in a patient with localization-related epilepsy with partial and secondarily generalized seizures and a hemiparesis due to a malformation of cortical development (MCD) in the right hemisphere by using EEG-triggered functional MRI (fMRI), diffusion tensor imaging (DTI), and chemical shift imaging

(CSI). fMRI revealed significant changes in regional blood oxygenation associated with interictal epileptiform discharges within the MCD. DTI showed a heterogeneous microstructure of the MCD with reduced fractional anisotropy, a high mean diffusivity, and displacement of myelinated tracts. CSI demonstrated low N-acetyl aspartate (NAA) concentrations in parts of the MCD. MR methods described functional, microstructural, biochemical characteristics of the epileptogenic tissue and pathophysiology of epilepsy [Bauewig et al.2001]. Recent focus of fMRI research is shifting towards integrated neurofunctional data acquisition such as electrophysiology (EEG), with simultaneous neurochemical mapping and diffusion tensor/molecular perfusion [Horwitz et al.2002; McDonald et al.2010; Matsumoto et al.2005; Vartiainen et al.2011]. However, success is awaited because of non-localized nature of diffusion tensor and fMRI sensitive brain functionality, wide variation in neurochemical changes in the same brain regions. In case of such possibility of integrated data acquisition, multimodal approaches such as fMRI/MRS/PET will be single step feasible one platform imaging method available in clinical neuroimaging in near future [Dale et al.2001]. The basis of imaging is Munro-Kellie doctrine principle to predict decline in cerebral venous blood volume secondary to an increase in cerebral arterial blood volume in fMRI identical to image blood flow by H_2O^{15}-PET [Fox et al.1984].

8.7 Multimodal methods of fMRI combined with adjuncts in localized neurodegeneration

The art of multimodal imaging approach is based on the fact that single platform can be used in one step imaging by using fMRI, EEG, diffusion MRI, MRS, PET, simultaneously in selected area of brain[Awojoyogbe et al. 2011]. Some notable examples are illustrated below.

Multiple Sclerosis: First author reported measurement of neurochemicals in growing MS lesions with MRSI. Gamma-aminobutyric Acid (GABA) was used as indicator of brain functionality [Sharma 2004; Sharma 2002]. Several reports indicated the value of fMRI as multimodal method combined with DTI, MRS, PET to assess cognitive impairment in multiple sclerosis. Such approach was based on the link between structural, metabolic and functional changes in multiple sclerosis [Filippi et al.2001]. It was interesting that neurochemicals and cognitive impairment in MS showed significant role [Tartaglia et al.2006]. This approach was further extended in other study based on the fact that cognitive impairment by fMRI was related with structural MRI changes and metabolic changes by PET [Sorensen et al.2006]. Overall, growing art of fMRI is now established in multiple sclerosis [Korsholm et al.2007]. Other investigators reported the lesions as a result of inflammatory demyelination which led to fMRI visible cognitive impairment [Rachbauer et al.2006]. Since the development of fMRI based multimodal imaging in evaluation of lesions, main obstacle remained coregistration and statistical data analysis [Fu et al.1996]. Now robust techniques of fMRI data analysis are available for structural and functional MRI correlation analysis to make evaluation of cortical reorganization in MS. We illustrate one example of T2*-weighted echo planar images acquired (64 · 64 matrix over a 24-cm field of view). These consisted of 25 consecutive, 4-mm thick axial sections, with TR/TE (repetition time/echo time) = 3000/50 ms, a 90_ flip angle and one excitation. [Peresedova et al.2009; Rocca et al.2009]. Motor task paradigm ('stop' and 'start') acoustic signals for hand motion was used for fMRI1 and 2 acquisition and voxel Z score analysis in x,y,z coordinates to make Talairach space by linear transformation as shown in Table 1.

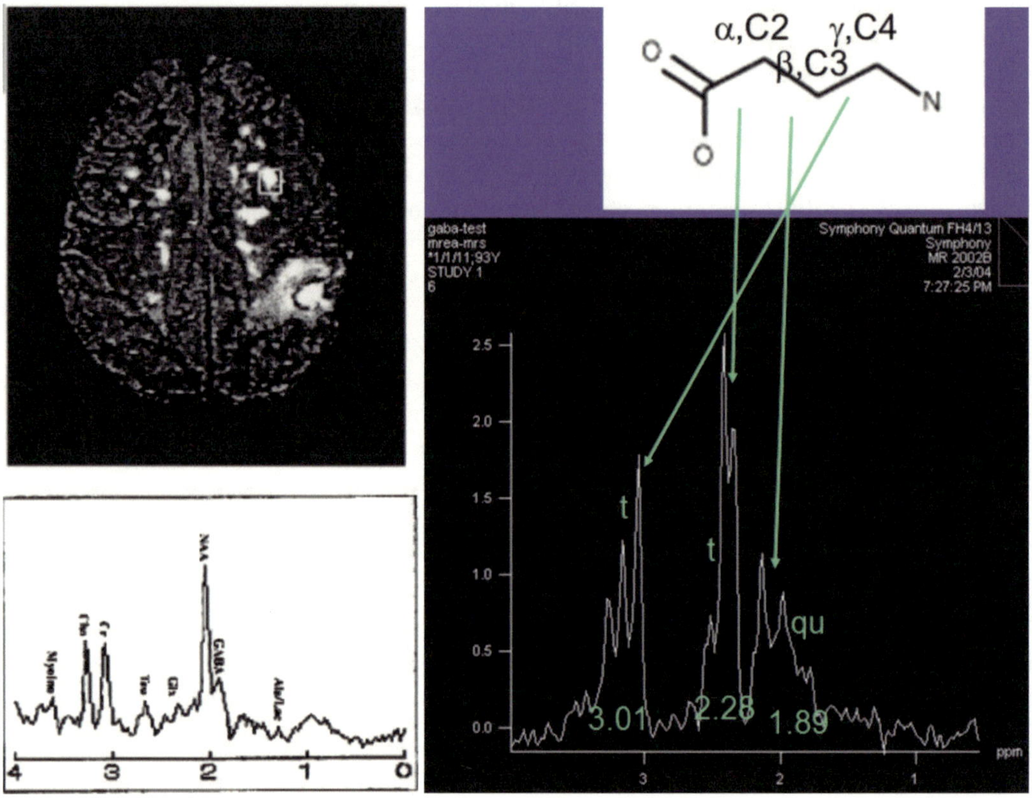

Fig. 21. A typical MS lesion rich voxel (upper panel) with respective spectral peaks is shown (panel at bottom), showing peak at 1.85 ppm for GABA metabolites (see enlarged panel on left at bottom and right) in 48 year old female patient. For simplicity, metabolites are labeled for lipids at 0.8-1.2 ppm, lactate-alanine at 1.2-1.33 ppm, NAA at 2.01 ppm, Cr at 3.0 ppm, Cho at 3.2 ppm, Myo-inositol at 3.6 ppm, Taurine at 2.8 ppm, Gltamine/Glutamate (Glx) , GABA peaks at 1.85, ethanolamine at 3.8 ppm, Glycine at 3.55 ppm, Threonine at 1.31 ppm (see panel on left at bottom). Reproduced with permission of reference Sharma 2004.

Alzheimer's Disease is a diffused injury due to neurofibrillary amyloid plaque formation affecting cortical and posterior cingulate region with fMRI visible cognitive impairment. Recently, multimodal imaging was established and reviewed to assess cognitive impairment using magnetic resonance spectroscopy, perfusion, and diffusion tensor properties [Zimmy et al.2011; Minati et al.2007]. However, other biophysical properties such as changes in biomagnetic, electrophysiological signals along with metabolite screening were established as link between neurochemical and magnetic interactions in brain during development of Alzheimer's Disease [Maesti et al.2005]. In quest of measuring these changes, deformable shape-intensity models were reported in Alzheimer's Disease, dementia [Zhu et al.2003; Gilberto et al.1996; Giacometti et al.1994].

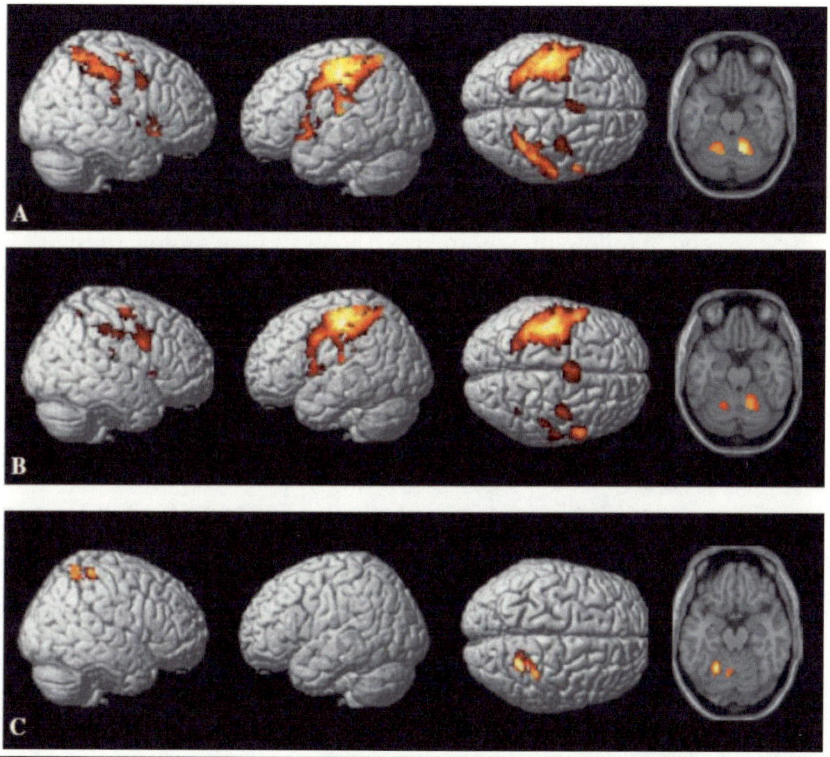

Brain area	Baseline		Follow-up	
	Talairach coordinates (x, y, z)	Z	Talairach coordinates (x, y, z)	Z
L sensorimotor cortex (BA 1-4)	-44, -19, 43	5.80	- 38, -19, 47	7.57
L inferior parietal lobule (BA 40)	- 46, -32, 52	5.24	-53, -30, 24	4.15
			-49, -38, 48	3.87
L lateral premotor cortex (BA 6)	-34, -5, -55	5.14	-59, 6, 32	6.69
L supplementary motor area (BA 6)	-2, -1, 55	4.27	-2, 1, 53	5.44
L lentiform nucleus	-12, -12, -1	5.22	-26, 3, 9	5.21
L thalamus	-12, -11,13	4.72	-16, -17, 3	5.09
L insula	-55, 12, 3	4.69	-49, -20, 16	5.65
L cerebellum	-18, -55, -17	5.17	– –	-----
R sensorimotor cortex (BA 1-4)	42, 0, 52	4.06	45, -27, 40	4.55
R inferior parietal lobule (BA 40)	32, -48, 54	5.23	40, -33, 40	4.63
			61, -2, 19	4.39
R lateral premotor cortex (BA 6)	30, -7, 57	5.08	61, 7, 29	5.77
	57, 8, 36	4.81	36, -11, 58	5.26
R superior parietal cortex (BA 7)	32, -48, 54	5.23	36, -52, 56	4.67
R lentiform nucleus	–	–	22, -2, 2	4.37
R thalamus	12, -7, 13	4.17	12, -6, 13	4.17
R insula	57, 19, -4	4.78	57, 16, 1	4.22
	47, 4, -1	3.91		
R cerebellum	18, 55, 17	6.59	18, -53, -18	6.22
Vermis	2, -67, -10	5.89	2, -50, -3	4.68

Z = voxel level.

Fig. 22. Group maps generated from random effect analysis showing (A) task-related activation at fMRI1, (B) task-related activation at fMRI2 and (C) task-related activity decrease between the two fMRI studies during right hand movement in 18 patients with multiple sclerosis. Significant areas of activation (in colour) are superimposed on 3D brain rendering and slices (z = -18). Areas of decreased activity (fMRI1 > fMRI2) (C) included the right (ipsilateral) sensorimotor cortex and the left (contralateral) cerebellum. One-sample t-test ($P < 0.05$) corrected at the cluster level. Images are displayed according to the neurological convention. Location of significant neuroactivations ($P < 0.05$ corrected at the cluster level) during right hand movement in 18 MS patients are shown in table (see at bottom) at baseline and at follow-up within group analysis (one sample t-test SPM99 using Talairach coordinates in images on top). Reproduced with permission from reference Pantano et al.2005.

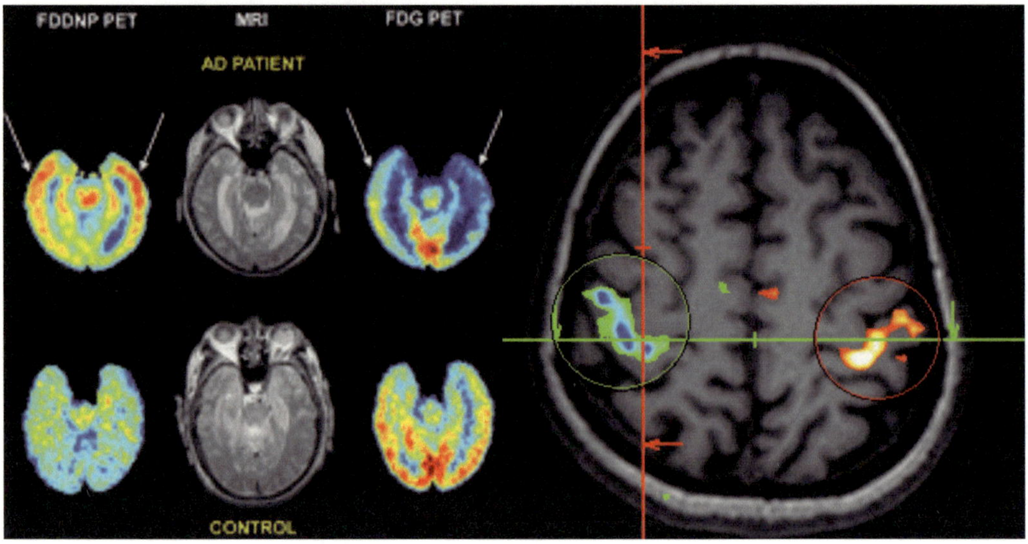

Fig. 23. Multimodal imaging is shown for fMRI combined with FDDNP-PET and FDG-PET to illustrate sites of high oxygen or high glycolysis metabolism (on left panel) and locations of neuroactivation (on right panel). Copyright material from webpage http://precedings.nature.com/documents/4317/version/1

Initial application of fMRI in epilepsy evaluation was exciting [Sullivan et al.2005]. However, epilepsy is considered as focal brain disease with possible regional changes in brain function, diffusion tensor properties, neurochemicals [Krakow et al.1999]. fMRI with simultaneous neurochemical measurement serves as noninvasive quantitative MR modality to assess the epileptogenic foci [Morales-Chacon 2001]. Diffusion tensor tractography and neurochemicals with fMRI pinpoint the location of motor neuron disease and schizophrenia[Nelles et al.2008; Steel et al.2001]. MRS and DTI methods have been developed to evaluate and assess the cerebral small vessel disease progress and its chemical nature [Nitkunan et al. 2006]. Being more sentive to electrophysiological response epilepsy is best evaluated by electrophysiology and use of electrodes [Guye et al.2002]. Now attempts were made in the direction of metabolic and oxygen changes during epileptogenic development in cortex using PET/MRI/DTI [Chandra et al.2006].

9. Conclusion

Present chapter introduces the concept of functional MRI and physiological basis of neuroactivation as a result of motor and sensory tasks to make change in blood oxygen and blood flow characteristics in some established neurodegenerative diseases with cognitive impairments in multiple sclerosis, Alzheimer's Disease, epilepsy. fMRI technique is offshoot of structural MRI with other adjunct imaging techniques and it serves as multimodal imaging to map out structural and functional changes in different brain areas simultaneously to decipher the information of neurochemical, anatomical, regional differences to make assessment of cognition impairment, brain recovery and brain functionality before and after disease or drug treatment. Major issues still remain unsolved of wide variability of fMRI sensitive neuroactive locations, fast acquisition, low resolution and rapid data analysis. With available robust and rapid techniques and software, it will be easier to map brain functions simultaneous with neurochemical and metabolic imaging.

10. Disclosure of interest

Authors have no conflict of interest. The chapter is based on the contents from a review article authored by authors of this chapter and cited as reference 108 in the reference list.

11. References

Amunts, K.., Schleicher, A., Ditterich, A., Zilles, K. (2003). Broca's region: Cytoarchitectonic Asymmetry and Developmental Changes. *The Journal of Comparative Neurology*, 465, pp72-89.

Awojoyogbe, O.B., Dada,M. (2011) Basis for the application of analytical models of the Bloch NMR flow equations for functional resonance imaging(fMRI): A review. Renet Patents on Medical Imaging.1,pp 33-67.

Bandettini, P.A., Ungerleider, L.G. (2001) From neuron to BOLD: new connections. Nature Neurosci. 4, pp864–866.

Bandettini, P.A., Cox, R.W. (2000) Event related fMRI contrast when using constant interstimulus interval: Theory and experiment. Magn Reson Med. 30, pp161–173.

Baudewig, J., Bittermann, H.J., Paulus, W., Frahm, J. (2002) Simultaneous EEG and functional MRI of epileptic activity: a case report. Clinical Neurophysiology,112(7), pp1196-1200.

Horwitz B, Poeppel D. How Can EEG/MEG and fMRI/PET Data Be Combined? Human Brain Mapping, 17, pp1–3.

Binkofski, F., Amunts, K., Stephen, K.M., Posse, S., Schormann, T., Freund, H.J., Zilles, K. & Seitz, R.J. (2000). Broca's Region Subserves Imagery of Motion: A Combined Cytoarchitectonic and fMRI Study. *Human Brain Mapping*, 11, pp273-285

Brewer, A.A., Press, W.A., Logothetis N.K., Wandell, B.A. (2002) Visual areas in macaque cortex measured using functional magnetic resonance imaging. J Neurosci. 22, pp10416–26.

Buchert, M., Greenle,e M.W., Rutschmann, R.M., Kraemer, F.M., Luo, F., Hennig, J. (2002) Functional magnetic resonance imaging evidence for binocular interactions in human visual cortex. Exp Brain Res. 145, pp334–9.

Buxton, R.B., Frank, L.R. (1997) A model for the coupling between cerebral blood flow and oxygen metabolism during neuronal stimulation. J Cereb Blood Flow Metab.17, pp 64–72.

Cachier, P., Mangin, J.F., Pennec, X., Riviere, D., Papadopoulos-Orfanos, D., Regis, J., Ayachi, N. (2001) Multipatient registration of brain MRI using intensity and geometric features. In: Niessan W, Vierever M, editor. Proceedings of MICCAI. LNCS 2208. pp. 734–742.

Cao, Y., Vikingstad, E. M., George, P. K., Johnson, A. F., & Welch, K. M. A. (1999). Cortical Language Activation in Stroke Patients Recovering From Aphasia With Functional MRI. *Stroke, 30,* pp. 2331-2340.

Caplan, D., Alpert, N., Waters, G. & Olivieri, A. (2000). Activation of Broca's Area by Syntactic Processing Under Conditions of Concurrent Articulation. *Human Brain Mapping*, 9, pp 65–71.

Chandra PS, Salamon N, Huang J, Wu JY, Koh S, Vinters HV, Mathern GW. FDG-PET/MRI coregistration and diffusion-tensor imaging distinguish epileptogenic tubers and cortex in patients with tuberous sclerosis complex: a preliminary report. Epilepsia. 2006;47(9):1543-9.

Cheng, K., Waggoner, R.A., Tanaka, K.. (2001) Human ocular dominance columns as revealed by high field functional magnetic resonance imaging. Neuron. 32, pp. 359–374.

Ciulla, C., Deek, F.P. (2002) Performance assessment of an algorithm for the alignment of fMRI time series. Brain Topogr. 14, pp. 313–32.

Cohen, E.R., Ugurbil, K., Kim, S.G. (2002) Effect of basal conditions on the magnitude and dynamics of the blood oxygenation level-dependent fMRI response. J Cereb Blood Flow Metab. 22, pp. 1042–53.

Cox, R.W., (1999) Jesmanowicz A. Real-time 3D image registration for functional MRI. Magn Reson Med. 42, pp.1014–1018.

Cox, R.W.(1996) AFNI: software for analysis and visualization of functional magnetic resonance neuroimages. Comput Biomed Res. 29,pp.162–73.

Dale, A.M., Halgren, E. (2001) Spatiotemporal mapping of brain activity by integration of multiple imaging modalities. Curr Opin Neurobiol. 11, 2, pp.202-8.

Di Russo, F., Martinez, A., Sereno,M.I., Pitzalis, S., Hillyard, S.A.(2002) Cortical sources of the early components of the visual evoked potential. Hum Brain Mapp.15, pp. 95–111.

Disbrow, E.A., Slutsky, D.A., Roberts, T.P., Krubitzer, L.A. (2000) Functional MRI at 1.5 Tesla: A comparison of the blood oxygenation level-dependent signal and electrophysiology. Proc Natl Acad Sci USA. 97, pp. 9718–9723.

Fadiga, L. & Craighero, L. (2006a). Hand actions and speech representation in Broca's area. *Cortex*, 42, pp. 486–490

Fadiga, L., Craighero, L., Desto, M. F., Finos, L., Cotillon-Williams, N. et al. (2006b). Language in shadow, *Social Neuroscience*, 1, pp.77–89

Filippi, M.(2001) Linking structural, metabolic and functional changes in multiple sclerosis. Eur J Neurol. 2001 Jul;8(4):291-7.

Fink, G.R., Manjaly, Z.M., Stephen, K.E., Gurd, J.M., Zilles, K., Amunts K., Marshall, J.C. (2006). A Role for Broca's Are Beyond Language Processing: Evidence from Neuropsychology and fMRI. In: *Broca's Region*. Amunts, K. & Grodzinsky, Y. (Eds). Oxford University Press, Oxford

Fischl, B., Sereno, M.I., Dale, A.M. (1999) Cortical Surface-based analysis I: Segmentation and Surface Reconstruction. Neuroimage. 9, pp. 195–207.

Fischl, B., Sereno, M.I., Dale, A.M. (1999) Cortical Surface-based analysis II: Inflation, Flattening, and a Surface-Based Coordinate System. Neuroimge. 9, pp.179–194.

Fischl, B., Salat, D.H., Busa, E., Albert, M., Dieterich, M., Haselgrove, C., van der Kouwe, A., Killiany, R., Kennedy, D., Klaveness, S., Montillo, A., Makris, N., Rosen, B., Dale, A.M. (2002) Whole brain segmentation: Automated labeling of neuroanatomical structures in the human brain. Neurone. 33, pp.341–355.

Fox, P.T., Mintun, M.A., Raichle, M., Herscovitch, P. (1984) A noninvasive approach to quantitative functional brain mapping with H_2O^{15} Positron Emission Tomography. J Cereb Blood Flow Metab, 4, pp.329-333.

Fransson, P., Kruger, G., Merboldt, K.D., Frahm, J. (1997)A comparative FLASH and EPI study of repetitive and sustained visual activation. NMR Biomed. 10, pp.204–7.

Friederici, A. (1998). The neurobiology of language comprehension, In: *Language Comprehension: A Biological Perspective,* Friederici, A.D. (Ed.),Springer, Berlin/Heidelberg/New York, pp. 263-301.

Friston, K.J., Glaser, D.E., Henson, R.N.A., Kiebel, S., Phillips, C., Ashburner, J.(2002) Classical and Bayesian inference in neuroimaging applications. Neuroimage. 16, pp.484–512.

Fu, L., Wolfson, C., Worsley, K.J., De Stefano, N., Collins, D.L., Narayanan S, Arnold, D.L.(1996) Statistics for investigation of multimodal MR imaging data and an application to multiple sclerosis patients. NMR Biomed. 9,8, pp.339-46.

Giacometti, A.R., Davis, P.C., Alazraki, N.P., Malko, J.A. (1994) Anatomic and physiologic imaging of Alzheimer's disease. Clin Geriatr Med.10,2, pp.277-98.

Gilberto González, R. (1996) Molecular and functional magnetic resonance neuroimaging for the study of dementia. Ann N Y Acad Sci. 777, pp.37-48.

Gokcay, D., Mohr, C.M., Crosson, B., Leonard, C.M., Bobholz, J.A. (1999) LOFA: software for individualized localization of functional MRI activity. Neuroimage. 10, pp.749–55.

Gold, S., Christian, B., Arndt, S., Zeien, G., Cizadlo, T., Johnson, D.L., Flaum, M., Andreasen, N.C. (1998) MRI statistical software packages: a comparative analysis. Hum Brain Mapp. 6, pp.73–84.

Goodyear, B.G., Menon, R.S.. (2001) Brief visual stimulation allows mapping of ocular dominance in visual cortex using fMRI. Human Brain Mapp. 14, pp.210–217.

Greewe, T., Bornkessel, I., Zysset, S., Wiese, R., von Cramon, Y.D., Schlesewsky, M. (2005). The Reemergence of the Unmarked: A New Perspective on the Language-Specific Function of Broca's Area. *Human Brain Mapping*, 26, pp.178–190.

Guye, M., Le Fur, Y., Confort-Gouny, S., Ranjeva, J.P., Bartolomei, F., Régis, J, Raybaud, C.A., Chauvel, P., Cozzone, P.J. (2002) Metabolic and electrophysiological alterations in subtypes of temporal lobe epilepsy: a combined proton magnetic resonance spectroscopic imaging and depth electrodes study. Epilepsia. 43,10, pp.1197-209.

Haslinger, B., Erhard, P., Kampfe, N., Boecker, H., Rummeny, E., Schwaiger, M., Conrad, B., Ceballos-Baumann, A.O.(2001) Event related functional magnetic resonance imaging in Perkinson's disease before and after levodopa. Brain. 124, pp.558–570.

Henson, R.N., Rugg, M.D., Friston, K.J. (2001) The choice of basis functions in the eventrelated fMRI. Neuroimage. 15, pp.83–97.

Hickok, G., Poeppel, D.(2007).The cortical organization of speech processing. *Nature Reviews Neuroscience*, 8, pp.393-402

Hong, L., Kaufman, A.E. (1999) Fast Projection-Based Ray-Casting Algorithm for Rendering Curvilinear Volumes. IEEE Trans Visual and Comp Graph. 5, pp.322–332.

Indovina, I., Sanes, J.N. (2001) Combined visual attention and finger movement effects on human brain representations. Exp Brain Res. 140, pp.265–79.

Jackson, G.M., Swainson, R., Mullin, A., Cunnington, R., Jackson, S.R. (2004) ERP correlates of a receptive language-switching task. Q J Exp Psychol A. 57, pp.223–40.

Jueptner, M., Weiller, C. (1995) Does measurement of regional cerebral blood flow reflect synaptic activity: implication for PET and fMRI. Neuroimaging. 2, pp.148–156.

Kiebel, S., Holmes, A., Poline, J.B., Kherif, F., Penny, W. (2004) The general Linear Model; Contrasts and classical inference. In: Frackowiak RSJ, Friston KJ, Frith CD, Dolan RJ, Price CJ, Jeki S, Ashburner J, Penny W, editor. Human Brain Function. Chapters 37 and 38. Elsevier Academic Press, London. pp. 749–779

Kim, D.S., Kim, M., Ronen, I., Formisano, E., Kim, K.H., Ugurbil, K., Mori, S., Goebel R.(2003) In vivo mapping of functional domains and axonal connectivity in cat visual cortex using magnetic resonance imaging. Magn Reson Imaging. 21, pp.1131–40.

Kim, D.S., Duong, T.Q., Kim, S.G. (2003) High resolution mapping of iso-orientation columns by fMRI. Nature Neurosci. 3, pp.164–169.

Kim, S.G., Rostrup, E., Larsson, H.B., Ogawa, S., Paulson, O.B. (1999) Determination of relative CMRO2 from CBF and BOLD changes: Significant increase of oxygen consumption rate during visual stimulation. Magn Reson Med. 41, pp.1152–1161.

Kim, S.G. (1995) Quantification of relative cerebral blood flow change by flowsensitive alternating inversion recovery (FAIR) technique: Application to functional mapping. Magn Reson Med. 34, pp.293–301.

Kim, D.S., Duong, T.Q., Kim, S.G. (2000) High-resolution mapping of iso-orientation columns by fMRI. Nature Neurosci. 3, pp.164–169.

Kiviniemi, V., Kantola, J.H., Jauhiainen, J., Tervonen, O. (2004) Comparison of methods for detecting nondeterministic BOLD fluctuation in fMRI. Magn Reson Imaging. 22, pp.197–203

Kleinschmidt, A., Thilo, K.V., Buchel, C. (2002) Neural correlates of visual-motion perception as object- or self-motion. Neuroimage. 16, pp.873–82.

Korsholm, K., Mathiesen, H.K., Lund, T.E. (2007) Functional magnetic resonance imaging in multiple sclerosis. Ugeskr Laeger. 169,26, pp.2518-20.

Krakow, K., Wieshmann, U.C., Woermann, F.G., Symms, M.R., McLean, M.A., Lemieux, L., Allen, P.J., Barker, G.J., Fish, D.R., Duncan, J.S.(1999) Multimodal MR imaging: functional, diffusion tensor, and chemical shift imaging in a patient with localization-related epilepsy. Epilepsia. 1999;40(10):1459-62.

Kutas, M., Federmeier, K.D., Coulson, S., King, J.W. & Münte, T.F. (2000). Language. In: *Handbook of Psychophysiology*, Cacioppo, J.T., Tassinary, L.G. & Berntson, G. (Eds). Cambridge University Press, Cambridge. pp. 576-601.

Kwong, K.K., Chesler, D.A., Weisskoff, R.M., Donahue, K.M., Davis, T.L., Ostergaard, L., Campbell, T.A., Rosen, B.R. (1995) MR perfusion studies with T1-weighted echo planar imaging. Mag Reson Med. 34, pp.878–887.

Landisman, C.E., Ts'o, D.Y. (2002) Color processing in macaque striate cortex: relationships to ocular dominance, cytochrome oxidase, and orientation. J Neurophysiol. 87, pp.3126–37.

Lee, S.P., Silva, A.C., Ugurbil, K., Kim, S.G. (1999) Diffusion-weighted Spin-echo fMRI at 9.4T: Microvascular/tissue Contribution to BOLD Signal Changes. Magn Reson Med. 42, pp.919–928.

Logothetis, N.K., Pauls, J., Augath, M., Trinath, T., Oeltermann, A. (2001) A neurophysiological investigation of the basis of fMRI signal. Nature. 412, pp.150–157.

Lohmann, G., Yves von Cramon, D. (1998) Automatic detection and labeling of the human cortical fields in magnetic resonance data sets. In: Buckhardt H, Neumann B, editor. In Computer Vision, Fifth European Conference, EECV Friburg, Germany. Springer-Verlag, Berlin, pp. 369–381.

Maclin, E.L., Gratton, G., Fabiani, M. (2001) Visual spatial localization conflict: an fMRI study. Neuroreport. 12, pp.3633–6.

Maess, B., Koelsch, S., Gunter, T., Friederici, A. (2001). Musical syntax is processed in Broca's area: an MEG study. *Nature Neuroscience*, 4, pp.540-545.

Maestú, F., García-Segura, J., Ortiz, T., Montoya, J., Fernández, A., Gil-Gregorio, P., Campo, P., Fernández, S., Viaño, J., Portera, A. (2005) Evidence of biochemical and biomagnetic interactions in Alzheimer's disease: an MEG and MR spectroscopy study. Dement Geriatr Cogn Disord. 20,2-3, pp.145-52.

Mandeville, J.B., Marota, J.J., (1999) Ayata C, Zaharchuk G, Moskowitz MA, Rosen BR, Weisskoff RM. Evidence of a cerebral post-arteriole windlissel with delayed compliance. J Cereb Blood Flow Metab. 19, pp.679–689.

Matsumoto, A., Iidaka, T., Haneda, K., Okada, T., Sadato, N. (2005) Linking semantic priming effect in functional MRI and event-related potentials. Neuroimage. 24,3, pp.624-34.

Mayville, J.M., Bressler, S.L., Fuchs, A., Kelso, J.A. (1999) Spatiotemporal reorganization of electrical activity in the human brain associated with a timing transition in rhythmic auditory-motor coordination. Exp Brain Res. 127, pp.371–381.

McDonald, C.R., Thesen, T., Carlson, C., Blumberg, M., Girard, H.M., Trong,netrpunya, A., Sherfey, J.S., Devinsky, O., Kuzniecky, R., Dolye, W.K., Cash, S.S., Leonard M.K., Hagler, D.J. Jr, Dale, A.M., Halgren, E. (2010)Multimodal imaging of repetition priming: Using fMRI, MEG, and intracranial EEG to reveal spatiotemporal profiles of word processing. Neuroimage. 53,2, pp.707-17.

Meinzer, M., Harnish, S., Conway, T., Crosson, B. (2011) Recent developments in functional and structural imaging of aphasia recovery after stroke. *Aphasiology*, 25,3, pp.271-290.

Meyer, F.G. (2003) Wavelet-based estimation of a semiparametric generalized linear model of fMRI time-series. IEEE Trans Med Imaging. 22, pp.315–22.

Miki, A., Liu, G.T., Englander, S.A., Raz, J., van Erp, T.G., Modestino, E.J., Liu, C.J., Haselgrove, J.C. (2001) Reproducibility of visual activation during checkerboard stimulation in functional magnetic resonance imaging at 4 Tesla. Jpn J Ophthalmol. 45, pp.151–5.

Minati, L., Grisoli, M., Bruzzone, M.G. (2007) MR spectroscopy, functional MRI, and diffusion-tensor imaging in the aging brain: a conceptual review. J Geriatr Psychiatry Neurol. 20,1, pp.3-21.

Morales-Chacón, L. (2001) Magnetic resonance spectroscopy and functional magnetic resonance images: non-invasive alternatives for identifying epileptogenic foci. Rev Neurol. 32,3, pp.234-6.

Moutoussis, K., Zeki, S. (2004) The Chronoarchitecture of the Human Brain: Functional Anatomy Based on Natural Brain Dynamics and the Principle of Functional Independence. In: Frackowiak RSJ, Friston KJ, Frith CD, Dolan RJ, Price CJ, Jeki S, Ashburner J, Penny W, editor. Human Brain Function. Chapter 13. Elsevier Academic Press, London, pp. 201–229.

Müller, H.P., Kassubek, J. (2007) Multimodal Imaging in Neurology: Special Focus on MRI Applications and MEG. Synthesis Lectures on Biomedical Engineering, 2,1, pp.1-75.

Munk, M.H., Linden, D.E., Muckli, L., Lanfermann, H., Zanella, F.E., Singer, W., Goebel, R. (2002) Distributed cortical systems in visual short-term memory revealed byevent-related functional magnetic resonance imaging. Cereb Cortex. 12, pp.866–76.

Nakada, T., Fujii, Y., Kwee, I.L. (2001) Brain strategies for reading in the second language are determined by the first language. Neurosci Res. 40, pp.351–35.

Nakahara, K., Hayashi, T., Konishi, S., Miyashita, Y.(2002) Functional MRI of macaque monkeys performing a cognitive set-shifting task. Science. 295, pp.1532–6.

Nakai, T., Matsuo, K., Kato, C., Okada, T., Moriya, T., Isoda, H., Takehara, Y., Sakahara, H. (2001) BOLD contrast on a 3T magnet: detectibility of the motor areas. J Comput Assit Tomogr. 25, pp.436–445.

Nelles, M., Block, W., Träber, F., Wüllner, U., Schild, H.H., Urbach, H. (2008) Combined 3T diffusion tensor tractography and 1H-MR spectroscopy in motor neuron disease. AJNR Am J Neuroradiol. 29,9, pp.1708-14.

Nichols, T., Holmes, A. (2004) Non parametric permutation tests for functional neuroimaging. In: Frackowiak RSJ, Friston KJ, Frith CD, Dolan RJ, Price CJ, Jeki S,

Ashburner J, Penny W, editor. Human Brain Function Chapters 46. Elsevier Academic Press, London. pp. 887–908.

Nitkunan, A., McIntyre, D.J., Barrick, T.R., O'Sullivan, M., Shen, Y., Clark, C.A., Howe, F.A., Markus, H.S.(2006) Correlations between MRS and DTI in cerebral small vessel disease. NMR Biomed. 19,5, pp.610-6.

Novick, J.M, Trueswell, J.C. & Thompson-Schill, S.L. (2010). Broca's Area and Language Processing: Evidence for the Cognitive Control Connection, *Language and Linguistics Compass*, 4,10, pp.906-924.

Nybakken, G.E., Quigley, M.A., Moritz, C.H. (2002) Test-retest precision of functional magnetic resonance imaging processed with independent component analysis. Neuroradiology. 44, pp.403–6.

Oga, T., Honda, M., Toma, K., Murase, N., Okada, T., Hanakawa, T., Sawamoto, N., Nagamine, T., Konishi, J., Fukuyama, H., Kaji, R., Shibasaki, H. (2002) Abnormal cortical mechanisms of voluntary muscle relxation in patients with writer's cramp: An fMRI study. Brain. 125, pp. 895–903.

Ogawa, S., Menon, R.S., Kim, S.G., Ugurbil, K. (1998) On the characteristics of functional MRI of the brain. Ann Rev Biophy and Biomol Struct. 27, pp.447–74.

Ogawa, S., Lee, T.M., Nayak, A.S., and Glynn, P. (1990). "Oxygenation-sensitive contrast in magnetic resonance image of rodent brain at high magnetic fields". Magnetic Resonance in Medicine 14 , 1, pp.68–78.

Optiz, B., Friederici, A.D. (2007). Neural Basis of Processing Sequential and Hierarchical Syntactic Structures. *Human Brain Mapping*, 28, pp. 585-592.

Pantano, P., Mainero, C., Lenzi, D., Caramia, F., Donenico lannetti, G., Piattella, M.C., Pestalozza, I., Legge, S.D., Bozzao, L., Pozzilli, C. (2005) A longitudinal fMRI study on motor activity in patients with multiple sclerosis. Brain, 128, pp. 2146-2153.

Patel, A. (2003). Language, music, syntax and the brain. *Nature Neuroscience*, 7, pp.674–681

Binkofski, F., Buccino, G. (2004). Motor functions of the Brocas region'. *Brain and Language*, 89, pp.362-369.

Peelen, M.V., Downing, P.E. (2011). The role of occipitotemporal body-selective regions in person perception. *Cognitive Neuroscience*,

Peresedova, A.V., Konovalov, R.N., Krotenkova, M.V., Zavalishin, I.A., Trifonova, O.V.(2009) Cortical reorganization in multiple sclerosis with movement disorders detected by functional MRI (own observations and literature data). Zh Nevrol Psikhiatr Im S S Korsakova. 109,7, Suppl 2, pp.38-43.

Preibisch, C., Haase, A. (1999) Functional MR imaging of the human brain using FLASH: influence of various imaging parameters. J Magn Reson. 140, pp.162–71.

Rachbauer, D., Kronbichler, M., Ropele, S., Enzinger, C., Fazekas, F. (2006) Differences in cerebral activation patterns in idiopathic inflammatory demyelination using the paced visual serial addition task: an fMRI study. J Neurol Sci. 244,1-2, pp.11-6.

Rajapakse, J.C., Priyaratna, J. (2001) Bayesian approach to segmentation of statistical parametric maps. IEEE Trans on Biomed Eng. 48, pp.1186–1194.

Reber, P.J., Siwiec, R.M., Gitleman, D.R., Parrish, T.B., Mesulam, M.M., Paller, K.A.(2002) Neural correlates of successful encoding identified using functional magnetic resonance imaging. J Neurosci. 22, pp.9541–8.

Rocca, M.A., Valsasina, P., Ceccarelli, A., Absinta, M., Ghezzi, A., Riccitelli, G., Pagani, E., Falini, A., Comi, G., Scotti, G., Filippi, M.(2009) Structural and functional MRI correlates of Stroop control in benign MS. Hum Brain Mapp. 30,1, pp.276-90.

Rohde, G.K., Aldroubi, A., Dawant, B.M. (2003)The adaptive bases algorithm for intensity-based nonrigid image registration. IEEE Trans Med Imaging. 22, pp.1470–9.

Rugg, M.D., Henson, R.N. (2002) Episodic memory retrival: an event-related functional neuroimaging perspective. In: Parker AE, Wilding EL and Bussey T, editor. In the Cognitive Neuroscience of Memory Encoding and Retrieval. Psychology Press, Hove. pp. 150–189.

Russ, M.O., Cleff, U., Lanfermann, H., Schalnus, R., Enzensberger, W., Kleinschmidt, A(2002) Functional magnetic resonance imaging in acute unilateral optic neuritis. J Neuroimaging. 12, pp.339–50.

Schmitt, F., Grosu, D., Mohr, C., Purdy, D., Salem, K., Scott, K.T., Stoeckel, B.(2004) 3 Tesla MRI: successful results with higher field strengths. Radiologe. 44, pp.31–47.

Sharma, R., Sharma, A. (2004) Physiological basis and image processing in functional magnetic resonance imaging: Neuronal and motor activity in brain. *BioMedical Engineering OnLine* 3,13 doi:10.1186/1475-925X-3-13

Sharma, R. (2002) Serial Amino-neurochemicals Analysis in Progressive Lesion Analysis of Multiple Sclerosis by Magnetic Resonance Imaging and Proton Magnetic Resonance Spectroscopic Imaging. Magn Reson Med Sci 1,3, pp.169-173.

Shibata, K., Osawa, M., Iwata, M. (2000) Visual evoked potentials in cerebral white matter hyperintensity on MRI. Acta Neurol Scand. 102, pp.230–5.

Singh, M., Kim, S., Kim, T.S. (2003) Correlation between BOLD-fMRI and EEG signal changes in response to visual stimulus frequency in humans. Magn Reson Med. 49, pp.108–14.

Sørensen, P.S., Jønsson, A., Mathiesen, H.K., Blinkenberg, M., Andresen, J., Hanson, L.G., Ravnborg, M. (2006) The relationship between MRI and PET changes and cognitive disturbances in MS. J Neurol Sci. 245,1-2, pp.99-102.

Steel, R.M., Bastin, M.E., McConnell, S., Marshall, I., Cunningham-Owens, D.G., Lawrie, S.M., Johnstone, E.C., Best, J.J. (2001) Diffusion tensor imaging (DTI) and proton magnetic resonance spectroscopy (1H MRS) in schizophrenic subjects and normal controls. Psychiatry Res. 106,3, pp.161-70.

Sarkissian, E., Bowman, K.W. (2003) Application of a nonuniform spectral resampling transform in Fourier-transform spectrometry. Appl Opt. 42, pp.1122–31.

Sasaki, Y., Murakami, I., Cavanagh, P., Tootell, R.H.(2002) Human brain activity during illusory visual jitter as revealed by functional magnetic resonance imaging. Neuron. 35, pp. 1147–56.

Schoenfeld, M.A., Heinze, H.J., Woldorff, M.G. (2002) Unmasking motion-processing activity in human brain area V5/MT+ mediated by pathways that bypass primary visual cortex. Neuroimage. 17, pp.769–79.

Sullivan, J.E. 3rd, Detre, J.A.(2005) Functional magnetic resonance imaging in the treatment of epilepsy. Curr Neurol Neurosci Rep. 5,4, pp.299-306.

Tartaglia, M.C., Arnold, D.L. (2006) The role of MRS and fMRI in multiple sclerosis. Adv Neurol. 98, pp.185-202.

Tegeler, C., Strother, S.C., Anderson, J.R., Kim, S.G. (1999) Reproducibility of BOLD based functional MRI obtained at 4 T. Hum Brain Mapp. 7, pp.267–283.

Thompson-Schill, S.L. (2005). Dissecting the Language Organ: A new Look at the Role of Broca's Area in Language Processing. In: *Twenty-First Century Psycholinguistics. Four Cornerstones*, Cutler A, (Ed.), Lawrence Erlbaum Associates, Mahwah, NJ.pp. 173-190.

Toma, K., Nakai, T. (2002) Functional studies in human motor control studies and clinical applications. Mag Reson Med Sci. 1, pp.109–120.

Turner, R., Jezzard, P., Wen, H., Kwong, K.K., Le Bihan, D., Zeffiro, T., Balaban, R.S.(1993) Functional mapping of the human visual cortex at 4 and 1.5 T using deoxygenation contrast EPI. Mag Reson Med. 29, pp.277–279.

Ugurbil, K. (2002) Magnetic Resonace Studies of Brain Function and Neurochemistry. Annu Rev Biomed Eng. 2, pp.633–60.

Vartiainen, J., Liljeström, M., Koskinen, M., Renvall, H., Salmelin, R.(2011) Functional magnetic resonance imaging blood oxygenation level-dependent signal and magnetoencephalography evoked responses yield different neural functionality in reading. J Neurosci. 31,3, pp.1048-58.

Vemuri, B.C., Ye, J., Chen, Y., Leonard, C.M. (2003) Image registration via level-set motion: applications to atlas-based segmentation. Med Image Anal. 7, pp. 1–20.

Villringer, A. (1999) Physiological changes during brain activation. In: Moonen CTW, Bandenitti PA, editor. In "Functional MRI". Springer-verlag, Berlin; pp. 3–13.

Vuilleumier, P., Henson, R.N., Driver, J., Dolan, R.J.(2002) Multiple levels of visual object constancy revealed by event-related fMRI of repetition priming. Nature Neurosci. 5, pp.491–9.

Wade, A.R., Wandell, B.A. (2002) Chromatic light adaptation measured using functional magnetic resonance imaging. Neurosci. 22, pp. 8148–57.

Yan, L., Zhuo, Y., Ye, Y., Xie, S.X., An, J., Aguirre, G.K., Wang, J.. (2009) Physiological origin of low-frequency drift in blood oxygen level dependent (BOLD) functional magnetic resonance imaging (fMRI) Magnetic Resonance in Medicine. 61,4, pp. 819–827.

Yoo, S.S., Talos, I.F., Golby, A.J., Black, P.M., Panych, L.P. (2004) Evaluating requirements for spatial resolution of fMRI for neurosurgical planning. Hum Brain Mapp. 21, pp.34–43.

Zaharchuk, G., Ledden, P.J., Kwong, K.K., Reese, T.G., Rosen, B.R., Wald, L.L. (1999) Multislice perfusion and perfusion territory imaging in humans with separate label with image coils. Magn Reson Med. 44, pp.92–100.

Zaini, M.R., Strother ,S.C., Anderson, J.R., Liow, J.S., Kjems, U., Tegeler, C., Kim, S.G. (1999) Comparison of matched BOLD and FAIR 4.0T-fMRI with [^{15}O] water PET brain Volumes". MedicalPhysics. 26, pp.1559–1567.

Zhu, X.P., Du, A.T., Jahng, G.H., Soher, B.J., Maudsley, A.A., Weiner, M.W., Schuff, N. (2003) Magnetic resonance spectroscopic imaging reconstruction with deformable shape-intensity models. Magn Reson Med. 50,3, pp. 474-82.

Zimny, A., Szewczyk, P., Trypka, E., Wojtynska, R., Noga, L., Leszek, J., Sasiadek, M.(2011) Multimodal Imaging in Diagnosis of Alzheimer's Disease and Amnestic Mild Cognitive Impairment: Value of Magnetic Resonance Spectroscopy, Perfusion, and Diffusion Tensor Imaging of the Posterior Cingulate Region. J Alzheimers Dis. PMID:21841260

Section 2

fMRI Methods in Evaluation of Brain Functions

3

fMRI Analysis of Three Concurrent Processing Pathways

Deborah Zelinsky
The Mind-Eye Connection, USA

1. Introduction

Biomarkers are useful measurements to monitor ranges of neurological and biochemical activity. They can be used as warning signs of poor adaptation to changes in either internal or external environments. The eye is an apt structure to use for obtaining biomarkers, since it interacts with multiple systems. For instance, pupil size and response during visual scanning tasks is being touted as a potential biomarker for autism (Martineau, Hernandez et al., 2011), the osmolarity in human corneal tear layer is thought to possibly be a biomarker for dry eye severity (Suzuki, Massingale et al., 2010) and disruptions in rapid eye movement during sleep is found to correlate with amounts of stress (Mellman, Bustamante et al., 2002).

This chapter proposes a use of functional magnetic resonance imaging (fMRI) to obtain a visual stress biomarker in processing pathways. This hypothesized biomarker would use the eye to indicate the relationship between internal adaptation (influenced by conscious and non-conscious filtering and decision-making networks) and external environmental changes. Section two of the chapter simplifies the big picture of brain function into cortical and subcortical interconnected networks that have three concurrent movement pathways; section three emphasizes the eye and how its complex circuitry connects with systems, including motor, sensory and attentional networks linked with those three pathways. Section four describes a proposed visual stress test that could show a dysfunction in the synchrony among those three pathways, thus detecting disease states even before structural changes occur. Implementation of this proposed test might be useful in assessing levels of brain injury, or in early identification of diseases affecting brain circuitry, such as seizure disorders, Alzheimer's, Parkinson's and multiple sclerosis.

Documentation of brain activity can be achieved by various methods, using both functional and anatomical landmarks, which will help to account for individual patient differences. For example, some methods quantify neuronal firing (via electrophysiological tools), others measure oxygen levels in blood (via hemodynamic responses) and still others assess metabolic changes (via optogenetic methods). (Optogenetic methods use genetically engineered proteins to regulate activity of specific types of cells by turning neural circuits on and off through light-activated channels. This new method observes and assesses local networks within the framework of global circuitry.) Often, two or more testing methods are used together to account for limitations in each (Dale and Sereno, 1993). For instance, fMRI maps *where* local neuronal activity is by measuring the hemodynamics of blood flow, and electroencephalograms (EEG) map *when* electrical activity occurs by measuring frequency oscillations of brainwaves. The fMRI and EEG together have high spatial resolution and temporal resolutions respectively, providing more information than either method alone. Combining optogenetics with fMRI technology into an optogenetic fMRI (ofMRI) allows scientists to assess both neuronal activity and its metabolic sequellae, helping to identify, and in some cases treat, underlying disease states (Lee, Durand et al., 2010; Zhang, Gradinaru et al., 2010; Cardin, Carlen et al., 2010).

Although the fMRI is a wonderful diagnostic tool, one limitation is the restriction on patient movement. To address this apparently unchangeable drawback, instead of the patient moving, the external environment can be altered and the patient's adaptation measured. The alterations can be done through the eye by stimulating the retina with lenses, prisms, filters and/or mirrors.

2. Survival functions to executive functions: Brain circuitry

Brain activation involves stimulation, modulation, feedback and feedforward mechanisms in two main groupings: subcortical functions and cortical processing. Each grouping is known to have multiple interconnections, with more pathways being discovered annually. These extensive feedforward and feedback systems allow for interconnectivity of individual structures as well as linkages between movements and thoughts.

Brain activity can be viewed in terms of arousal of, awareness of and attention to both the internal and the external environment. Subcortical activity, such as survival functions (circulation, digestion, respiration, etc.), remain beneath conscious awareness until altered by suprathreshold sensory stimuli, causing distracting cortical activity. An individual with a larger threshold of tolerance to sensory changes would not be burdened by those stimuli, thus allowing more efficient brain function.

In 1973, Ralph Luria wrote about functional systems in the brain that were not in isolation. (Luria, 1973) He proposed that the cortical brain was composed of both units and zones, which, when functioning properly, work together to regulate behaviors, senses and thinking. The units included information handling, tone and regulation of mental activity. The zones included a primary, for information gathering, a secondary, for information processing and programming, and a tertiary, for complex forms of integrated mental activity. He hypothesized that sensation and perception were intimately involved with movement, having afferent and efferent components. He also proposed that the eye, as an extension of the brain, is never passive, and is always actively searching to pick out essential clues from the environment. Now, almost forty years after Luria's theory was first presented, functional organization and anatomical connectivity of regions in the cerebral cortex have been documented through neuroimaging and other techniques.

In the brain, structures are grouped to accomplish specific types of tasks. For instance, in general movement networking, many interacting pathways are involved with the frontal cortices, basal ganglia and cerebellum as the "main players." The frontal cortices plan and organize movement, generating motor programs (with the prefrontal and the premotor regions contributing to different functions), the basal ganglia govern movement intention programs, and the cerebellum is involved in the coordinated adjustment (smoothing out) of movement quality. The prefrontal cortex sends voluntary commands to the basal ganglia so that appropriate movement is selected, and other cortical association areas send the basal ganglia information for acquired (automatized) movement. Sensory signals from cortical processing are sent to the matrix of the basal ganglia, while the striosomal portion of the basal ganglia attaches an "emotional valence" to that sensory information for the purpose of learning.

Fine motor tasks such as eye movements add more "players". The brainstem's oculomotor system receives direct projections from the various eyefields located in their own brain network. Frontal eye fields, parietal eye fields, prefrontal eye fields and supplementary eye fields, each have a region involved in either saccadic or smooth eye movements (Lynch and Tian, 2006; Cui, Yan et al., 2003). Neuroanatomical studies in non-human primates determined that there are several distinct regions in the cerebral cortex (designated eye fields) forming a cortico-cortical network guiding and executing decisions for voluntary, visually guided saccadic and pursuit eye movements. Some of the subcortical structures used in eye movement, for example, involve the superior colliculus and the frontal eye fields integrating information received by the geniculate-striate pathway and contributing to more thinking and movement decisions (Ding and Gold, 2011).

Anatomical patterns of new movements, from initial learning to automation, shift over time as the movement is practiced and developed. The retention of movement schema (praxicons) is in parietal/temporal-parietal circuits and connects with the cerebellum which refines the praxicons and innervatory programs by comparing predicted movement outcome with error. These comparisons are accomplished by the brain via two types of procedures, described by theoretical control models. Forward models predict movement outcomes by projecting signals to parietal and frontal motor regions, allowing for automation and bypassing direct (slower) sensory input. Inverse cerebellar models are initiated outside of conscious awareness and bypass premotor cortex commands, allowing automatic movements. Speed and precise accuracy of intentionally guided actions and predictions is thus developed (Imamizu and Kawato, 2009).

Movement is not in isolation from thoughts; it is one part of a network of functional circuits, each with its own pathway, synchronizing like an orchestra. Concurrent pathways form loops, including sensory stimuli, processing and motor reactions and responses. The processing can be analytical and intentional, or intuitive and habitual, leading to various brain networks, such as, visuo-spatial processing from the parietal lobe, visually guided action from the premotor cortex and navigation, imagination and planning for the future in the prefrontal cortex. (Kravitz, Saleem et al., 2011) Both the mind (cortical) and body (subcortical) systems have to adapt to continual environmental changes, at either a conscious or non-conscious level of awareness. Also, there is substantial integration between subcortical and cortical structures as well as interrelationships and interactions at micro-circuitry levels.

At any given moment, three movement types (reflex, developed and intentional) are the result of three processing pathways, activated by different amounts of stimulation at different speeds, capturing different amounts of attention. Figure 1 highlights the differences between how these movement types are generated. The distinctions are important to our purposes because of the interrelationships among the three separate pathways. Developed movements include learned-orienting and anticipatory pathways. However, orienting movements can also be reflexive. It is possible that during an fMRI, the three processing pathways can be analyzed to assess which one has more of an attentional demand at the expense of the others and determine the location(s) of brain activity occurring.

The following diagram (Figure 1) has much more extensive integration of cortical and subcortical structures than implied by the small arrow, but is a simplification in order to describe the framework of subcortical to cortical shifts in brain activity. All cortical areas have significant inputs and major feedforward and feedback connections to numerous subcortical structures. Some functional networks share similar pathways. For instance, auditory and visual reflexive spatial orienting are controlled by a common underlying neural substrate (Santangelo, Olivetti Belardinelli et al., 2007) and there are subspecialized areas, such as the middle temporal lobe (MT) which, in congenitally blind people, reacts to tactile motion, but in sighted people, reacts to either visual or tactile motion. (Sani, Ricciardi et al., 2010).

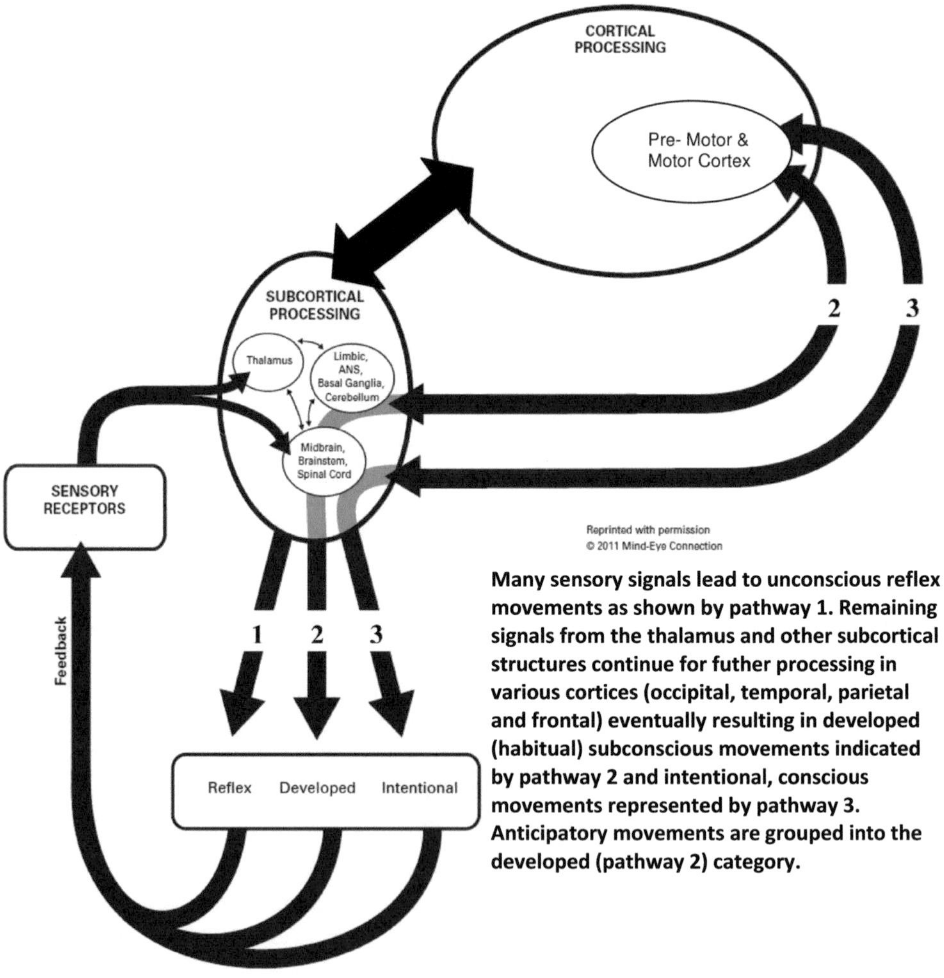

Fig. 1. Simplified Diagram of Three Concurrent Movement Pathways

Whether the paradigm used is anatomical, physiological, psychological, neurological, etc, there is only one brain with parallel systems in action. Below are some ways to view brain activity. Each is a continuum, with a constant two-way exchange of information.

Stimulus Location	Internal External
Processing Mode	Ambient Where Am I* Ambient Where is It?* Focal What is It*
Physiological Pathways	Magnocellular* Koniocellular* Parvocellular*
Anatomical Categories	Subcortical Cortical
Functional Networks	Survival Functions Executive Functions
Psychological Activity	Non-conscious Conscious
Perceptual Activity	Arousal Awareness Attention Intention
Brainwave Type	delta theta alpha beta gamma

Table 1. Simplified continuums in brain function analysis (*discussed in section 3)

Visual, auditory and somatosensory signals are transmitted partly through the thalamus and partly other subcortical regions. From the thalamus, auditory signals travel to the temporal lobe, and visual signals to the occipital lobe, later combining with proprioceptive and somatosensory information from the body in the parietal lobe for higher cortical processing (Williams, 2010).

The integration of somatosensory, auditory and visual inputs is one aspect of determining "Where am I?". There are also cognitive systems operating to assist in spatial orientation (Arthur, Philbeck et al., 2009). However when using MRI machines to assess brain activity and functional circuitry in thinking and movement pathways, body movement cannot be used because it is restricted. Similarly, auditory testing is difficult to use, because there is ambient noise. Therefore, the obvious choice would be the eye -- easily accessible and directly connected to the brain. It must be noted that recent studies suggest an effect upon the subject's vestibular system produced by the fMRI magnetic field (Roberts, Marcelli et al. 2011), which could possibly influence eye movement findings. However, the effect was noted during a resting state when the visual system was not provided any meaningful drive.

3. The mind-eye connection: Functional networks

Although eye movement is commonly assessed by fMRI, the complete depth of possibilities has not fully been explored. As has been shown above, the eye is much more than a visual sensory organ; it provides the entrance to a two-way street into the body and the mind. In this chapter, for the sake of simplicity, only three subsystems -- motor, sensory and attention -- will be addressed, while remaining aware that they are part of a much bigger, more complex cortical/subcortical loop with multiple feedback and feedforward channels in a continually adapting dynamic system of metabolic and neurological functional networks.

When the classically understood visual pathway from the eye to the visual cortex is engaged in a conscious activity (i.e. seeing), reflexive and responsive networks are also in use. For instance, the reading process comprises not only the cortical visual activity of seeing (letters on the page), but also a concurrent process creating the foundation for visualization and interpretation. In addition, the mind is on the alert for external and internal sensory signals which may shift mental attention. If a person is reading and a loud noise occurs, attention will tend to shift as many events take place. The head reflexively turns toward the perceived sound location, postural mechanisms maintain balance and respiration, digestion and circulation systems are momentarily disrupted, to name a few. All in all, if processing is disrupted, attention is often hindered.

There are numerous factors affecting visual processing such as internal health, attention, spatial awareness, emotional state, etc., each affecting the functional networking of reflexive, intuitive (developed) and analytical (intentional) processing pathways. If there is a problem in one or more functional networks, the issue could be due to structural damage or inefficient synchronization of systems. For instance, fMRI connectivity analysis demonstrates that auditory and visual cortices are linked; altering one affects the other (Eckert, Kamdar et al. 2008) . Recent studies propose that sensory systems might be able to be used to regulate timing of brainwaves (Hughes, 2008), implying that visual interventions could alter brain circuitry. fMRI testing revealed that in a resting state, activation in specific cortical networks differs between patients with Alzheimer's disease and healthy people. This distinguishing factor of decreased metabolism in certain brain structures can be a potential biomarker for Alzheimer's disease. (Greicius, Srivastava et al. 2004)

Each individual has a unique filtering process that includes simultaneous and sequential processing before decisions are made as to motor output. The mind continually filters external and internal stimuli, choosing how to respond, with a complex series of conscious and non-conscious thoughts and emotions, many of which affect brain networks connected with the eye. (Reactions, on the other hand, are more automatic, occurring without those "decision-making" processes). As will be shown, each of these decisions, reactions and responses can be thought of in terms of "clues, cues and cruise control" and related to the three processing pathways. Consciously used clues lead to intentional movements, inferences of cues accessed beneath conscious awareness lead to habitual responses, and automatic reflex systems on "Cruise Control" lead to reflex movements that function unconsciously.

(This is not a new concept. Dr. A.M Skeffington, the founding father of neuro-optometry, understood that patients' use of visual systems was not a simple, mechanical matter of seeing but instead was a patient's internal engagement with the external environment and desire to explore a spatial world around them. This was extremely evident to him by changes in the retinal reflex during optometric retinoscopy. Decades later, it was demonstrated that conscious perception of the external world activated fast brainwaves, different from the brain activity exhibited when perception of the external surroundings was not high attentional priority (Hughes, 2008).)

Subsections, 3.1, 3.2 and 3.3. describe those processing channels in terms of 1) movements, including eye movements, 2) sensory signal processing, including retinal signals, and 3) attentional factors, modulated by external and internal elements.

3.1 Movement networks: Reactions and responses

There are many measureable motor outputs from the eye, including pupillary reactions, ciliary body activity, eyelid and extraocular muscles (EOM) movement. The intraocular (pupil and ciliary body) and extraocular muscles each use different circuitry (Muri, Iba-

Zizen et al., 1996), often combining with feedback from eye muscle position (proprioceptors) in the eye and neck muscles. Because the purpose is to discuss intentional, habitual (developed) and reflexive movement pathways, this chapter is limited to the related extraocular muscles which can be moved reflexively, habitually (from developed skills) or intentionally. The eyelid will not be included because it is innervated by both smooth and skeletal muscles, and is therefore controlled by different functional networks.

Although the eyes can be moved voluntarily, most eye movements are reflexive (Weir, 2006).

Figure 2 shows reflexive reactions of extraocular muscles include the following, which share many of the same neuronal pathways:

- Vestibulo-Ocular Reflex (VOR) moves the eyes to counteract head movement, allowing the eyes to maintain fixation - a function critical for stabilizing the eyes while the head is moving.
- Optokinetic Nystagmus Reflex (OKN) pathways help eye stabilization during an involuntary fixation of moving objects (Swenson, 2006).
- Reflexive Saccadic eye movements - when the superior colliculus sends signals reflexively pointing the eyes to stimuli of interest, such as flashes of light or loud noises. The superior colliculus contains a spatial mapping of the external environment and receives visual, auditory and somatic sensation from many locations, including the spinal cord, the cerebral cortex and basal ganglia.

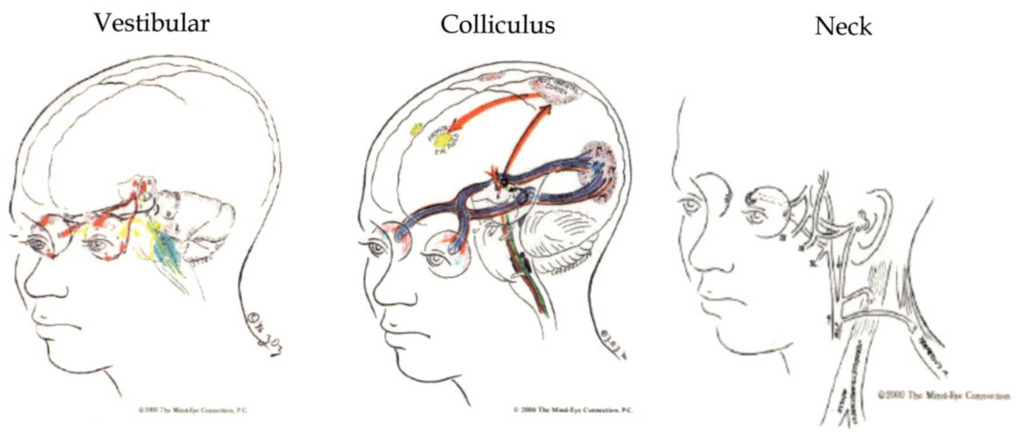

Fig. 2. Reflex pathways of eye movements

Cortical responses of extraocular muscles based on sensory input and attention:

- Non-reflexive saccadic eye movements
- Vergence eye movements - convergence and divergence, aiming the eyes toward a target on the z-axis.
- Smooth Pursuit eye movements - require the eyes to be fixated on a moving external target.
- Fixation eye movements - maintain target in line of central eyesight.

3.2 Sensory networks: Central and peripheral retinal signals

Other neurological sensory input in the visual system includes proprioceptors from the EOM. There are also chemical pathways in the eye that have feedback and feedforward input, such as the consistency of corneal tear layer which varies as the nervous system is stressed, and the chemical gradients in the optic nerve which vary with retinal activity.

The retina itself functions constantly, extraordinarily busy with metabolic and neurological activity, even during sleep. In fact, when eyelids are closed, regardless of the waking state, photic stimulation caused by ambient lighting affects retinal (and brain) processing. Concurrently, there is non-photic stimulation from metabolic activity. Of the multiple sensory networks in the eye, this section will focus on central and peripheral retinal stimulation. (Section 3.1 discussed retinal signals that were transmitted directly through the midbrain's superior colliculus to elicit reflex eye movements. This section emphasizes the retinal signals that synapse at the thalamus' lateral geniculate nucleus (LGN) and continue to the occipital lobe.)

Retinal stimulation occurs in at least three ways: from extrinsic illumination (light or lack of light), from intrinsic chemical changes via circadian rhythms (Tombran-Tink and Barnstable, 2008), or by mechanically induced pressure. The fact that extrinsic illumination stimulates the retina, in easily manipulated ways, will help establish the visual stress biomarker proposed in the beginning of the paper. During an fMRI, the visual stress test determines when the peripheral retinal stimulation reaches its threshold and distracts central retinal attention of details. Central stimulation occurs when the macular region receives light where attention is placed.

Chemically and electrically, there is a monumental amount of internal processing occurring in the retina via the main groups of retinal cells (bipolar, ganglion, horizontal, amacrine, photoreceptor and Mueller), which are subdivided into over a hundred cell types, each performing a different task. This cellular teamwork allows for such functions as luminous efficiency, sensitivities to spectral frequencies and gated signaling channels.

Retinal processing begins at the photoreceptor level when a photon of light is absorbed by the molecule rhodopsin, converting it into an activated state. Subsequently, a cascade of chemical changes occurs in the outer retina, leading to various ion channels opening and closing, eventually eliciting an electrical response in the inner retina, which is monitored by action potentials and calcium regulation pathways. The traveling signals eventually arrive in ganglion cells, continuing through the optic nerve and into the brain (Tombran-Tink and Barnstable, 2008) (See Figure 3).

The superior, inferior, temporal, nasal and macular portions of the retina are developed from completely different sets of chemical pathways and genetic codes, and each of those five geographical sections in the retina is regulated by different transcription factors and develops during different timeframes (DeGrip, Pugh et al., 2000; Tombran-Tink and Barnstable, 2008). This is important, because patterned neuronal activity in the early retina has a substantial influence on the retinotopic organization of the superior colliculus (Mrsic-Flogel, Hofer et al., 2005). Therefore, stimulating selected retinal portions with visual interventions can induce processing changes.

Retinal pathways differ not only in development, but also in function. This has been demonstrated by fMRI testing indicating that nasal and temporal regions vary in melatonin suppression (Ruger, Gordijn et al., 2005). Binasal occlusion on eyeglasses has been used for years to visually treat patients with crossed eyes and brain injuries. Perhaps this occlusion alters the chemical pathways, indirectly affecting neurological circuitry in eye movement control and thus perception of surrounding space (linking motor, sensory and attentional circuitry). Processing also differs between the inferior and superior hemifields of external space (Rubin, Nakayama et al., 1996). For instance, people are generally more attuned to visual information entering from the lower portion of external space (light coming upward stimulating the superior retina) than to light stimulating the inferior retina.

Alteration of retinal stimulation affects both subcortical and cortical processing. Visual processing has been documented in several hundred functional feedback and feedforward brain pathways encompassing almost fifty cortical regions (Klemm, 1996), and fMRI allows for better three dimensional spatial resolution of these pathways. When activated by light, the retina triggers activity at three concurrent levels of processing: analytical (conscious, simultaneous or sequential), intuitive (subconscious) and autonomic (unconscious). Eventually an fMRI database of normal functions can be accumulated so that functional changes during disease processes could be compared to normed data. fMRI usage can thus aid in the differentiation of pathways in concurrent systems during mental activity.

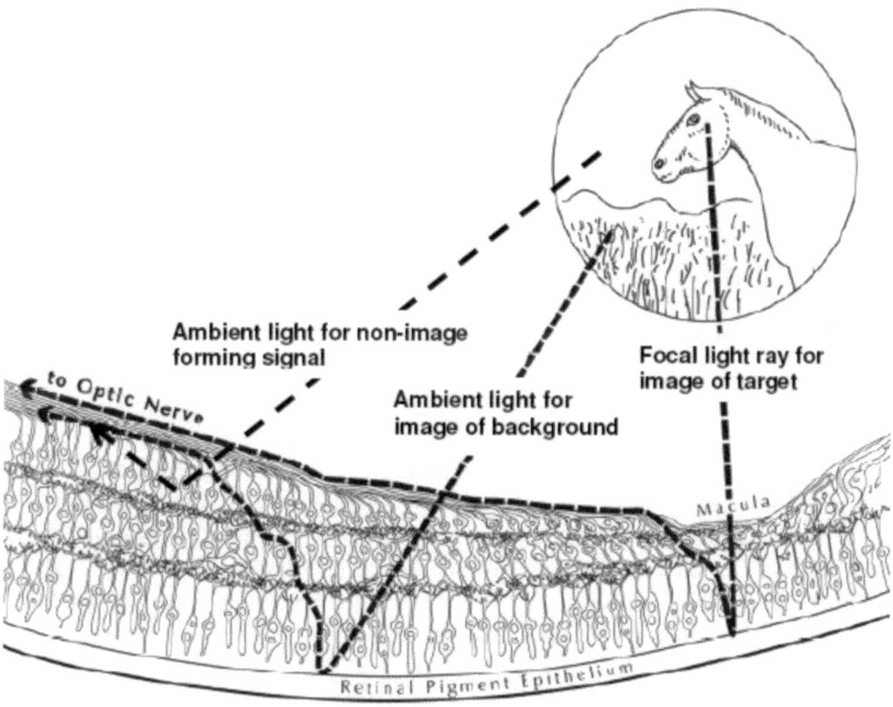

Fig. 3. Central and peripheral light rays striking the retina, exiting the optic nerve. ©2011 Mind-Eye Connection Reprinted with permission. For simplification, the dendrites are drawn in a line, but do vary in length.

3.3 Attentional networks

Retinal stimulation is, of course, only one portion of sensory input to the eye. There are many other sensory signals involved, such as proprioceptor information and signals from corneal receptors. Consider the effect of a small eyelash rubbing against the cornea. During the time when the eyelash is bothersome, reflex tearing occurs, the eyelid reflexively blinks, the extraocular muscles reflexively point the eyes away from the pain, the auditory system's awareness of the surroundings constricts, the pupils change size, etc. If the person wishes to continue to see, he must apply conscious effort. In a stressed condition or diseased state, the need to apply conscious attention will occur sooner and more frequently than under normal conditions. That painful sensory stimulus creates an attentional demand, diverting attention away from the external environment and eyesight. The sensory system and motor systems are not simply mechanical; they are inextricably linked with and influenced by attentional networks.

This process of sensory input via light striking the retina does not take place in a vacuum. Other events may influence the individual's perception, including which details are selectively filtered out from the available information at a given time. The level of awareness an individual is able to experience is dependent not only on the proper functioning of the retina and other structures of the eye, but also on the availability of the mind's attentional networks - neurological and chemical. This fact offers insight into patient function and dysfunction and also presents many possibilities for designing tests to define the normal parameters of conscious attention versus reflexive and habitual activity.

In 1911, an article commented on how retinal reflexes changed depending on attention factors and the angle of the light (Wilson, 1911). A hundred years later, in 2011, a more analytical research project demonstrated the validity of that concept in migraine sufferers (Huang, Zong et al., 2011).

In the 1930's, Dr. A.M. Skeffington, described "vision" as an emergent concept from four intertwining circles (Where am I? Where is it? What is it? and Speech/Auditory). The "Where am I?" relies mainly on subcortical processing, the "Where is it?" "What is it" and "Speech/Auditory" rely mainly on cortical processing. Dr. Skeffington spent years promoting his thoughts that the eye was part of the body, controlled by the brain, and that changing information which entered the eye would affect the entire body (Skeffington, 1957). This pioneering optometrist believed that sensory systems should be evaluated in total rather than in isolation. For instance, he believed that eye aiming and focusing be evaluated together as a team, termed a visual reflex, rather than separately as convergence and accommodation, since they are not separate. One responsibility of optometrists whose work emphasizes neuro-optometry is to measure the function or dysfunction of retinal circuitry. fMRI research demonstrates (decades after Dr. Skeffington's proposals) that the eyes do affect brain and body circuitry. (There is also interplay between an individual's genetic predisposition and their unique experiences, regulating brain circuitry.)

The sensory inputs of both eyes have magnocellular, koniocellular and parvocellular portions, arising from peripheral and central retinal stimulation. The magnocelluar portion is further divided into two smaller parts: non-conscious reflex and developed pathways. Testing the mental shift in attention from ambient processing (magnocellular pathways) to focal processing (parvocellular pathway) is important in differentiating movement pathways.

Magnocellular (M) system provides answers to "Where am I?" and "Where is It?" at a reflexive and a cortical level respectively, beneath conscious awareness, and the parvocellular (P) system answers the meaningful question of "What is It?" at the cortical level.

The fastest retinal signal pathway is the reflexive "Where am I?" portion of the magnocellular (M) pathway involving retinal signals that are processed subcortically. Of the retinal signals continuing through the optic radiations before arriving at the occipital cortex, some originate from macular stimulation (carrying information regarding color and detail) and others from peripheral retinal activation (carrying information regarding such factors as speed, location, size and shape). When entering the occipital lobe's striate cortex, the information is *spatially* based (externally controlled), with a point to point spatial representation of the external world mapped with pinpoint precision. However, upon exiting the occipital lobe, information is *attentionally* based (internally controlled), with the dorsal stream going on to the parietal lobe (carrying "Where is It?" signals of background information) and the ventral stream continuing to the temporal lobe (carrying "What is It?" signals of target information). Signals from the dorsal and ventral streams integrate, eventually arriving in the frontal lobe. From there, signals are transmitted to cranial nerves III, IV and VI which send signals to the extraocular muscles, resulting in eye movement.

In 2011, it was determined that a Koniocelluar (K) pathway activity might be gating the cortical circuits fed by the M and P pathways and hypothesized that the sensory streams can be adjusted to modify brain rhythms via parallel visual pathways (Cheong, Tailby et al., 2011). Also, each of the two cortical visual streams also have connections with subcortical nuclei (Webster, Bachevalier et al., 1995). These studies seem to provide validity to the concept of a visual stress biomarker.

In addition to the "Where am I?" (subcortical processing), "Where is It?" (dorsal stream) and "What is It?" (ventral stream), hypotheses for When and Why pathways emerged in 2003 (Krekelberg, 2003). In 2011, a study found a "When" pathway and demonstrated its connections between the visual cortex and the temporal lobe (Naya and Suzuki, 2011).

Sensory stimuli are filtered during processing, and decisions are made by the mind based on arousal, attention, awareness, emotions and memories. Conscious attention and awareness are often directed to different volumes of surrounding space which can be expanded or constricted depending on other internal and external signals, including general health and fatigue. Intra-cortical connections are responsible for routing information selectively to progressively higher and higher levels of processing. There is top-down processing from memory circuitry and bottom-up processing from retinal input, with the control of visual attention thought to be found in the pulvinar (the back section of the thalamus) (Olshausen, Anderson et al. 1993). The thalamus is also responsible for mediating the interaction between attention and arousal during perceptual and cognitive tasks (Portas, Rees et al., 1998; Saalmann and Kastner 2009, 2011). Dr. Selwyn Super, an optometrist whose work emphasizes neuro-optometry, discusses intention as a top-down executive function with feedforward and anticipatory circuitry and attention with both top-down and bottom-up connections, competing with each other. In the case of patients with attentional neglect, where internal awareness of surrounding space or of their body is not normal, some are deemed sensory-attentional, others motor-intentional and still others as having representational deficits (Super, 2005).

It is clear that controlled, subtle continual change in retinal stimulation will eventually cause shifts in attentional demands and brain activity as signals trigger shifts from arousal to awareness to attention. This type of controlled change can be produced by optometric methods.

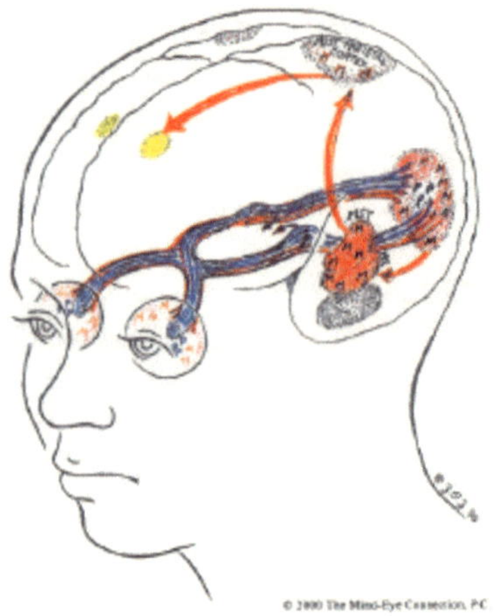

Fig. 4. Magnocellular "Where is It?" pathway signals traveling in middle temporal (MT) and medial superior temporal (MST) lobes.

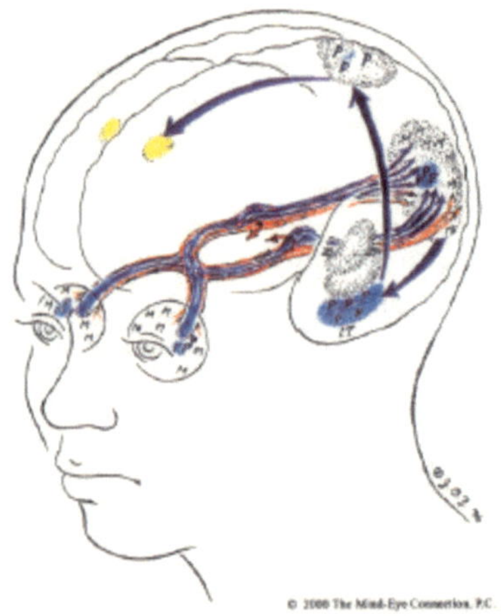

Fig. 5. Parvocellular "What is It?" pathway Signals traveling through the inferior temporal (IT) lobes.

4. Optometric changes to functional networks

Optometric tools, such as prisms, break light into frequencies and spatially distribute the light onto the retina. Each tool stimulates different areas of the retina, and as the eye moves, the optic flow sent to the brain is altered. By relying on the point to point brain mapping from the retina to the visual cortex, and the non-visual pathways from the retina to other brain circuitry, visual intervention could affect fMRI findings.

The visual changes could be accomplished by using combinations of lenses, prisms and filters (including occlusion) to alter entering light. The amount and direction of light input can be a controlled variable, and the patient's reactions to changing environmental stimuli can be measured to determine how well, and in what areas, the subcortical and cortical networks are interacting as well as its tipping point. Circuitry and pathways used for information processing can be identified and modified.

The visual spectrum has more to offer than eyesight alone. For instance, prisms and mirrors together are being developed to render objects invisible to the human eye (Zhang, Luo et al., 2011), and mirrors are being used in rehabilitations in patients with neglect from brain trauma (Ramachandran and Altschuler, 2009).

Intentional eye movements and retinal stimulation are often used to induce changes in brain activity during fMRI testing. Equally as valuable, is an assessment of a patient's adaptation to environmental change. Disruption of mechanisms can lead to disease. If there is significant variation from a normal database, eye movements can be used during fMRIs to detect deviations in information processing, perhaps identifying disease states before structural breakdowns occur.

Visual interventions can be in many forms, each stimulating the retina in a different way.

- Lenses - dispersing light toward the edges or the center of the retina. This change in light mainly alters the balance between central and peripheral circuitry by having the target and background occupy different percentages of the retinal input.
- Yoked Prisms - angling light toward one edge of the retina. This initially affects the body's positional sense, because reflexive eye movements will point the eyes toward the incoming light, triggering internal postural mechanisms in the hips for stability of balance, to counteract the eye movement. Depending on the stability of the person's sense of balance, attention may be then shifted to external targets.
- Non-yoked prisms - angling light toward either nasal or temporal retinal sensors. The eyes will also reflexively point toward the light, but this inward and outward movement stimulates different visual and postural mechanisms (shoulders rather than hips), pulling attention to the object location.
- Filters - altering either spatial or temporal retinal input, thus affecting processing.
- Tints - filtering out specific wavelengths of light, stimulating specific retinal cells, primarily altering internal sensations, via the autonomic nervous system.
- Mirrors - make targets appear farther away than the mirror frame, creating a sensory mismatch between the central (target) and peripheral (background).

Table 2. Optometric tools for non-invasive visual interventions

Movements, sensory inputs and attention can be considered within a broader framework of sensory integration. For instance, just because a person can hear and see does not mean he can simultaneously watch and listen to a moving target such as a teacher in a classroom. Using visual stress tolerated, as a biomarker for normal brain adjustments, will demonstrate adaptation ability (as long as the patient's individual tolerance level and overall physical and mental state is considered).

Eye stimulation can be used for both diagnostic and therapeutic purposes. When a person doesn't appropriately adapt to environmental changes, this proposed biomarker will be outside of a normal range. For instance, adaptation to specific spatial shifts in prisms led researchers to the conclusion that prism adaptation was processed in motor parts of the brain relating to action timing. Patients adapted to the prisms' spatial displacement independent of awareness of subjective timing (Tanaka, Homma et al., 2011).

5. Conclusion: A biomarker for usage of clues, cues and cruise control

The exploration of brain activity following changes in retinal inputs is fundamental for a better understanding of the basic principles governing large-scale neuronal dynamics. The hypo- and hypersensitivity of the retina, even through a closed eyelid, suggest a neurological basis for the diagnostic and therapeutic effect of lenses to consciously and non-consciously alter incoming sensory signals and influence brain processing.

Current functional magnetic resonance imaging vision research tends to focus on perception, or on eyesight and damage in eye structures, such as optic neuritis and macular degeneration. However, the eye offers much more. Its interactions and relationships within, between and among motor, sensory and attentional networks (as well as emotional and cognitive systems) can be documented by controlling external environmental changes and measuring internal adaptation, thus differentiating among the three concurrent processing pathways and movement outputs.

Assessment of the three different levels of eye movement and adaptation to change is important for diagnosis of systems' instability or dysfunction, with the ultimate goal to measure shifts in attention and compare to a normed database. Thoughts and movements are integrated via:

- Consciously used **clues**, leading to intentional **movements**
- Inferences of **cues** accessed beneath conscious awareness, leading to developed or habitual actions
- Automatic reflex systems on "**Cruise Control**" leading to movements that function unconsciously

Thus, visual systems involve not solely what the eyes see, but the integration of neural pathways. When observed during fMRI, eye motor responses offer insight into brain activity and can be helpful to further categorize and appropriately treat the increasing incidence of degenerative and other conditions. Specifically, a visual stress test can influence brain circuitry via alterations of retinal input during an fMRI procedure (using lenses, prisms, mirrors and/or filters) and can have the potential for revealing dysfunction in such pathways as information processing, attention, movement and other interconnected sensory systems. Imaging techniques are useful ways to demonstrate dysfunctional circuitry, both in grey and white matter, but sometimes the dysfunction has to be stressed before a breakdown can be observed. Clinical applications could include assessments of functional breakdowns in disease states, e.g., seizure disorders, memory deficits and visuo-cognitive abilities in patients with Alzheimer's disease and eye movement control and balance in patients with traumatic brain injuries or Parkinson's disease.

Retinal pathway changes and impairments have been noted in patients with epilepsy, Parkinson's and Alzheimer's along with other diseases (van Baarsen, Porro et al., 2009; Altintaş, Iseri, et al., 2008; Cubo,Tedeio, et al. 2010; Parisi V, 2003). Cortical atrophy in Alzheimer's patients can be seen years before cognitive impairment becomes evident (Dickerson, Stoub et al. 2011), yet cognitive impairment is not always the first symptom of Alzheimers disease (38% of people have vision, behavior or other warning signs (Balasa, Gelpi, et. al. 2011) and that the default network brain activity differs in people with Alzheimer's (Shin J., Kepe, V. et al., 2011). This paper hypothesizes that shifts in cognitive and attentional systems can be observed even earlier, using neuro-optometric interventions during fMRI, in combination with other testing methods, to measure an abnormal functional shift in either default attentional networks or cognitive networks, before the structural atrophy occurs. A defect in functional connectivity would be a valuable biomarker.

Embracing a viewpoint of brain circuitry and metabolism could shift optometry toward a profession of selective neurological and biochemical pathway stimulation. Using the eye as a portal to the nervous system, measurements of internal reactions and responses to external changes can be made, in hopes of providing a useful visual stress biomarker for future disease research and eventual interventions for preventive healthcare.

6. Acknowledgments

Credit must go to two optometrists who dedicate their lives to promoting neuro-optometric concepts. Dr. Albert A. Sutton, who continually applies and teaches Dr. Skeffington's visionary viewpoint and has allowed me the privilege of learning from him for years. Dr. Sutton's way of stimulating thinking led to the integration of concepts discussed above. Also, sincere thanks to Dr. Selwyn Super, practicing in California, for dedicating time to thought-provoking discussions with me regarding his groundbreaking work on intention, attention and inattention.

7. References

Altintaş O, Işeri P, et al. (2008). "Correlation between retinal morphological and functional findings and clinical severity in Parkinson's disease." Doc Ophthalmol. 2008 Mar;116(2):137-46. Epub 2007 Oct 26.

Arthur, J. C., J. W. Philbeck, et al. (2009). "Non-sensory inputs to angular path integration." *J Vestib Res* 19(3-4): 111-125.

Balasa, M, E. Gelpi, et al. (2011). "Clinical features and APOE genotype of pathologically proven early-onset Alzheimer disease." Neurology May 17, 2011 vol. 76 no. 20 1720-1725

Cardin, J. A., M. Carlen, et al. (2010). "Targeted optogenetic stimulation and recording of neurons in vivo using cell-type-specific expression of Channelrhodopsin-2." *Nat Protoc* 5(2): 247-254.

Cheong, S. K., C. Tailby, et al. (2011). "Slow intrinsic rhythm in the koniocellular visual pathway." *Proc Natl Acad Sci U S A.*

Cubo E, Tedejo RP, et al. (2010). "Retina thickness in Parkinson's disease and essential tremor." Mov Disord. Oct 30;25(14):2461-2. PMID:20669291

Cui D. M., Yan Y. J., and Lynch, J.C. (2003). Pursuit subregion of the frontal eye field projects to the caudate nucleus in monkeys. *J of Neurophysiol, 89*: 2678-2684.

Dale, A.M., Sereno, M.I. (1993) Improved localization of cortical activity by combining EEG and MEG with MRI cortical surface reconstruction: a linear approach. "*J of Cog. Neuroscience* 5(2): 162-176.

DeGrip, W. J., E. N. Pugh, et al. (2000). *Molecular mechanisms in visual transduction.* Amsterdam ; New York, Elsevier.

Dickerson, B. C., T. R. Stoub, et al. (2011). "Alzheimer-signature MRI biomarker predicts AD dementia in cognitively normal adults." *Neurology* 76(16): 1395-1402.

Ding, L. and J. I. Gold (2011). "Neural Correlates of Perceptual Decision Making before, during, and after Decision Commitment in Monkey Frontal Eye Field." *Cereb Cortex.*

Eckert, M. A., N. V. Kamdar, et al. (2008). "A cross-modal system linking primary auditory and visual cortices: evidence from intrinsic fMRI connectivity analysis." *Hum Brain Mapp* 29(7): 848-857.

Greicius, M. D., G. Srivastava, et al. (2004). "Default-mode network activity distinguishes Alzheimer's disease from healthy aging: evidence from functional MRI." *Proc Natl Acad Sci U S A* 101(13): 4637-4642.

Huang, J., X. Zong, et al. (2011). "fMRI evidence that precision ophthalmic tints reduce cortical hyperactivation in migraine." *Cephalalgia* 31(8): 925-936.

Hughes, J. R. (2008). "Gamma, fast, and ultrafast waves of the brain: their relationships with epilepsy and behavior." *Epilepsy Behav* 13(1): 25-31.

Imamizu, H. and M. Kawato (2009). "Brain mechanisms for predictive control by switching internal models: implications for higher-order cognitive functions." *Psychol Res* 73(4): 527-544.

Klemm WR. (1996). Understanding neuroscience. St. Louis (MO): Mosby; p.151–52.

Kravitz, D. J., K. S. Saleem, et al. (2011). "A new neural framework for visuospatial processing." *Nat Rev Neurosci* 12(4): 217-230.

Krekelberg, B. (2003). "Sound and vision." *Trends Cogn Sci* 7(7): 277-279.

Lee, J. H., R. Durand, et al. (2010). "Global and local fMRI signals driven by neurons defined optogenetically by type and wiring." *Nature* 465(7299): 788-792.

Luria, A.R. (1973). The working brain: an introduction to neuropsychology. Penguin Books

Lynch, J. C. and J. R. Tian (2006). "Cortico-cortical networks and cortico-subcortical loops for the higher control of eye movements." *Prog Brain Res* 151: 461-501.

Martineau, J., N. Hernandez, et al. (2011). "Can pupil size and pupil responses during visual scanning contribute to the diagnosis of autism spectrum disorder in children?" *J Psychiatr Res* 45(8): 1077-1082.

Mellman, T. A., V. Bustamante, et al. (2002). "REM sleep and the early development of posttraumatic stress disorder." *Am J Psychiatry* 159(10): 1696-1701.

Mrsic-Flogel, T. D., S. B. Hofer, et al. (2005). "Altered map of visual space in the superior colliculus of mice lacking early retinal waves." *J Neurosci* 25(29): 6921-6928.

Muri, R. M., M. T. Iba-Zizen, et al. (1996). "Location of the human posterior eye field with functional magnetic resonance imaging." *J Neurol Neurosurg Psychiatry* 60(4): 445-448.

Naya, Y. and W. A. Suzuki (2011). "Integrating what and when across the primate medial temporal lobe." *Science* 333(6043): 773-776.

Olshausen, B. A., C. H. Anderson, et al. (1993). "A neurobiological model of visual attention and invariant pattern recognition based on dynamic routing of information." *J Neurosci* 13(11): 4700-4719.

Parisi V. (2003). "Correlation between morphological and functional retinal impairment in patients affected by ocular hypertension, glaucoma, demyelinating optic neuritis and Alzheimer's disease." Semin Ophthalmol. Jun;18(2):50-7.

Portas, C. M., G. Rees, et al. (1998). "A specific role for the thalamus in mediating the interaction of attention and arousal in humans." *J Neurosci* 18(21): 8979-8989.

Ramachandran, V. S. and E. L. Altschuler (2009). "The use of visual feedback, in particular mirror visual feedback, in restoring brain function." *Brain* 132(Pt 7): 1693-1710.

Roberts, D.C., V. Marcelli, et al. (2011). "MRI magnetic field stimulates rotational sensors of the brain." Curr Biol 21(19): 1635-1640.

Rubin, N., K. Nakayama, et al. (1996). "Enhanced perception of illusory contours in the lower versus upper visual hemifields." *Science* 271(5249): 651-653.

Ruger, M., M. C. Gordijn, et al. (2005). "Nasal versus temporal illumination of the human retina: effects on core body temperature, melatonin, and circadian phase." *J Biol Rhythms* 20(1): 60-70.

Saalmann, Y. B. and S. Kastner (2009). "Gain control in the visual thalamus during perception and cognition." *Curr Opin Neurobiol* 19(4): 408-414.

Saalmann, Y. B. and S. Kastner (2011). "Cognitive and perceptual functions of the visual thalamus." *Neuron* 71(2): 209-223.

Sani, L., E. Ricciardi, et al. (2010). "Effects of Visual Experience on the Human MT+ Functional Connectivity Networks: An fMRI Study of Motion Perception in Sighted and Congenitally Blind Individuals." *Front Syst Neurosci* 4: 159.

Santangelo, V., M. Olivetti Belardinelli, et al. (2007). "The suppression of reflexive visual and auditory orienting when attention is otherwise engaged." *J Exp Psychol Hum Percept Perform* 33(1): 137-148.

Shin J., Vladimir Kepe, et al. (2011) Multimodal Imaging of Alzheimer Pathophysiology in the Brain's Default Mode Network SAGE-Hindawi Access to Research International Journal of Alzheimer's Disease Volume 2011, Article ID 687945, 8 pages doi:10.4061/2011/687945

Skeffington, A. M. (1957). "The totality of vision." *Am J Optom Arch Am Acad Optom* 34(5): 241-255.

Super, S. (2005). *Intention, attention, inattention & neglect*. Santa Ana, CA, Optometric Extension Program.

Suzuki, M., M. L. Massingale, et al. (2010). "Tear osmolarity as a biomarker for dry eye disease severity." *Invest Ophthalmol Vis Sci* 51(9): 4557-4561.

Swenson, R.S. (2006) Review of functional neuroscience Chapter 8D Eye movements Dartmouth medical school. Accessible at: http://www.dartmouth.edu/~rswenson/NeuroSci/chapter_8D.html

Tanaka, H., K. Homma, et al. (2011). "Physical delay but not subjective delay determines learning rate in prism adaptation." *Exp Brain Res* 208(2): 257-268.

Tombran-Tink, J. and C. J. Barnstable (2008). *Visual transduction and non-visual light perception*. Totowa, N.J., Humana Press.

van Baarsen K.M., Porro G.L., et al. (2009). "Epilepsy surgery provides new insights in retinotopic organization of optic radiations. A systematic review." Curr Opin Ophthalmol. Nov;20(6):490-4.

Webster, M. J., J. Bachevalier, et al. (1995). "Transient subcortical connections of inferior temporal areas TE and TEO in infant macaque monkeys." *J Comp Neurol* 352(2): 213-226.

Weir, C.R. (2006). "Proprioception in extraocular muscles." *J Neuroophthalmol* 26(2): 123-127.

Williams, A. L. and A. T. Smith (2010). "Representation of eye position in the human parietal cortex." *J Neurophysiol* 104(4): 2169-2177.

Wilson, J. A. (1911). "Retinoscopy without Atropine, and Some Observations on Ocular Headaches." *Br Med J* 2(2640): 258-259.

Zhang, B., Y. Luo, et al. (2011). "Macroscopic invisibility cloak for visible light." *Phys Rev Lett* 106(3): 033901.

Zhang, F., V. Gradinaru, et al. (2010). "Optogenetic interrogation of neural circuits: technology for probing mammalian brain structures." *Nat Protoc* 5(3): 439-456.

4

Neural Correlates of Rule-Based Perception and Production of Hand Gestures

Nobue Kanazawa[1], Masahiro Izumiyama[2], Takashi Inoue[3], Takanori Kochiyama[4], Toshio Inui[5] and Hajime Mushiake[1,6]

[1]*Department of Physiology, Tohoku University Graduate School of Medicine, Sendai*

[2]*Department of Neurology, Sendai Nakae Hospital, Sendai*

[3]*Department of Neurosurgery, Kohnan Hospital, Sendai*

[4]*Advanced Telecommunications Research Institute, Brain Activity Imaging Center, Kyoto*

[5]*Asada Synergistic Intelligence Project, ERATO, Japan Science and Technology Agency Kyoto University*

[6]*CREST, Japan Science and Technology Agency,Tokyo, Japan*

1. Introduction

Rule-based behavior is defined as flexible information processing that occurs across the sensory and motor domains. Recent studies on human and nonhuman primates have led to the identification of a set of brain regions that mediate flexible rule-guided behavior (White and Wise, 1999; Asaad et al., 2000; Hoshi et al., 2000; Wallis et al., 2001; Bunge et al., 2003; Sakai and Passingham, 2006, Bengtsson SL et al 2009). Hand gestures or postures have often been used as sensory signals and/or motor responses that are supposed to be produced under behavioral rules, each of which is unique to a behavioral context (Bunge, 2004). The number of possible hand gestures is virtually limitless, but a set of certain familiar hand gestures is often used in various cognitive contexts or under various behavioral rules. "Rock–paper–scissors" (RPS) is an example of a set of familiar hand gestures that has been used to make selections during games. The same hand postures in the RPS game are used for counting with fingers in a different context. On the other hand, observations of hand gestures or postures are known to activate the mirror neuron system, which include functions that are related to the imitation and/or understanding of actions (Iacoboni et al., 1999; Koski et al., 2002, 2003; Rizzolatti et al., 2004; Dinstein et al., 2007, 2008; Iacoboni and Dapretto, 2006; Iacoboni, 2009). When observers see a motor event that shares features with a similar motor event included in their motor repertoire, they are primed to repeat the same movement. Thus, given the natural tendency to imitate observed gestures, the brain regions involved in the observation and production of hand gestures guided by multiple rules has not been clear. To address this issue, we introduced a new rule-guided hand-gesture task that required subjects to produce an appropriate hand gesture in response to an observed hand posture according to two behavioral rules: the RPS-game rule and the number-based rule. Under these two different rules, the same hand gesture signified either rock–paper–

scissors or null–two–five. We hypothesized that performance of the hand-gesture task under guidance of multiple rules would require that the meanings of hand-gestures to be represented in a rule-specific manner and the supervisory or other control system must be recruited to balance the rule-guided behavioral systems with the mirror system to overcome a covert and automatic tendency to imitate observed hand postures.

2. Methods, results and discussion

2.1 Materials and methods

2.1.1 Subjects

Nineteen healthy right-handed male subjects (mean age: 22.2 years, age range: 22–28 years) volunteered to participate in this study. All subjects had normal vision, and none had a history of neurological or psychiatric illness. Written informed consent was obtained from each subject before their participation in this study. All procedures were conducted in accordance with the guidelines approved by The Office of Policy Coordination of the Tohoku University Graduate School of Medicine.

2.1.2 Rule-based hand-gesture task (Fig. 1)

The subjects wore a head-mounted display to view objects projected by a computer and pushed buttons embedded in a small box held in their right hands. Participants were asked to perform a task involving rule-based hand gestures, as described in detail in the following section. Before functional magnetic resonance imaging (fMRI) scanning, all participants were asked to perform a brief exercise as a pre-scanning task.

Subjects were asked to perform a task involving rule-based hand gestures (Fig. 1A). In each trial, participants were asked to gaze at a central fixation spot (white dot) that appeared on the screen for 1500–2500 ms. Next, one of three illustrations of hand shapes (rock, paper, or scissors) was presented on the screen as a sample stimulus for 500 ms (stimuli shown in Fig. 1B). After a delay of 2500–4500 ms, the subjects were asked to produce a hand gesture in response to instruction cues. Two rule conditions were used: the RPS-rule condition and the number-rule condition. Under the RPS-rule condition (rock beats scissors, scissors beats paper, paper beats rock), one of three instruction cues—"win," "draw," or "lose"—was presented to the subjects for 500 ms (Fig. 1B, right and middle rows). As shown in the example presented in Figure 1A, each subject was instructed to produce the scissors gesture after observing the paper stimulus in response to the instruction to win. Under the number-rule condition, rock represented null, scissors represented two, and paper represented five. The subject was asked to produce the hand gestures corresponding to the appropriate numbers according to three instruction cues: "more," "equal," or "less." For example, the subject was required to produce the scissors hand gesture (two) in response to the rock stimulus (null) when an instruction cue of "more" was given. Presented with a number depicted by simple hand gestures, the subjects were instructed to use hand gestures to indicate the next higher or next lower number. Under both conditions, the subjects were instructed to press a button after producing the hand gesture. The inter-trial interval was 3000 ms. All subjects practiced a short version of the task prior to scanning. The RPS-rule and number-rule conditions were blocked as shown in Figure1C.

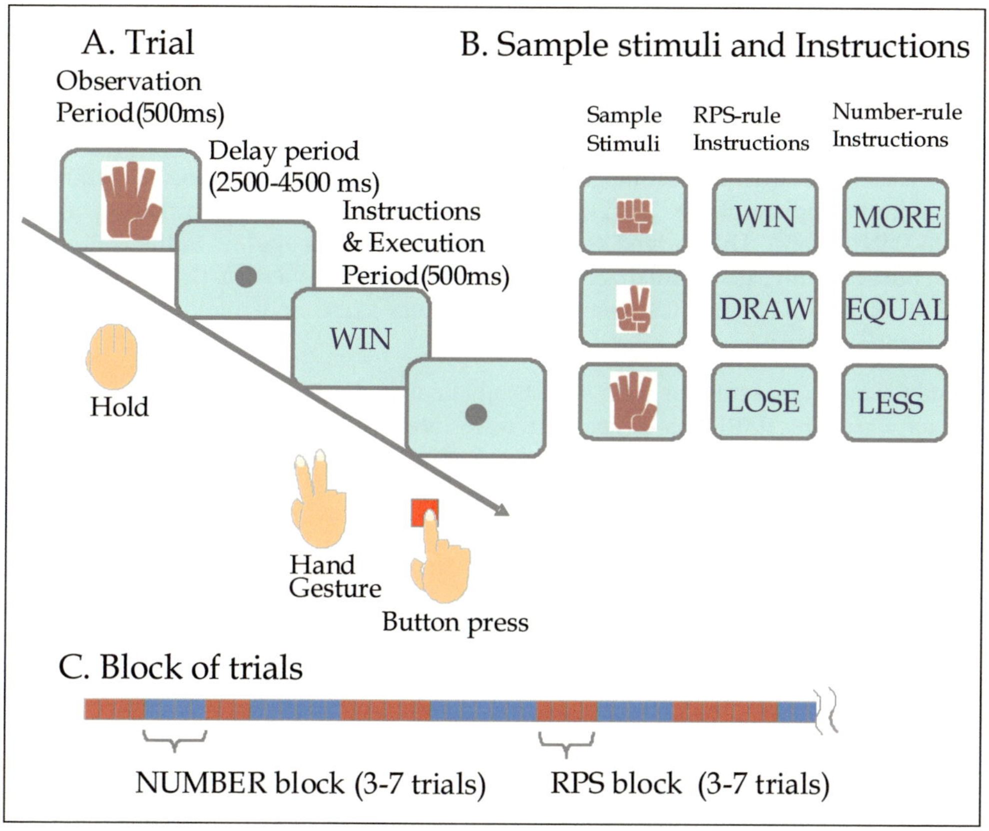

Fig. 1. Schematic diagram of Rule-based hand-gesture task. (A) Task sequence during fMRI scanning. During stimulus presentation, one of three illustrations of hand shapes was presented on a screen. During the instruction and execution periods, one of three instruction cues ("win," "lose," or "draw" under the Rock–Paper–Scissors-(RPS)-rule condition of the RPS block; or "more," "less," or "equal" under the number-rule condition of the number block) was presented on the screen. (B) Illustrations of hand shapes were used for sample stimuli and instruction cues used to guide the production of hand gestures. (C) A scanning session consisted of blocks of trials. Each block occurred under either the RPS- or number-rule condition and consisted of three to seven trials, yielding a total of 126 trials. The RPS block is represented in red and the number block is shown in blue.

2.1.3 MRI data acquisition

Images were obtained with a 3-Tesla MRI scanner (GE Signa Excite; GE Medical Systems, Milwaukee, WI, USA) equipped with echo-planar imaging capability. Functional MRI images were acquired using a gradient echo-planar sequence (repetition time = 3000 ms, echo time = 50 ms, field of view = 24 x 24 mm, matrix size = 64 x 64, flip angle = 90°, slice thickness = 7 mm (no interslice gap). We obtained 20 horizontal slices along the anteroposterior commissure AC-PC line, which encompassed the whole brain.

2.1.4 fMRI analysis

Image processing and statistical analyses of the fMRI data were performed using statistical parametric mapping (SPM5; Wellcome Department of Imaging Neuroscience, London, UK, http://www.fil.ion.ucl.ac.uk) and Matlab (MathWorks, Natick, MA, USA). The effect of head motion across the scans was corrected by realigning all scans according to the first one. A mean image created from the realigned echo-planar imaging (EPI) images was co-registered with the structural T1 image, and the structural images were normalized spatially to a standard template of $2 \times 2 \times 2\text{-mm}^3$ voxel size in the space (Montreal Neurological Institute (MNI) space). The derived spatial transformation was applied to the realigned EPI images. Subsequently, the normalized EPI images were smoothed spatially with an 8-mm full-width at half-maximum Gaussian filter to reduce noise and minimize the effects of normalization errors.

The data for individual subjects were statistically analyzed using the general linear model in SPM5 software. The fMRI time-series data were modeled by a series of events convolved with a canonical hemodynamic response function. Global changes were adjusted by proportional scaling, and the low-frequency confounding effects were removed using an appropriate high-pass filter.

Statistical analysis was accomplished within SPM. The design matrix for blocked analysis was computed to characterize regionally specific effects under the RPS- and number-task conditions using a kernel that approximated the hemodynamic response function. We calculated contrast with a boxcar reference waveform using a t-value (SPM{t}) at each voxel. The SPM{t} was transformed to the unit normal distribution SPM{Z}.

To examine the activity changes related to each behavioral event during the task phase, we conducted an event-related analysis for each subject and a random-effect analysis for data from multiple subjects. In the single-subject-level analysis, we estimated the activity changes in response to the onset of sample stimuli under each rule condition. We also estimated activity changes in response to the instruction cues under each condition. According to these instructions, the subjects produced hand gestures that were identical to the sample when cued with "equal" or "draw." These conditions were considered to represent imitations of observed hand postures. As noted later in the Results section, the reaction times (RTs) for these two instruction cues were very brief and similar to each other, suggesting the operation of a priming effect related to observing a sample.

To identify rule-selective regions, we excluded regions affected by common priming effects based on the tendency toward imitation. In this sense, we considered activity changes in response to these instructions as baseline activity under the control condition. We then obtained the following two contrasts from each subject to identify rule-selective areas: the response to "win" or "lose" (RPS-rule condition) minus the response to "equal" or "draw" (control condition), and the response to "more" or "less" (number-rule condition) minus the response to "equal" or "draw" (control condition). Thereafter, we also identified rule-nonselective regions by performing a conjunction analysis of cortical activations common to number-rule and RPS-rule conditions.

We computed the group effect with a random-effect model using a one-sample t-test. Voxels were given a threshold of $p < 0.05$ using a maximal false-discovery rate (FDR), a method of correcting for multiple comparisons. Additionally, we applied parametric modulation to investigate the region corresponding to performance (RT or trial frequency) using a between-block design. A voxel-level threshold of $p < 0.05$ (FDR) and an extent threshold of five voxels were reported in the parametric modulation. The MNI coordinates were nonlinearly converted into Talairach coordinates using the MNI2tal® conversion program (ftp://ftp.mrc-cbu.cam.ac.uk/pub/imaging/MNI2tal/mni2tal.m).

We used two types of software to identify anatomical and functional areas: the 'Talairach Daemon' client to identify Brodmann's areas (BAs) (http://ric.uthscsa.edu/ projects/ talairachdaemon.html) and the AAL plugin (http://www.cyceron.fr/web/aal anatomical_automatic_labeling.html) to identify functional activation maps.

2.1.5 Regions of interest (ROI) analysis

To quantitatively examine the context of the brain activities, we conducted an ROI analysis based on the statistical parametric map obtained by the event-related analysis. We hypothesized that activated brain regions were classified into rule-selective (number-rule or RPS-rule) areas for implementation of rule-dependent task sets and common areas for supervisory roles or active memory retrieval against the covert tendency to imitate observed hand postures. Under the number-rule condition, we selected first set of three areas [i.e., the superior parietal lobule (SPL), the intraparietal sulcus (IPS), and the premotor area (PMA)] in which number representations were found. Although subjects usually play RPS-games to win, subjects were asked to produce hand gestures even though a particular hand gesture resulted in a loss under our RPS condition. Thus, we selected second set of three areas [i.e., the orbitofrontal cortex (OFC), the anterior cingulated cortex (ACC), and the pre-supplementary area (pre-SMA)], which are involved in reward-based action selection or conflict resolution under the RPS-condition. We selected third set of three areas [i.e., the dorsolateral prefrontal cortex (DLPFC) for its role in executive functioning, the posterior cingulated cortex (PCC) for its role in the retrieval of memorized rules, and the supplementary motor area (SMA) for its role in memory-guided action selection] as nonselective areas common for both rules. We therefore defined the nine individual ROIs in each hemisphere of each subject.

The ROIs that reached a statistical threshold of $p < 0.05$ were presented as spheres centered on the peaks of clusters within a radius of 8 mm. The mean percentage of signal change (relative to a fixation period inserted between blocks) within each ROI was calculated for each subject and task using Mars Bar® (http://marsbar.sourceforge.net/).

2.2 Results

2.2.1 Behavioral data for the fMRI scanning task

To examine the effect of task condition on RTs, we plotted the averaged RTs and conducted statistical comparisons of the values obtained for these variables in response to each instruction cue (Fig. 2). Under the RPS-rule condition, the RTs in response to "draw" were significantly shorter than RTs in response to "win" [$t(339) = 4.21$, $p = 0$]. The RTs for "draw" were significantly shorter than RTs in response to "lose" [$t(351) = 7.11$, $p = 0$]. In contrast, under the number-rule condition, the RTs in response to "equal" were significantly shorter than those for "more" [t(329) = 8.03, p = 0]. The RTs for "equal" were significantly shorter than those for "less" [t(335) = 11.35, p = 0]. Means and standard errors for all conditions are listed in Table 1. The shorter RTs for the "draw" and "equal" instructions under each rule condition may have reflected the rapid production of a hand gesture identical to the sample, reflecting the difference between the process of imitation and that of rule-based selection as well as the impact of the priming effect on the imitation of observed hand postures.

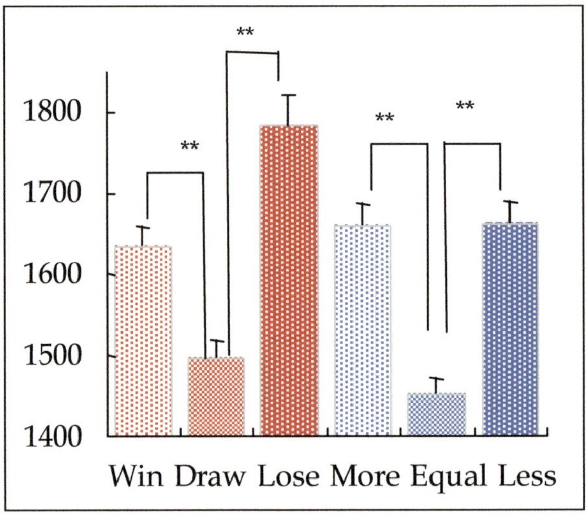

Fig. 2. Average response times of all subjects. (A) Plot of reaction times under six instruction conditions ("win," "draw," "lose," "more," "equal," and "less").

Instruction conditions	
RPS ruled	
Win	1634.67±23.43
Draw	1497.61±20.96
Lose	1784.8±38.35
Number ruled	
More	1661.36±24.43
Equal	1454.61±16.84
Less	1663.89±26.05
Values are means ±SE; msec.	

Table 1. The effect of instruction type on reaction time

2.2.2 Neural activity during the instruction and execution periods

We showed contrast activity changes in response to the instruction cues under the RPS-rule condition and the number-rule condition based on the event-related analysis explained in the Methods section. On the basis of these comparisons, instruction-related activity was classified into three categories: RPS-rule-selective activity, which showed significantly greater changes in activity under the RPS than under the number condition [p < 0.05 (FDR)]; number-rule-selective activity, which showed significantly greater changes in activity under the RPS condition than under the number condition [p < 0.05 (FDR)]; and nonselective activity, which showed similar changes in activity under both the RPS and number conditions. (Fig.3).

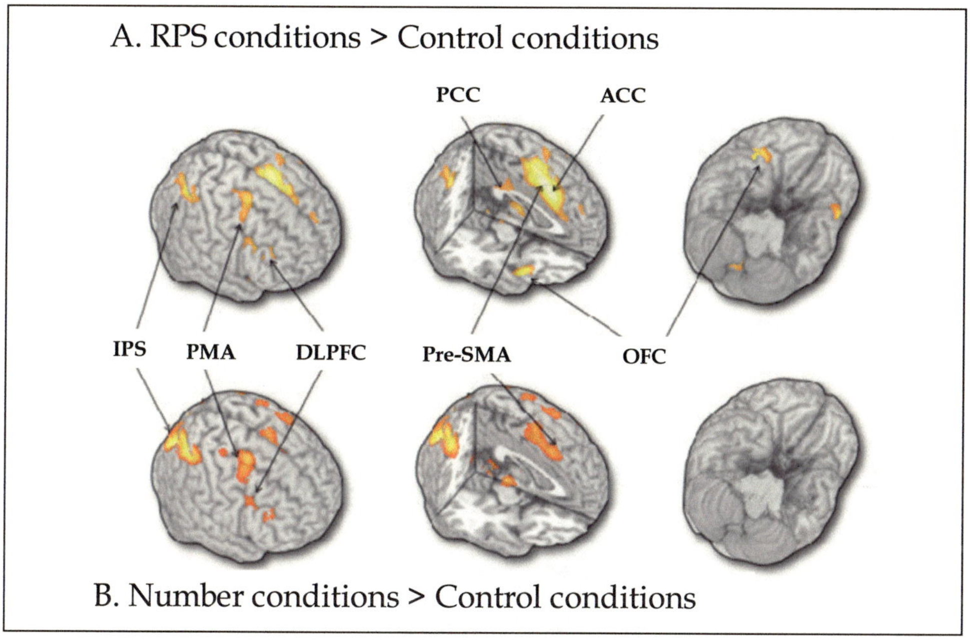

Fig. 3. Rule-selective activity during the execution period (A) Brain areas significantly activated in response to "win" or "lose" under the RPS-rule condition. (B) Brain areas significantly activated in response to "more" or "less" under the number-rule condition.

To quantitatively examine activation patterns, we performed a ROI-based analysis for the OFC, IPS, and DLPFC by extracting data on the mean percent signal changes at each ROI, as shown in 4A, 4B, and 4C, respectively. ROI analysis of rule-related activity during the execution period was listed in Table 2.

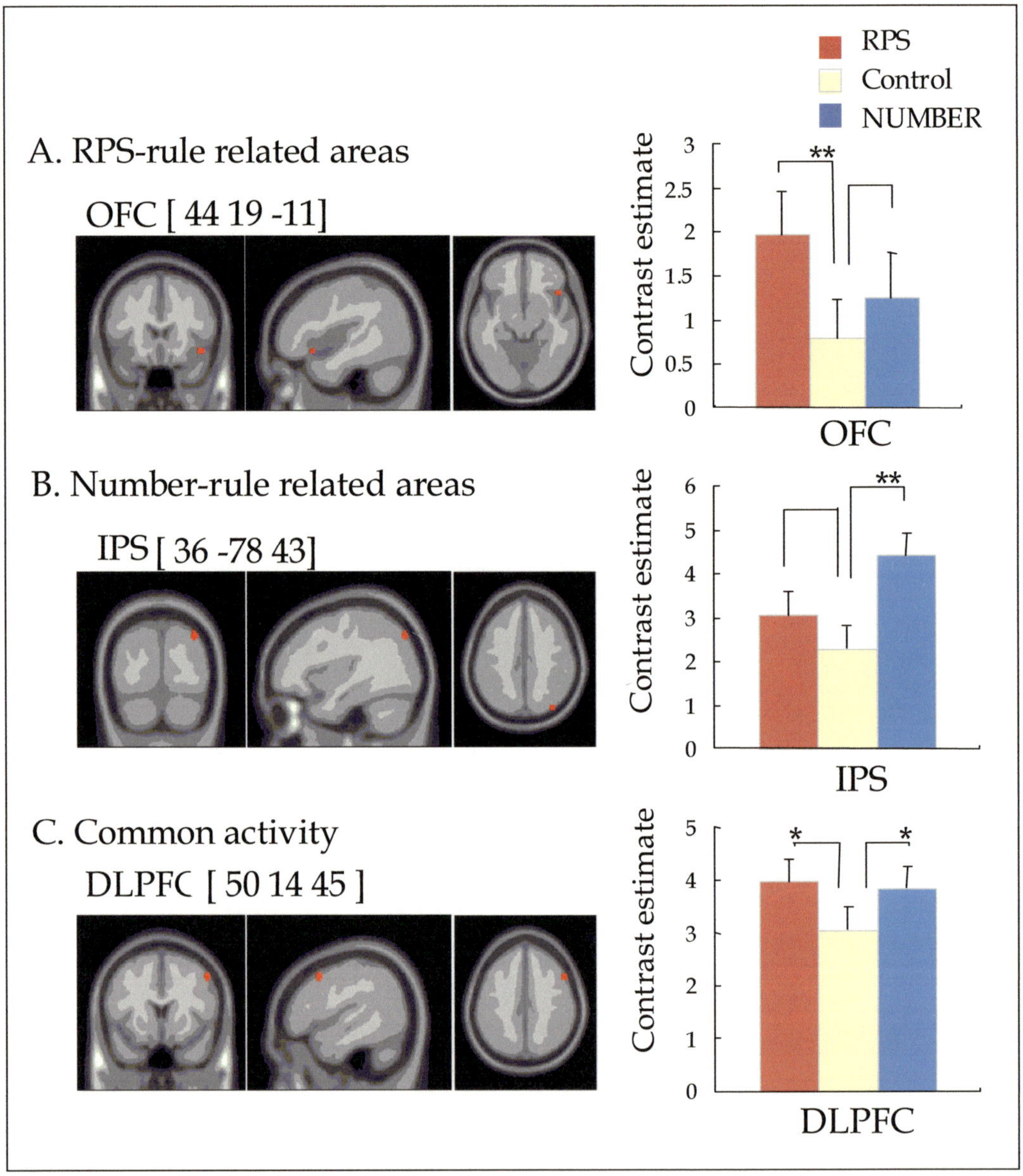

Fig. 4. Rule-related activity and ROI analysis. (A) The orbitofrontal cortex (OFC) was significantly more activated under the RPS-rule condition than under the control and number-rule conditions. (B) The intraparietal sulcus (IPS) was significantly more activated under the number-rule condition than under the control and RPS-rule conditions. (C) The dorsolateral prefrontal cortex (DLPFC) was significantly more activated under both the RPS- and number-rule conditions than under the control condition (Table 2).

Region of activation L/R Area			coordinates of peak activation			
			x	y	z	Z value
RSP > Number>ctrl						
ACC	L/R	24	4	-10	40	4.01
PreSMA	L/R	6	4	21	63	4.82
OFC	L/R	47	44	19	-11	4.51
Number >RPS> ctrl						
IPS	L/R	7/40	36	-78	43	4.22
PMA	L/R	6	-41	-2	62	3.71
SPL	L/R	40	-41	-54	60	3.96
Non-selective activity in RPS condition (Number > ctrl) and (RPS> ctrl)						
DLPFC	L/R	9	50	14	45	3.77
SMA	L/R	6	-4	-10	74	3.87
PCC	L/R	23	-4	-38	26	4.02
Non-selective activity in Number condition (Number > ctrl) and (RPS> ctrl)						
DLPFC	L/R	9	50	14	45	3.1
SMA	L/R	6	-4	-10	74	3.66
PCC	L/R	23	-4	-38	26	3.47

Table 2. ROI analysis of rule-related activity during the execution period

Furthermore, to quantitatively compare the rule-related activity in response to the "win" and "lose" instructions under the RPS-rule condition, we conducted a ROI analysis for the ACC (BA24) and OFC (BA47). We found that the "lose" and "win" cue elicited significantly greater changes in activity than the "draw" cue under the RPS condition (Fig. 5A). To quantitatively compare the instruction-related activity of the "more" and "less" cues under the number-rule condition, we also conducted a ROI analysis for the IPS (BA7/40) and the PMA (BA6). We found similar activity changes in response to "more" and "less" (Fig. 5B).

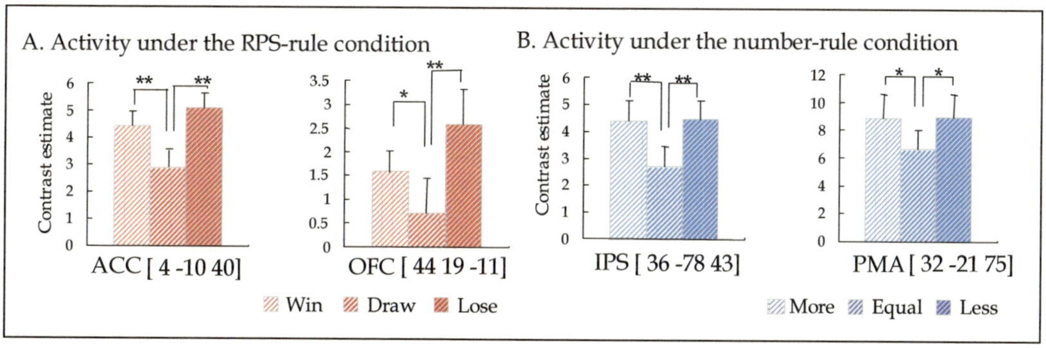

Fig. 5. ROI analysis of rule-related activity during the execution period. (A) The anterior cingulate cortex (ACC) and orbitofrontal cortex (OFC) were significantly more activated in response to "lose" and "win" than to "draw." (B) The intraparietal sulcus (IPS) and premotor area (PMA) showed similar activation in response to "more" and "less."

2.2.3 Neural activity during the observation periods

We examined brain activation during the observation period (Fig. 6) and in general found greater activation in various task-related areas under the number-rule condition than under the RPS-rule condition. Based on our findings of rule-selective activities in response to instructional cues and to sample hand shapes, we compared the rule selectivity for the two task periods. Areas showing number-rule selectivity during the instruction and execution periods were more active under the number-rule than under the RPS-rule condition during the observation period (Fig. 6B). However, areas showing RPS-rule selectivity during the instruction and execution periods were active under both conditions during the observation period (Fig. 6A). Several RPS-rule-selective brain areas were more active under the number-rule than under the RPS-rule condition.

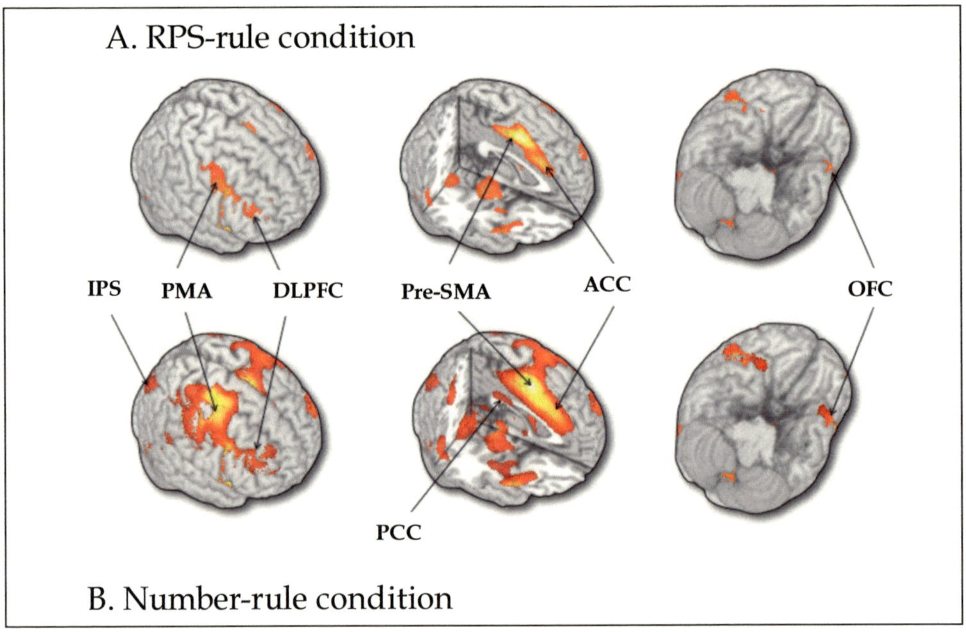

Fig. 6. ROI analysis of rule-related activity during the execution period. Brain areas activated in response to the hand-shape stimuli under the RPS-rule and number-rule conditions during the observation period. (A) Brain areas activated in response to the hand-shape stimuli under the RPS-rule condition. (B) Brain areas activated in response to the hand-shape stimuli under the number-rule condition.

To quantitatively examine changes in activity, we performed a ROI analysis on the IPS, PMA, ACC, and OFC. Both the IPS and PMA showed higher activation under the number-rule condition during the instruction, response, and observation periods (Fig. 7A). In contrast, the OFC was activated in response to the sample hand shape under both conditions. Unexpectedly, the ACC showed greater activation under the number-rule condition than under the RPS-rule condition even though this area was preferentially active under the RPS-rule condition during the instruction and execution periods and thus reflective of selective activity during the instruction and execution periods (Fig. 7B).

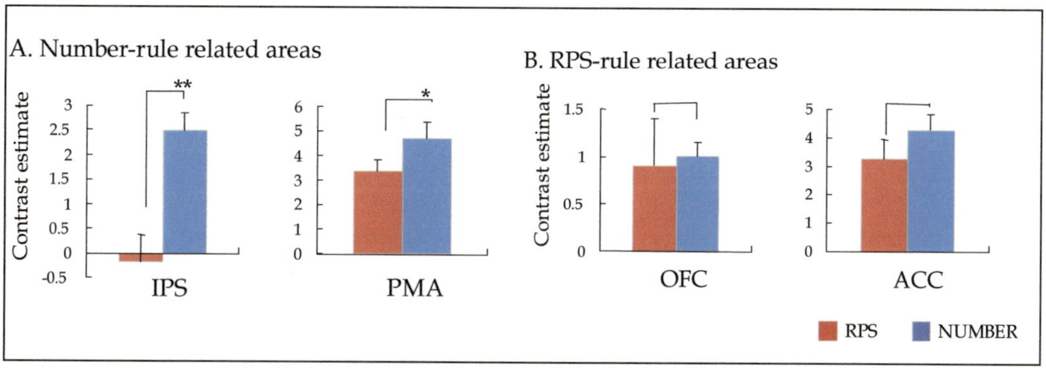

Fig. 7. ROI analysis of rule-related activity in the observation period. (A) IPS and PMA showed greater activation under the number-rule condition than under the RPS-rule condition during the observation and execution periods. (B) OFC and ACC showed greater activation under the number-rule condition than under the RPS-rule condition even though they are classified as RPS-selective areas.

2.3 Discussion

We defined the brain regions recruited for recognition and production using two behavioral rules. Rule one was based on the RPS game in which subjects were required to produce hand gestures in response to the observed sample hand postures according to one of three instructions: "win", "draw", or "lose" (RPS rule). The other rule two was based on number gestures in which subjects were required to produce number gestures by hand for the value of the observed hand posture in response to one of three instructions: "more", "equal", or "less" (number rule). A closed fist, extended index and middle fingers, and extensions of all fingers were gestures common to both rules, denoting rock, scissors, and paper, respectively, under the RPS-rule condition and null, two, and five, respectively, under the number-rule condition. We found that production of the same hand gestures recruited activation of different brain regions and that the IPS and the PMA exhibited distinct activation when subjects observed the sample hand shapes and produced the hand gestures according to the instructions under the number-rule condition. We also found that the ACC and the OFC exhibited distinct activation when the subjects produced the hand gestures under the RPS-rule condition. Under both "equal" and "draw" conditions, reaction times were shorter and rule-selective activities decreased compared to other conditions. These findings clearly demonstrated that observation of hand shapes evoked a priming effect for the mirror system Furthermore, both the ACC and OFC were active when the subjects observed the sample hand shapes, irrespective of the current rule condition. This finding indicated that observation of hand shapes also evoked covert activations in RPS rule-selective areas. The lateral prefrontal cortex (LPFC) was active under both rule conditions, suggesting a role coordinating the mirror and rule-guided gesture systems as a supervisory controller.

2.3.1 Mirror system, rule-based perception, and production of hand gestures

Rapid reproduction of the hand gestures representing equal in the number-rule and draw under the RPS-rule conditions suggested the priming effect of the mirror system. Observers are primed to repeat a motor event that shares features with a similar motor event present in their motor repertoire upon encountering it. It means the greater the similarity between the observed event and the previous motor event, the stronger will be the priming effect (Prinz, 2002). Decreases in rule-selective activities also supported the covert effect of the mirror system.

A human mirror system has been elucidated by a substantial number of studies that focused on reactions to the observation of actions performed by others (Iacoboni et al., 1999; Koski et al., 2002, 2003; Rizzolatti et al., 2004; Dinstein et al., 2007, 2008; Iacoboni and Dapretto, 2006; Iacoboni, 2009). This mirror system forms a complex network consisting of an anterior area in the IFC that encompasses the posterior inferior frontal gyrus (IFG) and the adjacent ventral premotor cortex (PMC) as well as a posterior area in the rostral part of the inferior parietal lobule (IPL) (Iacoboni et al., 1999; Koski et al., 2002, 2003; Rizzolatti et al., 2004; Brass and Heyes, 2005; Dinstein et al., 2007, 2008; Iacoboni and Dapretto, 2006; Iacoboni, 2009). The rule-selective areas, such as the ACC and OFC, under the RPS-rule condition and the PMA (PMd) and IPS were not included in the conventional mirror neuron system (Gazzola V and Keysers C. 2009). One hypothesis about the functional role of mirror neurons is that mirror-neuron activity mediates imitation. Subjects in our study were required to observe hand shapes and execute hand gestures according to the two behavioral rules. In this task, subjects selected hand gestures that differed from the observed hand postures except in response to "equal" under the number-rule condition and "draw" under the RPS-rule condition. Indeed, our study identified rule-selective brain regions by noting areas characterized by significantly greater activations than those during the imitation of gestures following instructions of "draw" or "equal". We then calculated the contrasts in the activations associated with producing hand gestures that differed from those that were observed. Decreased activity in rule-selective brains regions suggested greater contributions of the mirror system for gestures following instructions of "draw" or "equal". Rule-guided system for arbitrary mapping sensory and motor events and the mirror neuron system for imitation based on direct sensory-motor mapping function competitively.

2.3.2 RPS-rule-related areas

We found that RPS-rule-selective activities in the ACC and OFC were involved in associating and integrating stimuli and rewards (Paus,2001;Schultz, 2004; Ridderinkhof et al 2004;Kringelbach, 2005; Coricelli et al., 2007; Rushworth et al., 2007; Wallis, 2007; Rolls and Grabenhorst, 2008; Seymour and McClure, 2008; Buelow and Suhr, 2009; Mainen and Kepecs, 2009). According to Wallis (2007), the OFC determines the potential reward outcome. Although a reward was not associated with any response or stimulus in our experiment, the subjects may have anticipated a potential reward because the RPS game is frequently related to rewards in daily life. Also, the ACC has been proposed to participate in conflict monitoring (Botvinick et al., 1999,2004; van Veen and Carter, 2005; Kerns, 2006). Under our RPS-rule condition, RTs in the "lose" situation were longer than those in the "win" situation. This asymmetrical distribution of RTs suggested that the subjects were biased toward selecting hand gestures associated with winning and wanted to do so even when the instruction was to lose. This tendency was associated with response conflict and activated the ACC. Furthermore, a meta-analysis of neuroimaging data has suggested that the ACC and OFC were often co-activated when behavioral conflict was detected and behavioral change was required (Kringelbach, 2005).

This type of biased activation was not observed in comparisons of responses to the "less" and "more" cues. Indeed, the RTs under the "less" and "more" instructions did not statistically differ, and subjects did not show biases for either response. Based on this finding of biased responses, one can hypothesize that the instruction to lose frequently caused conflict because of a desire to win and led to a greater delay in the selection response than the instruction to win under the RPS-rule condition. The instructions to win or lose involved potential reward and/or conflict. In contrast, under the number-rule condition, more and less involved merely quantitative judgments about size and neutral decision-making about hand gestures.

Unexpectedly, RPS-selective areas such as the ACC and OFC, defined based on instruction-related activities, were covertly active under both the number and RPS conditions during the execution period. This pattern differed from that observed for the number-rule-selective areas, in which rule selectivity was maintained throughout the experiment. At least two possible interpretations for this pattern of activity can be proposed. One involves the implicit activation of RPS-related areas due to a stronger tendency to produce hand gestures in the RPS game than under the number-rule condition. Finger counting is often used in preschool education, but it is not used in the everyday lives of most adults. However, even adults use the RPS game. This difference in familiarity may cause the implicit activation of RPS-related areas even under the number-rule condition. Another possible interpretation concerns the behavioral conflict associated with the two behavioral rules. As mentioned in the previous section, the ACC and OFC were often co-activated in situations involving behavioral conflict. When hand shapes were presented to the subjects before the instructions, they may have experienced conflict between the two behavioral rules, one a relatively familiar RPS rule and the other a neutral number rule. According to both interpretations, observation of hand shapes elicited not only visual but also cognitive responses related to rule-based action selection.

2.3.3 Number-rule–related areas

Consistent with previous functional imaging studies showing that mental arithmetic activated the IPS bilaterally (Roland and Friberg, 1985; Dehaene et al., 1996, Piazza 2007), we found number-rule-selective activities in the IPS and PMC. Indeed, recent fMRI studies have revealed number-related parietal activation irrespective of the ways in which number stimuli were presented (e.g., sets or series of dots) (Piazza et al., 2004; Cantlon et al., 2006; Castelli et al., 2006; Piazza et al., 2006; Nieder and Dehaene, 2009). The PMC has also been reported to include number-related areas (Fridman et al., 2006; Kansaku et al., 2006, 2007). The number-rule-related areas were also active when the shape of the hand was presented as a sample stimulus under the number-rule condition. This anticipatory activation of number-related areas suggested that number-rule-selective areas were multimodal and related to perception and production of hand gestures when the rule mediating between stimulus and response was based on quantity.

2.3.4 Nonselective rule-related areas

We found that the LPFC was activated under both the RPS- and number-rule conditions. The LPFC has been implicated in rule retrieval in both nonhuman and human primates (Murray et al., 2000; Passingham et al., 2000). Human imaging studies have shown that the LPFC was active when individuals retrieved the meanings of rules and retained them over several seconds (Poldrack et al., 1999; Brass and von Cramon, 2002, 2004; Bunge et al., 2003). Thus, the LPFC is involved in rule retrieval and maintenance. Furthermore, the LPFC may be involved in suppressing the priming of the mirror system, which causes observers to reproduce observed hand postures. The LPFC is important to establish a cognitive set required for each rule condition (Sakai and Passingham,2006;Bengtsson et al 2009). It may also play an important role in rule switching and coordinating with the medial PFC including the pre-SMA (Rushworth et al., 2002; Wallis, 2007).

2.3.5 Limitations of present study and approaches to resolve difficulties

One of limitations of present study was that we did not able to show the results of functional connectivity among regions of interests. Main reason was because the number of subjects was not sufficient to draw firm conclusions. According to the previous study by Sakai K and Passingham RE.2006, activity of the LPFC reflected the process of implementing the rule for subsequent cognitive performance and showed rule-selective interactions with areas involved in execution of the specific rule-guided behavior. In our task, the LPFC may be involved in not just implmenting each behavioral rule, but also in controling production process of hand gestures primed by the mirror system but guided by multiple behavioral rules. For aapproaches to resolve difficulties about evaluation of multiple interactions among task related areas, we should collect more data and examine interactions between the mirror system and rule-guided system by using dynamic causal modeling which enables us to infer the causal architecture of task-related areas as coupled or distributed dynamical systems.

3. Conclusion

3.1 Major findings

To examine the brain areas involved in flexible rule-based perception and the hand gestures produced according to our covert tendency to imitate observed hand postures, we measured brain activation using functional magnetic resonance imaging while participants performed hand gestures based on the multiple behavioral rules of Rock–Paper–Scissors (RPS). Using this familiar practice, which involves multiple uses of the same set of hand gestures, subjects were asked to produce one of three hand gestures—rock (null), paper (five), or scissors (two)—in response to a sample hand shape and according to the instructions "win," "draw," or "lose" under the RPS-rule condition and according to the instructions "more," "equal," or "less" under the number-rule condition.

We found that the intraparietal sulcus (IPS) and the premotor area (PMA) exhibited distinct activation when the subjects observed the sample hand shapes and produced the hand gestures according to the instructions under the number-rule condition. We also found that the anterior cingulate cortex (ACC) and the orbitofrontal cortex (OFC) exhibited distinct activation when the subjects produced hand gestures under the RPS-rule condition. Under both the equal and draw conditions, reaction times were shorter and rule-selective activities decreased compared to those under other conditions, suggesting that the priming effect of the mirror system influenced rule-guided behaviors. Furthermore, both the ACC and OFC were active when the subjects observed the sample hand shapes, irrespective of the current rule condition. These findings demonstrated that the observation of hand shapes evoked a priming effect such as that demonstrated by a mirror system and elicited covert activations in rule-selective areas. The lateral prefrontal cortex was also recruited in coordinating the mirror and rule-guided gesture systems.

3.2 Implication and summary diagram

Figure 8 presents a diagrammatic depiction of our two hypothesized rule-guided systems, the mirror and the supervisory systems. According to this diagram, observation of hand postures initially evokes the priming effects of the mirror-system. Rule-guided behavior systems, with the help of top-down signals from the DLPFC, seem to override mirror-system priming in the imitation of observed hand gestures. In two rule-guided systems, observation of hand gestures preferentially activates the ACC and OFC, which are selective for RPS-rule behavior during the execution period but are activated under both conditions during the observation periods. Top-down signals from the DLPFC in involved in

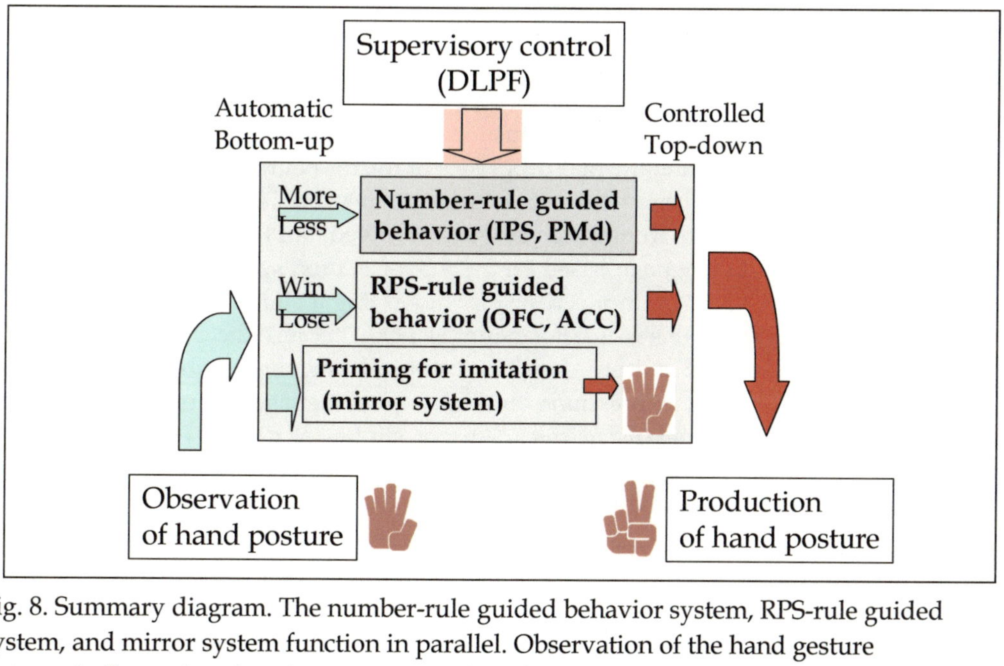

Fig. 8. Summary diagram. The number-rule guided behavior system, RPS-rule guided system, and mirror system function in parallel. Observation of the hand gesture automatically evokes the mirror system and preferred rule condition (RPS) in a bottom-up manner. When a rule-guided behavior is specified by instruction cues, a supervisory control signal adjusts the flow of information via top-down signalling. In the case depicted, some instructions specify the number-rule condition and others are guided by the number-rule system.

coordinating not only mirror system but also two rule-guided systems. During the execution periods, subjects are able to select appropriate hand gestures under the supervisory control of the DLPFC. In summary, observation of hand postures evoke automatic parallel activation of rule-related structures based on its preference in a bottom up manner, then appropriate hand gestures were produced based on the current status of the valid rule with the help of controlled top-down signal from the DLPFC.

3.3 New developments and future prospective

As we mentioned in introduction, the number of possible hand gestures is virtually limitless, but a set of certain familiar hand gestures is often used in various cognitive contexts or under various behavioral rules. In current studies, we examined brain regions related to observation and productions of simple hand gestures and postures without complicated spatiotemporal structures. However, hand gestures are often produced in space and in a sequential manner. Well-controlled studies using non-human primate have revealed many cortical motor areas, especially medial frontal motor areas, involved in control of sequential motor actions (Mushiake et al 1992; Hikosaka et al 1999;Shima K, Tanji J.2000;Tanji J.2001). Numerous functional imaging studies have found active foci in the cerebral cortex including the medial frontal cortex associated with the performance of a variety of sequential movements by human subjects (Shibasaki et al 1993; Deiber et al 1999;Kansaku et al 2006). The mirror system may contribute to imitation and understanding of complicated actions such as sequential movements performed by others (Rizzolatti et al., 2004; Iacoboni and Dapretto, 2006; Iacoboni, 2009). According to our current study, the dorsal premotor areas may contribute to rule-guided behaviours. A question arise which areas are involved in observation and production of rule based sequential hand gestures. Furthermore on the basis of fundamental properties of mirror neurons, Rizzolatti and Arbib (1998) proposed a hypothesis that the mirror neuron system represents the neurophysiological mechanism from which language evolved. But there are still explanatory gap between gestures and language based on the mirror neuron system (Hickock 2010). To narrow this explanatory gap, brain mechanisms underlying a sign language may provide important information about this issue (Poizner et al 1990), because the sing language is the visual-gestural language and a fully developed natural language with highly complex grammatical rules. Complex expressions through sign language include the recursive application of hierarchically organized rules. Further studies of rule based hand gesturers will provide more comprehensive view of neural mechanisms underlying observation and production of action for communication.

4. Acknowledgments

We thank M. Kurama and Y. Takahashi for their technical assistance and the radiology technologists of Kohnan Hospital and Sendai Nakae Hospital for assisting with the fMRI experiment. This study was supported by the Japan Science and Technology, Global Center of Excellence Program, and a Grant-in-Aid for Scientific Research on Priority Areas (Integrative Brain Research) from the Ministry of Education, Culture, Sports, Science and Technology, Japan, the Core Research for Evolutional Science and Technology, and the Japan Science and Technology Agency.

5. References

Asaad WF, Rainer G, Miller EK. 2000. Task-specific neural activity in the primate prefrontal cortex. J Neurophysiol 84, 451–459.

Bengtsson SL, Haynes JD, Sakai K, Buckley MJ, Passingham RE. 2009. The representation of abstract task rules in the human prefrontal cortex. Cereb Cortex 19, 1929–1936.

Botvinick M, Nystrom LE, Fissell K, Carter CS, Cohen JD. 1999. Conflict monitoring versus selection-for-action in anterior cingulate cortex. Nature 402, 179–181.

Botvinick MM, Cohen JD, Carter CS. 2004. Conflict monitoring and anterior cingulate cortex: an update. Trends Cogn Sci 8, 539–546.

Brass M, von Cramon DY. (2002) The role of the frontal cortex in task preparation. Cereb Cortex. 12, 908-914.

Brass M, von Cramon DY. (2004) Selection for cognitive control: a functional magnetic resonance imaging study on the selection of task-relevant information. J Neurosci. 24, 8847-8852.

Brass M, Heyes C. 2005. Imitation: is cognitive neuroscience solving the correspondence problem? Trends Cogn Sci 9, 489–495 (Review).

Buelow MT, Suhr JA. 2009. Construct validity of the Iowa Gambling Task. Neuropsychol Rev 19, 102–114.

Bunge SA. 2004. How we use rules to select actions: a review of evidence from cognitive neuroscience. Cogn Affect Behav Neurosci 4, 564–579 (Review).

Bunge SA, Kahn I, Wallis JD, Miller EK, Wagner AD. 2003. Neural circuits subserving the retrieval and maintenance of abstract rules. J Neurophysiol 90, 3419–3428.

Cantlon JF, Brannon EM, Carter EJ, Pelphrey KA. 2006 Functional imaging of numerical processing in adults and 4-y-old children. PLoS Biol. 4:e125.

Castelli F, Glaser DE, Butterworth B. 2006. Discrete and analogue quantity processing in the parietal lobe: a functional MRI study. Proc Natl Acad Sci USA 103, 4693–4698.

Coricelli G, Dolan RJ, Sirigu A. 2007. Brain, emotion and decision making: the paradigmatic example of regret. Trends Cogn Sci 11, 258–265.

Dehaene S, Tzourio N, Frak V, Raynaud L, Cohen L. 1996. Cerebral activations during number multiplication and comparison: a PET study. Neuropsychologia 34, 1097–1106.

Deiber MP, Honda M, Ibanez V, Sadato N, Hallett M. 1999. Mesial motor areas in self-initiated versus externally triggered movements examined with fMRI: effect of movement type and rate. J. Neurophysiol. 81:3065–77

Dinstein I, Hasson U, Rubin N, Heeger DJ. 2007. Brain areas selective for both observed and executed movements. J Neurophysiol 98, 1415–1427.

Dinstein I, Gardner JL, Jazayeri M, Heeger DJ. 2008. Executed and observed movements have different distributed representations in human aIPS. J Neurosci 8, 11231–11239.

Fridman EA, Immisch I, Hanakawa T, Bohlhalter S, Waldvogel D, Kansaku K, Wheaton L, Wu T, Hallett M. 2006. The role of the dorsal stream for gesture production. Neuroimage 29, 417–428.

Gazzola V, Keysers C. 2009. The observation and execution of actions share motor and somatosensory voxels in all tested subjects: single-subject analyses of unsmoothed fMRI data. Cereb Cortex 19, 1239–1255. Epub 19 Nov. 2008.

Hickok G.2009 The functional neuroanatomy of language. Phys Life Rev. 6:121-43.

Hikosaka O, Nakahara H, Rand MK, Sakai K, Lu X, Nakamura K, Miyachi S, Doya K.1999 Parallel neural networks for learning sequential procedures.Trends Neurosci. 22:464-71.

Hoshi E, Shima K, Tanji J. 2000. Neuronal activity in the primate prefrontal cortex in the process of motor selection based on two behavioral rules. J Neurophysiol 83, 2355–2373.

Iacoboni M. 2009. Imitation, empathy, and mirror neurons. Annu Rev Psychol 60, 653–670 (Review).

Iacoboni M, Dapretto M. 2006. The mirror neuron system and the consequences of its dysfunction. Nat Rev Neurosci 7, 942–951 (Review).

Iacoboni M, Woods RP, Brass M, Bekkering H, Mazziotta JC, Rizzolatti G. 1999. Cortical mechanisms of human imitation. Science 286, 2526–2528.

Kansaku K, Johnson A, Grillon ML, Garraux G, Sadato N, Hallett M. 2006. Neural correlates of counting of sequential sensory and motor events in the human brain. Neuroimage 31, 649–660.

Kansaku K, Carver B, Johnson A, Matsuda K, Sadato N, Hallett M. 2007. The role of the human ventral premotor cortex in counting successive stimuli. Exp Brain Res 178, 339–350.

Kerns JG. 2006. Anterior cingulate and prefrontal cortex activity in an FMRI study of trial-to-trial adjustments on the Simon task. Neuroimage 33, 399–405.

Koski L, Wohlschlager A, Bekkering H, Woods RP, Dubeau MC, Mazziotta JC, Iacoboni M. 2002. Modulation of motor and premotor activity during imitation of target-directed actions. Cereb Cortex 12, 847–855.

Koski L, Iacoboni M, Dubeau MC, Woods RP, Mazziotta JC. 2003. Modulation of cortical activity during different imitative behaviors. J Neurophysiol 89, 460–471.

Kringelbach ML. 2005. The human orbitofrontal cortex: linking reward to hedonic experience. Nat Rev Neurosci 6, 691–702.

Mainen ZF, Kepecs A. 2009. Neural representation of behavioral outcomes in the orbitofrontal cortex. Curr Opin Neurobiol 19, 84–91.

Murray EA, Bussey TJ, Wise SP. 2000 Role of prefrontal cortex in a network for arbitrary visuomotor mapping. Exp Brain Res., 133, 114-129.

Mushiake H, Inase M, Tanji J.1991 Neuronal activity in the primate premotor, supplementary, and precentral motor cortex during visually guided and internally determined sequential movements. J Neurophysiol. 66:705-18.

Nieder A, Dehaene S. 2009. Representation of number in the brain. Annu Rev Neurosci 32, 185–208 (Review).

Passingham RE, Toni I, Rushworth MF 2000 Specialisation within the prefrontal cortex: the ventral prefrontal cortex and associative learning. Exp Brain Res., 133, 103-13.

Paus T. 2001. Primate anterior cingulate cortex: where motor control, drive and cognition interface. Nat Rev Neurosci 2, 417–424 (Review).

Piazza M, Izard V, Pinel P, Le Bihan D, Dehaene S. 2004. Tuning curves for approximate numerosity in the human intraparietal sulcus. Neuron 44, 547–555.

Piazza M, Mechelli A, Price CJ, Butterworth B. 2006. Exact and approximate judgements of visual and auditory numerosity: an fMRI study. Brain Res 1106, 177–188.

Piazza M, Pinel P, Le Bihan D, Dehaene S. 2007. A magnitude code common to numerosities and number symbols in human intraparietal cortex. Neuron 53, 293–305.

Poizner H,Klima ES, Bellugi U 1990 what the hands reveal about the brain MIT press

Poldrack RA, Selco SL, Field JE, Cohen NJ. 1999 The relationship between skill learning and repetition priming: experimental and computational analyses. J Exp Psychol Learn Mem Cogn. 25, 208-235.

Prinz W. 2002. Experimental approaches to imitation, pp. 143–162 in Meltzoff AN, Prinz W (eds). The Imitative Mind. Development, Evolution and Brain Bases. Cambridge, UK: Cambridge University Press.

Ridderinkhof KR, Ullsperger M, Crone EA, Nieuwenhuis S. 2004. The role of the medial frontal cortex in cognitive control. Science 306, 443–447.

Rizzolatti G, ArbibMA.1998. Language withinour grasp. Trends Neurosci. 21:188–94

Rizzolatti G, Craighero L. 2004 The mirror-neuron system. Annu Rev Neurosci.;27:169-92.

Roland PE, Friberg L. 1985. Localization of cortical areas activated by thinking. J Neurophysiol 53, 1219–1243.

Rolls ET, Grabenhorst F. 2008. The orbitofrontal cortex and beyond: from affect to decision-making. Prog Neurobiol 86, 216–244.

Rushworth MF, Hadland KA, Paus T, Sipila PK. 2002. Role of the human medial frontal cortex in task switching: a combined fMRI and TMS study. J Neurophysiol 87, 2577–2592.

Rushworth MF, Behrens TE, Rudebeck PH, Walton ME. 2007. Contrasting roles for cingulate and orbitofrontal cortex in decisions and social behaviour. Trends Cogn Sci 11, 168–176.

Sakai K, Passingham RE. 2006. Prefrontal set activity predicts rule-specific neural processing during subsequent cognitive performance. J Neurosci 26:1211–1218.

Schultz W. 2004. Neural coding of basic reward terms of animal learning theory, game theory, microeconomics and behavioural ecology. Curr Opin Neurobiol 14, 139–147 (Review).

Seymour B, McClure SM. 2008. Anchors, scales and the relative coding of value in the brain. Curr Opin Neurobiol 18, 173–178. 1626–1633.

Shibasaki H, Sadato N, Lyshkow H, Yonekura Y, Honda M, et al. 1993. Both primary motor cortex and supplementary motor area play animportant role in complex finger movement.Brain 116:1387–98

Shima K, Tanji J.2000 Neuronal activity in the supplementary and presupplementary motor areas for temporal organization of multiple movements. J Neurophysiol. 84:2148-60.

Tanji J.2001 Sequential organization of multiple movements: involvement of cortical motor areas.Annu Rev Neurosci. 2001;24:631-51. Review.

Van Veen V, Carter CS. 2005. Separating semantic conflict and response conflict in the Stroop task: a functional MRI study. Neuroimage 27, 497–504.

Wallis JD. 2007. Orbitofrontal cortex and its contribution to decision-making.Annu Rev Neurosci 30, 31–56 (Review).

Wallis JD, Anderson KC, Miller EK. 2001. Single neurons in prefrontal cortex encode abstract rules. Nature 411, 953–956.

White IM, Wise SP. 1999. Rule-dependent neuronal activity in the prefrontal cortex. Exp Brain Res 126, 315–335.

5

Neural Cognitive Correlates of Orthographic Neighborhood Size Effect for Children During Chinese Naming

Hong-Yan Bi and Qing-Lin Li
Key Laboratory of Behavioral Science, Institute of Psychology, Chinese Academy of Sciences, Beijing, China

1. Introduction

A lot of researchers are concerned of orthographic neighborhood (N) effect (Andrews, 1989, 1992; Carreiras et al., 1997; Laxon et al., 1988; Peereman & Content, 1995; Sears et al., 2006), which can reflect how the potential word candidates with similar orthography affect the word naming task. In alphabetic writing systems, orthographic neighborhood refers to a word pool, which is consisted by changing one letter of a given word while keeping other letters unchanged (Coltheart et al., 1977). Behavioral researches with naming tasks have reported a facilitatory effect of N size (Andrews, 1989, 1992; Carreiras et al., 1997; Peereman & Content, 1995; Sears et al., 1995), which the presence of many orthographic neighbors facilities phonological retrieval of the target word, and such facilitation would be more prominent for low-frequency words (Andrews, 1989, 1992; Peereman & Content, 1995). This large N advantage is also found as orthographic distinctiveness effect in memory (Glanc & Greene, 2007; 2009). Modeling researches suggested that the facilitation of large N arises from the overlapping phonemes of their neighbors (Coltheart et al., 2001) and the feedback activations from orthographic units to feature units strengthen the phonological retrieval (Reynolds & Besner, 2002). Recently, Fiebach et al. (2007) examine the neural mechanisms of N size effect using fMRI. Their results demonstrated the interactions of lexicality and N size in mid-dorsolateral and medial prefrontal cortex, suggesting domain general processes during word recognition.

Another important lexical factor related to orthographic neighbors is neighborhood frequency (N frequency). Researchers have found that the presence of neighbors which have a higher word frequency would facilitate naming processing in French (Grainger, 1990) and Spanish (Carreiras et al., 1997), whereas no influences in English (Sears et al., 2006). One possible reason of these different results is language characteristics. As well known, Spanish and French are both of shallow orthography, and words in the same orthographic neighborhood tend to be phonological neighbors, speeding up phonological activation of the target word. In comparison, English is a kind of language with deeper orthography, in which there are some orthographic neighbors with different pronunciation with the target word, resulting in the null effect.

Chinese is known as a typical logographic writing system (Tan et al., 2001), complex visual-spatial information exits in the form of each character (Li & Kang, 1993). Chinese with a deeper orthography has no grapheme-to-phoneme correspondence (GPC), similar orthographic structures arbitrarily correspond to different phonological information. Based on the above definition of N size in alphabetic languages, there is no N in Chinese without individual letters, but over 81% Chinese characters are compound characters (Li & Kang, 1993), consisting of phonological and semantic radicals. Generally speaking, phonetic radical provides the pronunciation of the whole character, and semantic radical indicates its meaning. Bi et al. (2006) defined the neighborhood of Chinese characters as the characters with the same phonetic radical because they focused the phonological processing. For example, [璜(huang2, upholster), 簧(huang2, reed), 磺(huang2, sulfur), 横(heng2, across)] is a orthographic neighborhood with the same phonetic radical 黄(huang2, yellow). Bi et al. (2006) reported a surprising result that target characters with more neighbors would produce a slower naming latency than those with few neighbors. This result is inconsistent with the finding in alphabetic researches, the authors inferred that the large N disadvantages in Chinese naming resulted from the phonological interference of neighbors. Due to the low level of phonological consistency, there would be some different sounds in a given neighborhood. The different phonologies of neighbors would be activated to inhibit phonological retrieval of target. Recently, researchers explored the N effect in Chinese character naming in details, and the large N advantages in Chinese naming was found, the inhibitory effect in Bi et al. (2006) was accounted by the uncontrolled N frequency (Li et al., 2011), just like what found by Huang et al. (2005) that characters with higher-frequency neighbors induced an inhibitory effect in RT and elicited more N400 than those with no higher frequency neighbors (Huang et al. 2005). Li et al. (2011) argued that the presence of many neighbors with the same orthographic structure facilitates characters' recognition and phonological retrieval when there is no higher-frequency neighbors, higher-frequency neighbors with different phonologies would interfere the target word naming due to their higher level of static activation, there are more high-frequency neighbors in large neighborhoods, so, the inhibitory N effect appeared in Chinese naming. Following Neuroimaging study supported these opinions. Researchers (Li et al., 2010) found that target characters with smaller Ns elicited greater activation in left middle frontal gyrus, while those with larger Ns induced more prominent activation in right middle occipital gyrus in silent naming tasks in without- higher-frequency neighbor conditions. The authors argued that right middle occipital gyrus was associated with orthographic facilitation, which the activated visual form information of neighbors facilitated the target character recognition and further processing, left middle frontal gyrus reflected the difficulty of mapping visual forms to phonemes, the target character from smaller neighborhood needed more involving of this area to search information for such mapping. In addition, the authors also revealed a main effect of N frequency, which target characters with higher-frequency neighbors induced more activation in bilateral inferior frontal gyrus suggesting phonological competition and the inhibition of wrong information.

For the development of N size effect in alphabetic languages, only a few researches consistently showed that such N effect exited in English (Laxon et al., 1988) and Spanish (Dunabeitia & Vidal-Abarca, 2008) beginning readers, but for Chinese children, the cognitive characteristics and neural basis of N effect were still not explored.

The purposes of this research were two, one was to examine whether there is N size effect in Chinese children reading just like findings in alphabetic languages, and if it exists, whether N size effect in Chinese children reading is the same as what found in Chinese adults reading (Li, et al., 2011); the other was to explore the neural basis responsible for N size effect in Chinese children reading.

2. Behavioral study

2.1 Materials and methods

2.1.1 Participants

Forty students of grade 3 from Beijing normal primary schools (mean age=9.5, range: 9.2-9.9, n=20 males) participated in this study. All the children are native Chinese speakers with normal or corrected normal vision, right-handed.

2.1.2 Stimuli

There were 34 characters, 17 characters were for large neighborhood size and 17 characters for small neighborhood size. Following Bi et al. (2006), the orthographic neighbors of a character refer to the characters sharing its phonetic radical. As described in Li & Kang (1993), the characters were selected so that there were 2-7 neighbors for the small size, and 10-16 neighbors for the large size. The characters selected were just learnt by the students in the recent two years.

Following Li et al. (2011), the criteria for selection of stimuli were: All stimuli were compound characters with the structures proceeded from left to right, phonetic radicals were on the right-hand side, the phonetic radicals were single characters, no two characters shared the same phonetic radical, each had its own meaning, none of the characters were polyphones, stroke number and consistency level had no significant differences between two conditions. The information of stimuli was shown in Table 1.

According to Fang et al. (1986), the consistency level (con) was calculated from the ratio of the number of neighbors with the same pronunciation (n) and N size (con=n/N). The 'same pronunciation' refers to the same initial consonant and compound vowels, tones were not considered here. For example, in the neighborhood including the phonetic radical 及 (ji2, and), the neighbors are 圾 (ji1, garbage), 汲 (ji2, draw), 极 (ji2, pole), 笈 (ji2,book), 岌 (ji2, danger), 级 (ji2, class), 吸 (xi1, absorb), and 靸 (sa3, shoes) (N=8). There are six neighbors with the pronunciation of ji: 圾 (ji1,garbage), 汲 (ji2, draw), 极 (ji2, bally), 笈 (ji2, danger), 岌 (ji2, danger), 级 (ji2, class, n=6), so the consistency level of the pronunciation ji in this neighborhood is produced as .75 by con=n/N=6/8.

Neighborhood size					
Large			Small		
Number of neighbors	Consistency level	Stoke number	Number of neighbors	Consistency level	Stoke number
14.9	0.33	9.5	4.6	0.30	8.2

Table 1. Information of stimuli

2.2 Procedure

All the stimuli were presented by E-Prime professional 2.0 on an IBM laptop computer. The viewing distance was of 45 cm, subtending a visual angle of approximately 3°×3°. The characters were presented in a randomized order, each for 2000 ms. A fixation cross was displayed for 500 ms in the interval between the presentation of two characters. Participants were tested individually and instructed to read the characters aloud as accurately and quickly as possible to activate the voice-key. The voice-key was connected between the computer and the SRBOX to record reaction times. The character disappeared upon response, or at the end of the 2000 ms response window. The reaction times longer than 2000 ms or that the voice-key activated by other sounds were excluded from analysis.

Practice was conducted for all children before the normal study in order to make them familiar with the study. The practice contained 20 characters different from the stimuli in real experiment.

2.3 Results

The data of 9 children with error rate more than 50% in one condition were eliminated. Thus, the data from 31 participants were included for further analysis. Incorrect responses and response latencies out of the range of three standard deviations were excluded from analysis. Mean latencies for correct responses and average error rates (see Table 2) were submitted to one-way ANOVA (N size: large/small).

The analysis of reaction times revealed a significant facilitatory neighborhood size effect ($F(1, 30) = 8.25$, $p<.008$), participants responded faster to characters with large Ns than to characters with small Ns. And the analysis of error rates showed that there was less error to characters with large Ns than to characters with small Ns ($F(1, 30)=12.29$, $p<.002$).

Neighborhood size			
Large		Small	
RT(ms)/SD	ER (%)/SD	RT(ms)/SD	ER (%)/SD
712.0/123.4	3.1/1.2	739.3/117.3	4.6/1.4

Table 2. Mean reaction latencies (RT, in ms) and error rates (ER, in %) in behavioral study

2.4 Discussion

Both the results of naming time and error rate revealed a significant facilitatory N effect for participants of grade 3. The large-N advantage for participants suggested that facilitation of similar orthographic structures exited in children with early reading experience, which is consistent with the results of developmental studies in alphabetic languages (Laxon et al., 1988; Dunabeitia & Vidal-Abarca, 2008). Such results suggested that at early stage of reading, neighbors with similar orthographic structure would facilitate character recognition and phonological retrieval. That is to say, similar visual forms of characters would help naming processing for children. After re-analysis the stimulus characters, we found that there were more than 88% target characters having higher-frequency neighbors with different pronunciations in each experimental condition. In this circumstance, according to the finding from adults (Li, et al., 2011), inhibitory N size effect is expected for the reason of phonological interference from higher-frequency neighbors, but the present result is different. The interferences of higher-frequency neighbors were not found for grade-3 students. One possible reason is that the potential higher-frequency neighbors might not be learned by the participants at their age, so the pronunciation of these higher-frequency neighbors didn't affect the target character naming; Another possible reason is that these higher-frequency neighbors were not of higher frequency indeed for grade-3 children, because we judge the frequencies of characters including target words and their neighbors by the criterion of the character frequency of adults, the frequency information may not be formed due to their limited reading experience.

3. fMRI study

3.1 Materials and methods

3.1.1 Participants

Eleven students of grade 3 from a Beijing normal primary school (mean age=9.3, range: 9.1-9.4, n=7 males) were scanned, these children also participated in behavioral study. All the participants are native Chinese speakers with normal or corrected normal vision, right-handed. The study was approved by the ethics committee of the Institute of Psychology, Chinese Academy of Sciences, China. Written consent for participation was obtained from the children's parents as well as their school teachers.

3.1.2 Stimulus characteristics

The stimuli were the same as what used in behavioural study. The fMRI Procedure was the same as the paradigm in behavioral study, except that children were instructed to read the characters silently as soon as each character was presented. After fMRI scanning, participants were asked to perform a post naming test. Post-naming test was a typical naming task, the experimental set and the stimulus characters was the same as in the behavioural study. What's more, there are 20 buffer trials in this session in order to counteract practicing effect.

3.1.3 Image collection

Hemodynamic responses were acquired on a 3T Siemens Trio MR system (Siemens Trio Magnetic Resonance Imaging system, Germany). All the participants were instructed to keep still, and their heads were aligned to the center of the magnetic field.

For each participant, a high resolution, three-dimensional anatomical data set was acquired, using Siemens' magnetization-prepared rapid acquisition gradient echo (MPRAGE) sequence (Repetition time/TR=2s, 30 contiguous axial slices, 1.33 mm thick,TE= 30 ms, flip angle = 90°, 256 mm field of view). A BOLD-sensitive gradient echo-plane imaging (EPI) sequence was acquired (30 contiguous axial slices, 1.33 mm thick TR=2000 ms, TE=30 ms, matrix=64×64, 200 mm field of view).

3.1.4 Data preprocessing and statistical analyses

Data processing and statistical analyses were conducted using the AFNI software package (Cox, 1996, Cox & Hyde, 1997, http://afni.nimh.nih.gov/afni/). For each dataset of individual child, slice timing correction, motion correction and temporal filtering of functional images were performed. The magnetization-prepared rapid acquisition gradient echo anatomical scan was then normalized to the Talairach space (Talairach and Tournoux, 1988). The Talairach-aligned dataset was spatially smoothed using a 7-mm full-width half-maximum Gaussian kernel. General linear models were used for single-subject analysis with deconvolution analysis, producing the hemodynamic response function for each condition. A group mask was created to remove voxels falling outside the brain, made by multiplying masks from each participant to include only voxels with valid signals for all participants.

N size effect analysis was performed by direct comparison between the statistical images of different neighborhood size using paired t-test, uncorrected.

3.2 Results

Brain activations relative to the resting baseline are shown in Table 3 and Fig 1, revealing common network regions for children reading, including left fusiform gyrus, right middle occipital gyrus, left precentral gyrus, left inferior frontal gyrus, and left middle frontal gyrus.

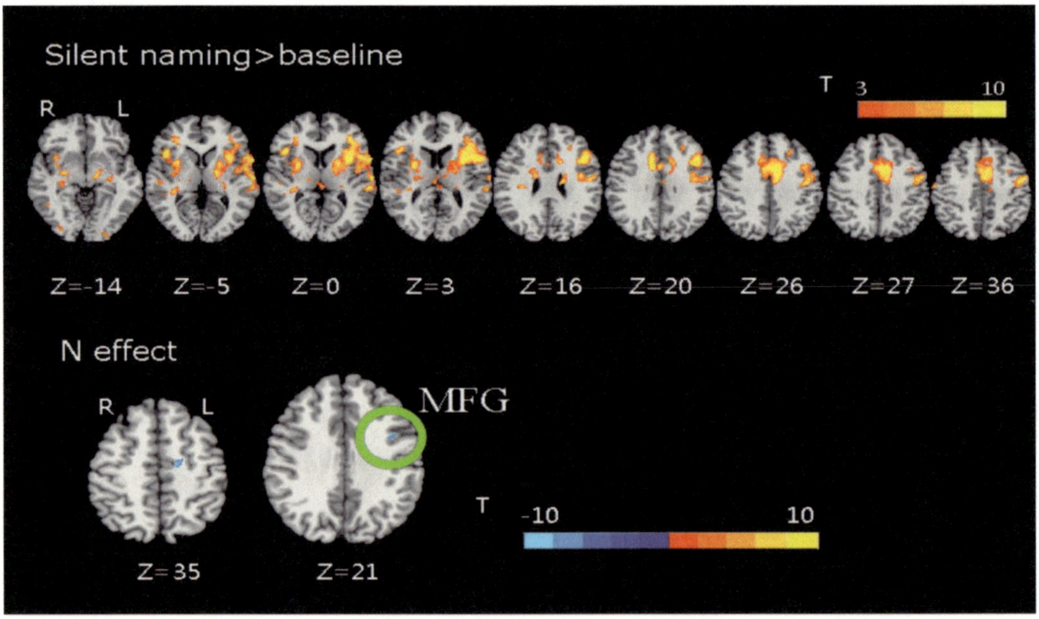

Fig. 1. Brain activations of silent naming contrast to rest baseline and ON size effect

Contrast	Brain area	X	Y	Z	Volume	t
Silent naming>baseline						
	R middle occipital gyrus/fusiform gurus	30	-78	-4	2048	6.993
	L middle occipital gyrus/fusiform gyrus	-32	-79	-8	4774	5.680
	L inferior frontal gyrus/middle frontal gyrus	-32	32	2	2829	5.542
	L precentral gyrus	-46	6	7	184	9.982
	L medial frontal gyrus	0	14	44	4800	7.417
	R precentral gyrus	31	-8	24	288	4.235
	R inferior frontal gyrus	28	21	9	757	5.153
	L inferior parietal lobule/supramaginal gyrus	27	49	39	443	4.064
	L middle temporal gyrus	-37	-53	0	278	5.531
N effect (large>small)						
	L cingulate gyrus	-14	-12	46	163	-4.954
	L middle frontal gyrus	-35	2	35	126	-4.453

Table 3. Summary information for brain activations. Note: 'Silent naming>baseline' means naming performance contrast to rest baseline, in this section the areas activated were reported, 'N effect (large>small)' refers to the contrast of targets from large neighborhoods to that from small neighborhoods. X, Y and Z are coordinates in Talairach space of the peaks. Targets from small N induced more activation on left middle frontal gyrus and left cingulate gyrus than those from large N for children. While there was no activated area accounting for large N advantage.

3.3 Discussion

The fMRI imaging results showed the neural net-works involved phonological processing in Chinese children. The activated brain areas by the contrast between silent naming and baseline include: left fusiform gyrus, right middle occipital gyrus, left precentral gyrus, left inferior frontal gyrus, and left middle frontal gyrus. These results are in line with previous imaging studies on Chinese children reading process (Bitan et al., 2007; Bookheimer et al., 1995; Booth et al., 2002; Booth et al., 2006; Cao et al., 2009; Herbster et al., 1997).

Children showed significant activation in left middle frontal gyrus for characters with small Ns than for characters with large Ns, and this result is similar with adults' in Li et al. (2010). Left middle frontal gyrus are reported highly involved in Chinese reading (Booth et al., 2006; Chee et al., 2004; Kuo et al., 2004; Perfetti et al., 2005; Tan et al., 2005; Tan et al., 2001; Tan et al., 2003). Other previous research (Li et al., 2010) revealed that left middle frontal gyrus was partially responsible for the facilitation of large ON, more activity in this area reflected more difficulty in integrating orthography to phonology. Present results suggested that children with early reading experience could already take advantages from orthographic neighbors as adults did.

In present study, we didn't found greater activation for large-neighborhood characters compared with small-neighborhood characters in left inferior frontal gyrus and right inferior frontal gyrus. These two areas were reported to be related to higher-frequency neighbors in the previous study (Li et al., 2010). That is, the greater activation in bilateral inferior frontal gyrus reflected the automatic phonological activation of higher-frequency neighbor and the inhibition of uncorrected sound. As mentioned above, more than 88% target characters had higher-frequency neighbors. However, we didn't found the effect of higher-frequency neighbors as adults, and this result was supported by the findings in the first behavioral experiment. So, it is understandable that the neural networks for the effect of higher-frequency neighbors haven't formed.

Till now, we can conclude that the grade-3 children can be facilitated by the similar orthographic forms in character reading, but not be influenced by the frequency information of orthographic neighbors.

We have strong desire to determine the precise time of activation among different regions and the relationship relative to different brain areas during N effect for children, however, due to the low temporal resolution of fMRI, the BOLD signal peaks about 5s after neuronal firing, it is difficult to interpret the effects in different locations of brain in real-time.

4. Acknowledgements

This research was funded by the National Science Foundation of China (30770726, 30970910).

5. References

Andrews, S. (1989). Frequency and neighborhood effects on lexical access: activation or search? *Journal of Experimental Psychology: Learning, Memory, and Cognition*, 15, 5, pp. 802-814, ISSN 0278-7393.

Andrews, S. (1992). Frequency and neighborhood effects on lexical access: lexical similarity or orthographic redundancy? *Journal of Experimental Psychology: Learning, Memory, and Cognition*, 18, 2, pp. 234-254, ISSN 0278-7393.

Bi, H.Y., Hu, W. & Weng, X.C. (2006). Orthographic neighborhood effects in the prounciation of Chinese words (in Chinese). *Acta Psychologica Sinica*, 38, 6, pp. 791-797, ISSN 0439-755X.

Bitan, T., Cheon, J., Lu, D., Burman, D.D., Gitelman, D.R., Mesulam, M.M. & Booth, J.R. (2007). Developmental changes in activation and effective connectivity in phonological processing. *NeuroImage*, 38, 3, pp. 564-575, ISSN 1053-8119.

Bookheimer, S.Y., Zeffiro, T.A., Blaxton, T., Gaillard, W. & Theodore, W. (1995). Regional cerebral blood flow during object naming and word reading. *Human Brain Mapping*, 3, 2, pp. 93-106, ISSN 1065-9471.

Booth, J.R., Lu, D., Burman, D.D., Chou, T.L., Jin, Z., Peng, D.L., Zhang, L., Ding, G.S., Deng, Y. & Liu, L. (2006). Specialization of phonological and semantic processing in Chinese word reading. *Brain Research*, 1071, 1, pp. 197-207, ISSN 0006-8993.

Booth, J.R., Burman, D.D., Meyer, J.R., Gitelman, D.R., Parrish, T.B. & Mesulam, M.M. (2002). Functional anatomy of intra- and cross-modal lexical tasks. *NeuroImage*, 16, 1, pp. 7-22., ISSN 1053-8119

Cao, F., Peng, D., Liu, L., Jin, Z., Fan, N., Deng, Y. & Booth, J.R. (2009). Developmental differences of neurocognitive networks for phonological and semantic processing in Chinese word reading. *Human Brain Mapping*, 30, 3, pp. 797-809, ISSN 1065-9471.

Carreiras, M., Perea, M. & Grainger, J. (1997). Effects of orthographic neighborhood in visual word recognition: cross-task comparisons. *Journal of Experimental Psychology: Learning Memory and Cognition*, 23, 4, pp. 857-871, ISSN 0278-7393.

Chee, M. W., Soon, C. S., Lee, H. L. & Pallier, C. (2004). Left insula activation: a marker for language attainment in bilinguals. *Proceedings of the National Academy of Sciences of the United States of America*, 101, 42, pp. 15265-15270, ISSN 0027-8424.

Coltheart, M., Davelaar, E., Jonasson, J.T. & Besner, D. (1977). Access to the internal lexicon. In: *Attention and performance VI*, S. Dornic, (Ed.), 535-555. Erlbaum, ISBN 0-470-99120-8, Hillsdale, USA.

Coltheart, M., Rastle, K., Perry, C., Langdon, R. & Ziegler, J. (2001). DRC : A Dual Route Cascaded Model of visual word recognition and reading aloud. *Psychological Review*, 108, 1, pp. 204-256, ISSN 0033-295X.

Dunabeitia, J.A. & Vidal-Abarca, E. (2008). Children like dense neighborhoods: Orthographic neighborhood density effects in novel readers. *The Spanish Journal of Psychology*, 11, 1, pp. 26-35, ISSN 1138-7416.

Fiebach, C. J., Ricker, B., Friederici, A. D. & Jacobs, A. M. (2007). Inhibition facilitation in visual word recognition: Prefrontal contribution to the orthographic neighborhood size effect. *NeuroImage*, 36, pp. 901-911, ISSN 1053-8119.

Fang, S.P., Horng, R.Y. & Tzeng, O.J.L. (1986). Consistency effects in the Chinese character and pseudo-character naming tasks. In: *Linguistics, Psychology, and the Chinese Language*, H. S. R. Kao, & R. Hoosain (Eds.), 11−21, Hong Kong: Centre of Asian Studies, ISBN 962-7103-01-2, Hong Kong, China.

Glanc, G. A., Greene, R. L. (2007). Orthographic neighborhood size effects in recognition memory. *Mem Cognit*, 35(2):365-71.

Glanc, G. A., Greene, R. L. (2009). Orthographic neighborhood size effects and associative recognition. *Am J Psychol*,122(1):53-61.

Grainger, J. (1990). Word frequency and neighborhood frequency effects in lexical decision and naming. *Journal of Memory and Language*, 29, 2, pp. 228-244, ISSN 0749-596X.

Herbster, A. N., Mintun, M. A., Nebes, R. D. & Becker, J. T. (1997). Regional cerebral blood flow during word and nonword reading. *Human Brain Mapping*, 5, 2, pp. 84-92, ISSN 1065-9471.

Huang, H. -W., Lee, C. -Y., Lee, C. -L., Tsai, J. - L., Hung, D. L., & Tzeng, O. J. -L. (2005). An Electrophysiological study of the orthographic neighborhood frequency effect in Chinese word recognition. The 12th annual meeting of Cognitive Neuroscience Society (CNS), New York, USA.

Kuo, W.J., Yeh, T.C., Lee, J.R., Chen, L.F., Lee, P.L., Chen, S.S., Ho, L.T., Hung, D.L., Ovid Tzeng, J.L. & Hsieh, J.C. (2004). Orthographic and phonological processing of

Chinese characters: an fMRI study. *NeuroImage*, 21, 4, pp. 1721-1731, ISSN 1053-8119.

Laxon, V.J., Coltheart, V. & Keating, C. (1988). Children find friendly words friendly too: Words with many orthographic neighbours are easier to read and spell. *British Journal of Educational Psychology*. 58, 1, pp. 103-119, ISSN 0007-0998.

Li, Q.L., Bi, H.Y., Wei, T.Q. & Chen, B.G. (2011). Orthographic neighborhood size effect in Chinese character naming: Orthographic and phonological activations. *Acta Psychologica*, 136, pp. 35-41, ISSN 0001-6918.

Li, Q.L., Bi, H.Y. & Zhang, J.X. (2010). Neural correlates of the orthographic neighborhood size effect in Chinese. *European journal of Neuroscience*, 32, pp. 866-872, ISSN 1460-9568.

Li, Y. & Kang, J.S. (1993). The research on phonetic-radical of modern Chinese phonetic-semantic compound. In: Information Analysis of Modern Chinese Characters (in Chinese), Y. Chen, (Ed.), 5-294. Shanghai Education Publishing House, ISBN 7-5320-3138-1, Shanghai, China.

Peereman, R. & Content, A. (1995). Neighborhood size effect in naming: lexical activation or sublexical correspondences? Journal of Experimental Psychology: Learning, Memory, and Cognition, 21, 2, pp. 409-421, ISSN 0278-7393.

Perfetti, C.A., Liu, Y. & Tan, L.H. (2005). The lexical constituency model: some implications of research on Chinese for general theories of reading. *Psychological Review*, 112, 1, pp. 43-59, ISSN 0033-295X.

Reynolds, M. & Besner, D. (2002). Neighbourhood density effects in reading aloud: new insights from simulations with the DRC model. *Canadian Journal of Experimental Psychology*, 56, 4, pp. 310-318, ISSN 1196-1961.

Sears, C.R., Campbell, C.R. & Lupker, S.J. (2006). Is there a neighborhood frequency effect in English? evidence from reading and lexical decision. *Journal of Experimental Psychology: Human Perception and Performance*, 32, 4, pp. 1040-1062, ISSN 0096-1523.

Sears, C.R., Hino, Y. & Lupker, S.J. (1995). Neighborhood size and neighborhood frequency effects in word recognition. *Journal of Experimental Psychology: Human Perception and Performance*, 21, 4, pp. 876-900, ISSN 0096-1523.

Talairach, J. & Tournoux, P. (1988). Co-Planar Stereptaxic Atlas of the Human Brain. Georg Thieme Verlag, ISBN-10: 0865772932, Stuttgart. Germany

Tan, L.H., Laird, A.R., Li, K. & Fox, P.T. (2005). Neuroanatomical correlates of phonological processing of Chinese characters and alphabetic words: a meta-analysis. *Human Brain Mapping*, 25, 1, pp. 83-91, ISSN 1065-9471.

Tan, L.H., Liu, H.L., Perfetti, C.A., Spinks, J.A., Fox, P.T. & Gao, J.H. (2001). The neural system underlying Chinese logograph reading. *NeuroImage*, 13, 5, pp. 836-846, ISSN 1053-8119.

Tan, L.H., Spinks, J.A., Feng, C.M., Siok, W.T., Perfetti, C.A., Xiong, J., Fox, P.T. & Gao, J.H. (2003). Neural systems of second language reading are shaped by native language. *Human Brain Mapping*, 18, 3, pp. 158-166, ISSN 1065-9471.

6

Brain Plasticity Induced by Constraint-Induced Movement Therapy: Relationship of fMRI and Movement Characteristics

Urška Puh
University of Ljubljana, Faculty of Health Sciences
Slovenia

1. Introduction

Following stroke, the disturbed motor control results in subsequent movement disorders. Recovery means gradual returning of the specific function, after a deficit caused by a central nervous system damage (Held, 2000). The recovery of upper extremity movement following a stroke is generally poor. Three months after stroke its function remains totally or partially impaired in as much as 80 % of stroke survivors (Parker et al., 1986). Basmajian et al. (1982) reported that only 5% of stroke patients regained a total function of the upper extremity, and in 20% it remained totally non-functional. Majority of the reports indicated that in patients with initially markedly impaired upper extremity function, the recovery is minimal (Basmajian et al., 1982; Wade et al., 1983; Nakayama et al., 1994). In this group, a useful function of the upper extremity was regained in only 15% (Parker et al., 1986) or 18% of patients (Nakayama et al., 1994). It seems, however, that patients with initially partially impaired upper extremity function have a good potential for recovery. In this group, total recovery was reported in as much as 79% of patients (Nakayama et al., 1994).

Although there is evidence from the animal models that at least some of the recovery can be attributed to brain reorganization, the mechanisms of motor recovery after stroke in humans are not clear yet. During the first three to four weeks after stroke a combination of the brain spontaneous recovery processes (oedema and necrotic tissue absorption, collateral blood flow activation), and reorganisation of the neural mechanisms, the so called plasticity (unmasking of unused neuronal pathways, dendritic branching, synaptogenesis) influence the recovery. Later, only plasticity occurs (Lee & van Donkleaar, 1995). To understand the recovery after stroke in humans, a great number of functional imaging studies, using positron emission tomography (PET) and functional magnetic resonance imaging (fMRI) have been conducted. In general, a greater activation of the motor-related brain regions is reported during stroke-affected upper extremity motor tasks as compared to healthy subjects. Additionally, an increased recruitment of non-motor areas is shown consistently. In the 1st to 6th week after stroke, the activation was moved to the *contralesional* hemisphere. In the 3rd to 12th month after stroke the activation moved back to the *ipsilesional* hemisphere, which was concomitant with motor recovery, or stayed in the contralesional hemisphere (for review see: Calautti & Baron, 2003; Baron et al., 2004; Schaechter, 2004). The functional role of the ipsilateral activation was, however, under debate both in healthy subjects (Salmelin et al., 1995; Kawashima et al., 1998) and patients after stroke (Chollet et al., 1991; Turton et al., 1996; Netz et al., 1997; Marshall et al., 2000) without a clear answer.

Better understanding of the neurophysiological processes underlying brain reorganization and concomitant studying of the effects of the therapeutic techniques which were established to stimulate the brain plasticity may increase their effectiveness and thus improve the outcome of rehabilitation in patients after stroke.

2. Treatment-induced recovery of brain function and movement

It is not known yet if differences in the motor cortex areas between individuals are consequences of inherited genetic differences or of different experiences. It seems that the competition between the neurons for synaptic connections depends on their use. Sensory and motor areas of the brain cortex are constantly changing, depending on the amount of their activation through periphery inputs, environment, motor tasks, experiences, etc. (Jenkins et al., 1990; Shumway-Cook & Woollacott, 2007). In monkeys, a new learned task induced certain long-effecting changes in motor cortex areas (Jenkins et al., 1990; Nudo et al., 1996). However, attention should be paid to the fact that plastic changes can also be negative. Immobilisation of the two fingers, for example, obliterated the boundaries between the areas for an individual finger (Clark et al., 1988). Some reorganisation (adaptation) of the brain cortex always occurs after a stroke. It is assumed, however, that reorganisation can be affected with the experiences or sensory inputs and motor reactions, which are demanded after the lesion, especially in the process of rehabilitation (Carr & Shepherd, 2000). On the other hand, several weeks of inactivity would have a consequence in reorganisation of the brain cortex reflecting non-use (Shumway-Cook & Woollacott, 2007). The possibilities for functional recovery exist, but the methods and mechanisms of how to affect these processes need to be discovered (Lee & van Donkleaar, 1995).

Some authors speculated that there is a certain period of time, in which plastic changes of the brain after stroke can be influenced by therapeutic interventions (Lee & van Donkleaar, 1995). Mainly as a consequence of the brain spontaneous recovery (Hallett, 2001), the greatest possibility for the upper extremity movement recovery is during the first month (Kwakkel et al., 2003) or the first three months after stroke (Nakayama et al., 1994; Parker et al., 1986; Wade et al., 1983). However, after this period a recovery is not complete. The evidence of significant movement recovery in patients involved in constraint-induced movement therapy (CIMT), more than one year (to 20 years) after a stroke exist (Kunkel et al., 1999; Sterr et al., 2002; Taub et al., 2006; Wolf at al., 1989). This evidence was the main proof that neuroplastic changes induced by physiotherapy are possible in the chronic stage after stroke (Blanton et al., 2008). In spite of the assumptions that movement training can have a positive effect regardless of the time period in which a patient received it, because the brain is plastic throughout the whole life (Shumway-Cook & Woollacott, 2007) and the evidence on no time limit for recovery, the first three to six months after stroke seem to be the most important (European Stroke Initiative [EUSI], 2003). It should be emphasised, however, that studies, which reported better recovery included stroke patients involved in an active and task-related training (Buterfisch et al., 1995; Dean & Mackey, 1992; Mudie & Matyas, 1996), for which at least partial ability of the upper extremity function is required.

The examples of therapeutic techniques which have been established to promote recovery of the upper extremity movement through facilitating the brain plasticity in different ways are CIMT, bimanual training, and mirror therapy. They are supplementing or emphasising the concept of task-related training. A tendency of greater upper extremity movement recovery and greater sensory-motor cortex activation of the ipsilesional hemisphere were reported in a group of stroke patients included in the intensive task-related training (Nelles et al., 2001) or bimanual training (Luft et al., 2004) in comparison to the groups receiving conventional rehabilitation. Similar positive effects were reported in other studies investigating task-related training (Carey et al., 2002; Jang et al., 2003) and CIMT (see section 2.1.1). In general, results of all these studies show positive relationship between the ipsilesional hemisphere cortex activation and greater motor recovery, although the return of the activity back to the ipsilesional hemisphere did not occur in all subjects.

2.1 Constraint-induced movement therapy

Deficiency of the majority of therapeutic approaches which facilitate the normal movement is an insufficient amount of the affected upper extremity use in comparison to the unaffected extremity use during the whole day. CIMT is an additional therapeutic technique that is performed for a short period of time, most frequently for two weeks. The aim of CIMT is to prevent or reduce a learned non-use of the affected upper extremity (Van der Lee, 2001) which is frequently developed in patients after stroke. CIMT implies the forced use and the massed practice of the affected upper extremity. It is based on the following two principles: (1) from six to eight hours of restraining the use of the unaffected upper extremity (with a splint, sling or mitten) and thus forcing the use of the affected upper extremity during intensive training and activities of daily living; and (2) intensive massed practice - more than three hours of task-related training with the affected upper extremity. Therefore different therapeutic concepts can be used, including shaping, motor re-learning, and proprioceptive neuromuscular facilitation. Modified versions of CIMT (mCIMT) with shorter restraining (i.e. 5-6 hours) and training periods (3 hours or less) per day and longer treatment periods (i.e. 4 or 10 weeks) were also developed. Through proper and sufficient feedback information, CIMT contributes to a motor learning and thus through facilitation of the brain plasticity influences the affected upper extremity movement recovery.

CIMT is currently experimentally and clinically the most established therapeutic technique for facilitating the movement recovery following stroke (Blanton et al., 2008). Meta-analyses of the currently available randomized clinical trials (RCTs) show that CIMT has a significant effect on increasing upper extremity (arm) function (Langhorne et al., 2009; van Peppen et al., 2004), and has a moderate effect on increasing performance of the activities of daily living immediately following treatment (Sirtori et al., 2009). However, its effects on increasing hand function (Langhorne et al., 2009) were found to be inconsistent, and there was not enough evidence on the long-term effects (Sirtori et al., 2009). The existing evidence suggests that CIMT is a promising intervention for upper extremity function in patients after stroke (Langhorne et al., 2009). The optimal dose of constraint and practice needs further investigation. The identification of integrated approaches combining CIMT and other techniques which facilitate the brain plasticity is a direction for future research.

2.1.1 Studying the effects of CIMT using fMRI

Since CIMT is relatively well defined and more easily administered than longer duration treatment protocols, it seems to be a more practicable way of studying plasticity. The number of brain imaging studies investigating its effect on brain plasticity, including fMRI studies, has emerged since 2001 when the first fMRI study was conducted (Levy et al., 2001). In the first review paper, Mark et al. (2006) concluded that CIMT has been repeatedly associated with significant plastic brain changes in a variety of studies using fMRI and other brain imaging techniques. However, the authors emphasised several uncertainties /unanswered questions. Later, several studies of the effects of CIMT with fMRI were published.

Observations of the 16 currently published studies investigating the effects of CIMT on brain activity using fMRI are summarized in Tables 1 and 2. In three of these studies transcranial magnetic stimulation (TMS) was also performed (Liepert et al., 2004; Hamzei et al., 2006, 2008). The effects of the original form of CIMT (duration two weeks) were investigated in 11 studies (Azpiroz et al., 2005; Butler & Page, 2006; Dong et al., 2006, 2007; Hamzei et al., 2006; Kim et al., 2004; Langan & van Donkelaar, 2008; Levy et al., 2001; Liepert et al., 2004; Schaechter et al., 2002; Sheng & Lin, 2009). In other studies, different types of mCIMT were investigated, varied from three (Lin et al., 2010; Wu et al., 2010) to ten (Szaflarski et al., 2006) weeks of treatment duration. An important deficiency of the majority of the previous studies is the absence of a control group. A control was included only in three studies of the effects of CIMT in patients after stroke using TMS (Grotta et al., 2004; Liepert et al., 2001; Wittenberg et al., 2003) and PET (Wittenberg et al., 2003), and in three studies using fMRI (Table 2). Butler & Page (2006) investigated the effects of CIMT, mental practice, and combination of both in four patients altogether. Later, two RCTs were conducted, comparing the effects of mCIMT with a bilateral training (Wu et al., 2010) and traditional rehabilitation (Lin et al., 2010), respectively.

In the 16 studies with fMRI (Tables 1 and 2), only 72 subjects after stroke who participated in CIMT or its modifications (mean: 4.6 subject per study) and 13 subjects after stroke who participated in the control groups were included. Altogether, male subjects were included in 74.2 % (16 females and 46 males). However, in four studies the subjects' gender was not reported (Dong et al., 2006; Kim et al., 2004; Langan & van Donkelaar, 2008; Liepert et al., 2004). The age of all included subjects after stroke varied from 23 (Azpiroz at al., 2005) to 80 years (Hamzei et al., 2006), with a greatest range of 51 years in the study of Langan & van Donkleaar (2008). However, the age was not reported in two studies (Butler & Page, 2006; Liepert et al., 2004).

In majority of the studies, only patients with right-hand dominance before a stroke appearance were included (Azpiroz et al., 2005; Dong et al., 2007; Hamzei et al., 2006, 2008; Langan & van Donkelaar, 2008; Lin et al., 2010; Schaechter et al., 2002), with the exception of the first two studies (Levy et al., 2001; Johansen-Berg et al., 2002) wherein each one patient with left-hand dominance was included. However, in many studies this subjects' characteristic was not reported (Butler & Page, 2006; Dong et al., 2006; Kim et al., 2004; Liepert et al., 2004; Sheng & Lin, 2009; Szaflarski et al., 2006; Wu et al., 2010).

It is assumed that in majority of the studies, patients after first stroke were included. Although this was specified by few authors only (Dong et al., 2007; Hamzei et al., 2006, 2008;

Johansen-Berg et al., 2002; Schaechter et al., 2002), but Langan & van Donkelaar (2008) included one patient with a second stroke. Patients with ischemic (Dong et al., 2007; Hamzei et al., 2006, 2008; Johansen-Berg et al., 2002; Schaechter et al., 2002) and hemorrhagic types of stroke (Azpiroz et al., 2005; Butler & Page, 2006; Dong et al., 2007; Levy et al., 2001; Wu et al., 2010) were included. However, many authors did not specify the type and/or event of stroke (Butler & Page, 2006; Dong et al., 2006; Kim et al., 2004; Langan & van Donkelaar, 2008; Liepert et al., 2004; Lin et al., 2010; Sheng & Lin, 2009; Szaflarski et al., 2006; Wu et al., 2010).

Study	CIMT type/ duration (weeks)	N	Gender	Age (years)	Time after stroke	Affected body side
Levy et al., 2001	CIMT / 2	2	1 F, 1 M	48, 49	4,5 & 9 months	2 L
Johansen-Berg et al., 2002	mCIMT / 2	7	2 F, 5 M	44-61	6 months – 7 years	4 R, 3 L
Schaechter et al., 2002	CIMT / 2	4	1 F, 3 M	36-77	7-20 months	3 R, 1 L
Kim et al., 2004	CIMT / 2	4	Not reported	43-64	9-38 months	2 R, 2 L
Liepert et al., 2004	CIMT /2	3	Not reported	Not reported	6 months <	Not reported
Azpiroz et al., 2005	CIMT / 4	3	1 F, 2 M	23-66	48-72 months	3 L
Dong et al., 2006	CIMT / 2	8	Not reported	66±9	3 months <	Not reported
Hamzei et al., 2006	CIMT / 2	6	1 F, 5 M	63-80	1.5-10 years	6 L
Szaflarski et al., 2006	mCIMT / 10	4	2 F, 2 M	54-68	22-178 months	3 R, 1 L
Dong et al., 2007	CIMT / 2	4	1 F, 3 M	25-57	3 months <	3 R, 1 L
Hamzei et al., 2008	mCIMT / 4	8	3 F, 5 M	38-69	2-6 years	Not reported
Langan & van Donkelaar, 2008	CIMT / 2	8	Not reported	25-76	6 months <	4 R, 4 L
Sheng & Lin, 2009	CIMT / 2	1	1 M	71	4 months	1 L

Table 1. Treatment and subjects' characteristics in the studies investigating the effects of constraint-induced movement therapy (CIMT) and its modifications (mCIMT) using the functional magnetic resonance imaging in patients after stroke without a control group. Legends are shown as: N, number of subjects; F, females; M, males; L, left-side hemiparesis; R, right-side hemiparesis.

Time after stroke at inclusion to the study varied from more than three months (Butler & Page, 2006; Dong et al., 2006, 2007; Sheng & Lin, 2009), more than six months (Johansen-Berg et al., 2002; Langan & van Donkelaar; 2008 Liepert et al., 2004), to more than a year (Azpiroz et al., 2005; Hamzei et al., 2006, 2008; Szaflarski et al., 2006). In many cases patients from various stages of recovery after stroke were included to the same study (Butler & Page, 2006; Johansen-Berg et al., 2002; Kim et al., 2004; Levy et al., 2001; Schaechter et al., 2002; Wu et al., 2010).

Study	Experimental group (N) / CIMT type	Control group (N) / treatment	Duration (weeks)	Gender	Age (years)	Time after stroke	Affected body side
Butler & Page, 2006	3 = 1 CIMT + 2 CIMT & mental practice	1 / mental practice	2	1 F, 3 M	Not reported	3-16 months	Not reported
Lin et al., 2010	5 / mCIMT	8 / traditional rehabilitation	3	2 F, 11 M	average: 49	average: 18.3 months	6 R, 7 L
Wu et al., 2010	2 / mCIMT	4 / bilateral training	3	1 F, 5 M	45-68	9-40 months	4 R, 2 L

Table 2. Treatment and subjects' characteristics in the studies investigating the effects of constraint-induced movement therapy (CIMT) and its modifications (mCIMT) using the functional magnetic resonance imaging in patients after stroke, including control group/subject. Legends are shown as: N, number of subjects after stroke; F, females; M, males; L, left-side hemiparesis; R, right-side hemiparesis.

In four studies, only subjects with left-side hemiparesis were included (Azpiroz et al., 2005; Hamzei et al., 2006; Levy et al., 2001; Sheng & Lin, 2009). In others, subjects with right- and left-side hemiparesis were included (Dong et al., 2007; Johansen-Berg et al., 2002; Kim et al., 2004; Langan & van Donkelaar, 2008; Lin et al., 2010; Schaechter et al., 2002; Szaflarski et al., 2006; Wu et al., 2010), giving the common ratio of subjects with the left-side hemiparesis 53.2 % (right-side: 29; left-side: 33). In four studies this probably important subjects' characteristic was not reported (Butler & Page, 2006; Dong et al., 2006; Hamzei et al., 2008; Liepert et al., 2004). Langan & van Donkelaar (2008), however investigated the differences in recovery between the patients with right and left-side hemiparesis, and reported no significant difference in the brain cortex activations and results of the clinical motor function tests/measures between the two groups in their responses to CIMT.

The most commonly performed movement tasks during fMRI were different kinds of active finger flexion-extension or finger-tapping tasks (Azpiroz et al., 2005; Buler & Page, 2006; Dong et al., 2007; Johansen-Berg et al., 2002; Levy et al., 2001; Lin et al., 2010; Schaechter et al., 2002; Sheng & Lin, 2009; Szaflarski et al., 2006; Wu et al., 2010). Other active tasks included finger-thumb opposition without (Kim et al., 2004) or with compression (Dong et al., 2006), and making a fist/power grip without (Kim et al., 2004) or with compression (Langan & van Donklear, 2008). Some authors in the CIMT studies (Hamze et al., 2006, 2008; Liepert et al., 2004) performed passive wrist joint flexion-extension movement, and other studies (Buler & Page, 2006) also imagined finger flexion-extension task. It has been shown, however, that in patients after stroke the brain cortex activation may differ between simple and complex motor tasks (Puh et al., 2007).

In four studies, fMRI was performed also on healthy subjects. The aim of those studies was to test the reproducibility of fMRI activation (Dong et al., 2006) or to provide data regarding typical activation patterns in response to the movement task performed during fMRI (Dong et al., 2007; Schaechter et al., 2002; Szaflarski et al., 2006). Schaechter et al. (2002) reported similar activation pattern in either hand of healthy subjects and of the unaffected hand of stroke patients. The activation was predominantly in the contralateral/contralesional hemisphere (primary motor cortex (M1), pre-motor cortex (PMC), supplementary motor area (SMA), and somatosensory cortex) and ipsilateral cerebellum; more modest and variable activation was reported for the ipsilateral/ipsilesional brain hemisphere. Before initiating CIMT, the affected hand movement resulted in activation in the same brain regions, although activation in the ipsilesional hemisphere was typically increased (Schaechter et al., 2002). In comparison to healthy subjects, Dong et al. (2007) reported higher activation in the ipsilesional M1 during performance with the affected hand before and after CIMT.

For the affected hand movement during fMRI the results of all studies investigating the effects of CIMT or mCIMT have shown varied patterns of cortical reorganisation after treatment (Table 3). Increased activations in the ipsilesional (Berg et al., 2002; Dong et al., 2007; Hamzei et al., 2006; Johansen-Berg et al., 2002; Kim et al., 2004; Levy et al., 2001; Szaflarski et al., 2006), the contralesional (Kim et al., 2004; Lin et al., 2010; Schaechter et al., 2002; Szaflarski et al., 2006) or in both hemispheres (Azpiroz et al., 2005; Butler & Page, 2006; Levy et al., 2001; Sheng & Lin, 2009; Wu et al., 2010) were reported after treatment. On the contrary, in some studies decreased activation in either hemisphere (Azpiroz et al., 2005; Dong et al., 2006; Kim et al., 2004; Liepert et al., 2004; Schaechter et al., 2002; Szaflarski et al., 2006) was reported after treatment. Some authors (Dong et al., 2006, 2007; Levy et al., 2001; Lin et al., 2010; Schaechter et al., 2002; Wu et al., 2010) calculated the laterality index between the hemispheres, but its changes are also inconsistent (Table 3). In many studies the hemispheric changes and/or changes in cortical regions were not consistent across subjects (Azpiroz et al., 2005; Butler & Page, 2006; Dong et al., 2007; Hamzei et al., 2006; Kim et al., 2004; Langan & van Donkelaar, 2008; Levy et al., 2001; Schaechter et al., 2002; Szaflarski et al. 2006).

In parallel with the decreased activation in the ipsilesional sensori-motor cortex (SM1) after CIMT, Liepert et al. (2004) reported decreased inhibition of the affected hand (measured using TMS). In the following studies (Hamzei et al., 2006, 2008) the effect of the cortico-spinal tract integrity on increase or decrease of SM1 activation after CIMT was established. Stroke lesions in M1 or its cortico-spinal tract have been shown to have consequences in increased ipsilesional SM1 activation, and were accompanied by decreased intracortical excitability; and lesions outside M1 or the cortico-spinal tract had consequences in decreased ipsilesional SM1 activation which was parallel with an increase in intracortical excitability (Hamzei et al., 2006, 2008).

During CIMT procedure, one hand (the affected) is forced to be used and movement of the other hand (the unaffected) is constrained, therefore brain plasticity would be expected during performance of each hand. However, the brain cortex activation during movement of the unaffected hand was analysed only in some studies, in which different, sometimes opposite findings were reported (Dong et al., 2006; Johansen-Berg et al., 2002; Langan & van Donkelaar 2008; Szaflarski et al., 2006). After CIMT, for example, Langan & van Donkelaar (2008) reported significant changes in the total cortex activation for performance with the affected hand, and no changes for performance with the unaffected hand. For the unaffected hand Dong et al. (2006) also reported no difference in M1 activation across time. For one subject after CIMT, Sheng & Lin (2009) reported differences in the brain cortex activation during movement of the affected (see Table 3), but also during movement of the unaffected hand (decreased activation in the ipsilesional SM1). In the RCT by Lin et al. (2010) following mCIMT, activation in the contralesional hemisphere during movement of the affected (see Table 3) and unaffected hand (SM1) increased significantly. For the control group receiving traditional rehabilitation, a decrease in SM1 cortex activation of the ipsilesional hemisphere during movement of the affected hand, and no changes of the laterality indexes were reported (Lin et al., 2010). In the RCT by Wu et al. (2010), the total activation of each hemisphere during the affected and unaffected hand movement increased after treatment in both, mCIMT and bilateral training groups. During the affected hand movement in the mCIMT group, the laterality index decreased, but in the bilateral group it increased after treatment. For the unaffected hand movement, changes in laterality index were opposite (Wu et al., 2010).

In some studies, the activation in cerebellum was investigated. During the performance of the affected and the unaffected hand, an increased activation in the cerebellar hemispheres bilaterally was reported after CIMT (Johansen-Berg et al., 2002). During bilateral elbow movement, both CIMT patients showed decreased cerebellar activation, whereas three out of four bilateral training patients showed increased bilateral cerebellum activation after treatment (Wu et al., 2010)

Besides the measurements before and after CIMT performed in all 16 studies (Table 3), in some studies measurements were conducted in other periods. Langan & van Donkelaar (2008) performed double baseline measurements (2-3 weeks and 4 days before the start of CIMT). Dong et al. (2006) investigated the brain cortex activation in the middle of the two-week CIMT. For the performance with the affected hand the authors reported four patterns of laterality index evolution for M1 across time (n = 8). The long-term effects on the brain cortex activation after CIMT were investigated only in the three studies (Dong et al., 2007; Schaechter et al. 2002; Sheng & Lin, 2009). Two weeks after CIMT, a decrease of extensive cortex activation of each hemisphere and focus to the ipsilesional cortex during the affected hand movement was reported for one patient (Sheng & Lin, 2009). For the affected hand performance, Schaechter et al. (2002) reported a persistent trend toward a reduced laterality index at six months after CIMT, with differences on an individual basis. Also six months after CIMT, Dong et al. (2007) reported a decrease of activation in ipsilesional M1 (one patient) and contralesional M1 (both patients), which was followed by increased activation in M1 of each hemisphere at 12 months after CIMT.

In summation, an increase or decrease of activity in the motor related brain areas and the inclusion of other new areas in the ipsilesional and contralesional hemisphere were reported after CIMT (Table 3). The results about inclusion of new brain areas are rather inconsistent. The studies are inconsistent also with respect to whether the reorganisation changes occur more in the ipsilesional or contralesional hemisphere, as was already established earlier (Mark et al. 2006).

Study	Ipsilesional hemisphere	Contralesional hemisphere	Laterality
Levy et al., 2001	P1: increase near the lesion, association motor cortex; P2: increase near the lesion	P1: increase association motor cortex, M1	Inconsistent
Johansen-Berg et al., 2002	Increase PMC, secondary somatosensory cortex	/	/
Schaechter et al., 2002	Decrease M1 P1: decrease M1, SMA;	P3:increase SMA; P4: increase M1, PMC	Trend of decreased LI
Kim et al., 2004	P1,2: increase M1, PMC, SMA; P4: increase SMA, decrease M1	P3: increase M1, SMA;	/
Liepert et al., 2004	3/3: decrease SM1	/	/
Azpiroz et al., 2005	P1: increase M1, PMC, SMA, PF, dorsolateral; P2,3: decrease activation		/
Butler & Page, 2006	CIMT: increase motor and premotor areas; CIMT + mental practice: 1/2P more focal M1	CIMT: increase motor and premotor areas	/
Dong et al., 2006	/	Decrease M1	M1 -LI inconsistent
Hamzei et al., 2006	Intact M1 & cortico-spinal tract lesions: decreased SM1; M1 & cortico-spinal tract lesions: increase SM1; 5/6P decrease PC; 1P increase, 1P decrease SMA; 2P increase, 1P decrease PMC	1P decrease PC; 1P increase PMC	/
Szaflarski et al., 2006	P1: decrease precentral gyrus, increase cortical and subcortical areas; P2,4: no changes	P1: decrease pre- and postcentral gyrus; P3: decrease inferior frontal gyrus, increase middle frontal gyrus; P2,4: no changes	/
Dong et al., 2007	3P: increase M1; 1P: decrease M1	2P: increase M1; 2P: decrease M1	Increase M1-LI
Hamzei et al., 2008	Group 1: decrease SM1; Group 2: increase SM1	/	/
Langan & van Donkelaar, 2008	Significant change across subjects (total); Cortical regions not consistent across subjects.		/
Sheng & Lin, 2009	Increase apical, fontal lobe	Increase apical, fontal lobe	/

Study	Ipsilesional hemisphere	Contralesional hemisphere	Laterality
Lin et al., 2010	Not significant	Increase PMC and total	Decrease SMA-LI, total-LI
Wu et al., 2010	Increase total hemisphere activation (sum of SM1, PM, and SMA)		Decrease LI

Table 3. Summary of the functional magnetic resonance imaging results: changes in active voxel counts or image commentaries by the study authors from before to after constraint-induced movement therapy (CIMT) or its modifications in patients after stroke. Legends are shown as: P, patient; M1, primary motor cortex; PMC, pre-motor cortex; SMA, supplementary motor area; LI, laterality index; SM1, sensori-motor cotex; PF, prefrontal cortex.

2.1.2 Relationship of fMRI changes and movement recovery

It is assumed that increased affected arm use during CIMT will induce cortical reorganisation and have effects on motor recovery of the upper extremity. Therefore a relationship between movement recovery measured with various clinical motor function tests/measures and changes in brain activation measured by fMRI is expected. It was ascertained already in the review paper by Mark et al. (2006) that in some instances, the initial degree of brain reorganization occurred in parallel with the improvement in spontaneous, real-world use by the affected hand, which in spite of inconsistency of the studies regarding the level of changes in the ipsilesional vs. contralesional hemisphere, suggests that plastic brain changes in some manner support therapeutic effects.

In the studies investigating the brain cortex reorganisation after CIMT or its modifications, the upper limb movement function improved significantly in some (Azpiroz et al., 2005; Kim et al., 2006; Langan & van Donkelaar, 2008; Schaechter et al., 2002; Wu et al., 2010) or all of the investigated parameters (Butler & Page, 2006; Dong et al., 2006, 2007; Hamzei et al., 2006, 2007; Levy et al., 2001; Liepert et al., 2004; Lin et al., 2010; Sheng & Lin, 2009; Szaflarski et al., 2006) (see Table 4), and was accompanied/related with the brain cortex plasticity change after treatment. However, improvement of the affected upper limb function was not reported for all of the patients in the studies (Butler & Page, 2006; Kim et al., 2006; Szaflarski et al., 2006; Wu et al., 2010). Dong et al. (2007) reported that long-term functional gains at six and 12 months after CIMT paralleled with decrease of activation in ipsilesional M1 in both of the two patients.

Correlational analyses to assess the relationship between results of clinical tests/measures of motor function and cortical activation or their changes were performed in few studies only, but the results were rather inconsistent. In the three studies they did not result in any statistically significant outcomes (Dong et al., 2007; Langan & van Donkelaar, 2008; Lin et al., 2010). For example, in the RCT by Lin et al. (2010), significantly greater improvement in the FMA and MAL was reported for the mCIMT group in comparison to the control group. However, an examination of the relationships between functional gains on the clinical measures and the changes in brain activation revealed no significant correlation (Lin et al., 2010). On the other hand, statistically significant correlations ($r = 0.91$-0.96) were reported for improvements in hand grip strength and increases in the ipsilesional hemisphere (see Table 3) and the cerebellum activity during performance of the affected hand (Johansen-

Berg et al. 2002). The authors chose grip strength ratio as the primary behavioural measure and did not calculate correlations with the other two measures (Table 4). Dong et al. (2006) reported no correlation between pre- to post- change in WMFT and change in activation in M1 or dorsal PMC of each hemisphere, except for pre- to mid- change in contralesional M1 voxel count, which correlated with the change in mean WMFT time (pre- to post-) (r = 0.82). The midpoint M1 laterality index anticipated post-treatment change in time to perform WMFT (Dong et al., 2006).

Study	Clinical tests/measures of motor function
Levy et al., 2001	MAL#, WMFT#
Johansen-Berg et al., 2002	Motricity index, Jebsen arm test, grip strength (difference not tested)
Schaechter et al., 2002	MAL*, WMFT*, FMA*, grip strength**, frequency of finger flexion, EMG
Kim et al., 2004	FMA*, 9-hole peg test, Jebsen arm test
Liepert et al., 2004	MAL*
Azpiroz et al., 2005	FMA*, Motricity index*, Modified Ashworth scale*, FIM*, Barthel index
Butler & Page, 2006	MAL# (2/3P), WMFT# (2/3P)
Dong et al., 2006	WMFT*
Hamzei et al., 2006	MAL*, WMFT*
Szaflarski et al., 2006	MAL# (3/4P), ARAT# (3/4P), FMA# (3/4P)
Dong et al., 2007	FMA#, WMFT#
Hamzei et al., 2008	MAL*, WMFT*
Langan & van Donkelaar, 2008	MAL*, WMFT, grip strength*, 9-hole pegboard task*
Sheng & Lin, 2009	Upper extremity function test#, Simple test for evaluating hand function#
Lin et al., 2010	FMA*, MAL*
Wu et al., 2010	FMA#, ARAT#, MAL (3/6P)

Table 4. Improvement of the affected hand movement characteristics or its use is shown after constraint-induced movement therapy or its modifications in patients after stroke. Legends are shown as: MAL, Motor activity log; # improvement, statistics not calculated; WMFT, Wolf motor function test; * statistically significant improvement; FMA, Fugl-Meyer assessment; EMG, electromyography; FIM, Functional independence measure; P, patient; ARAT, Action research arm test).

3. Conclusion

The preliminary findings of studying the effects of CIMT using fMRI indicate that brain plasticity may be modulated by specific therapeutic approaches, such as CIMT, although generalisation of the fMRI findings is limited by characteristics of the studies (sample size, control group, etc.). Limitations and future perspectives are as follows.

3.1 Limitations and current developments

Current fMRI findings of post stroke cortical reorganisation studies illustrate the lack of consensus regarding the type of cortical plasticity that is concomitant with movement recovery after CIMT. Some of the differences may be a consequence of small sample sizes, different lesion locations and studying in different periods post stroke, mostly six months or even several years after stroke. An important deficiency of the majority of the current studies is the absence of a control group, which would enable identification of the treatment effects of CIMT from the other influences on brain plasticity. In spite of the greatest possibility for a movement recovery during the first three months after stroke, no currently published study investigated the effects of CIMT on the brain plasticity measured by fMRI in this period. However, two studies with a control group performed in the first month after stroke are in a process (Kwakkel et al., 2008) or waiting for publication (Puh et al., in publication).

Is seems that the fMRI data following a successful CIMT (with improved hand function) support two patterns of the brain reorganisation, as it was already suggested by some authors (Azpiroz et al., 2005; Hamzei et al., 2008). This would be: 1) increased or more spatially extensive activation area, indicating a recruitment of new brain areas; and 2) decreased or spatially reduced activation area, indicating more focused activation. Some evidence indicates that these patterns within the affected SM1 may depend on the integrity of the cortico-spinal tract from the M1 cortex (Hamzei et al., 2006, 2008).

The relationship between brain activation and functional gains needs further investigation. It is possible that correlations would be easily detected with the use of more objective or more direct measures of a specific movement recovery, as was in the case of hand grip strength (Johansen-Berg et al. 2002), and not in measures represented by scales or common scores.

3.2 Future perspectives

The heterogeneity of the fMRI findings underscores the need for further studies examining the mechanisms of cortical plasticity with the challenge to control the confounding factors. The effects of CIMT on brain reorganisation during movement of the affected and the unaffected hand should be analysed. A combination of fMRI and other techniques in brain imaging research, such as TMS and diffusion tensor imaging should be used to investigate the influence of the cortico-spinal tract integrity changes on the activation patterns seen with fMRI and might help to understand the functional significance of the contralesional brain hemisphere activity. The main challenge for the future is to identify the specific correlates between different clinical measures of the movement recovery achieved post-treatment and the fMRI data.

There is a need for common methodology of analysing and reporting the fMRI data. Clear presentation of the patients' characteristics such as gender, age, hand dominance before a stroke, type and event of stroke, and lesion location will enable investigations of their influence. More resemble sample characteristics, with emphasise on a time after stroke at inclusion to the same study may contribute to the homogeneity of the brain activation results and to establishment of the optimal time after stroke for CIMT application. The effects of different active and/or passive motor paradigms used during fMRI should not be ignored and need further investigation. Controlling the confounding factors may enable better comparisons and interpretations of the results between studies, aiming to understand and plan the effective treatment programs for patients after stroke based on brain plasticity principles. However, the most important seem to be an increase of sample size and inclusion of the control groups (with traditional rehabilitation or no treatment in this short study period), and execution of statistical analysis on the fMRI data.

Studies using fMRI may precede clinical studies of the optimal dose of constraint and practice in CIMT (comparison of different types of CIMT and mCIMT) which needs further investigation, including investigation of the long-term effects. In future, a comparison of the effects of different therapeutic techniques on the brain cortex reorganisation and upper extremity recovery, and identification of optimal integrated approaches combining CIMT and other techniques which facilitate the brain plasticity is necessary.

4. Acknowledgement

The work was supported by the research grant P3–0019 from the Research Agency of the Republic of Slovenia, and by the Faculty of Health Sciences at University of Ljubljana.

5. References

Azpiroz, J., Barrios, F., Carrillo, M., Carrillo, R., Cerrato, A., Hernandez, J., Leder, R., Rodriguez, A., & Salgado, P. (2005). Game motivated and constraint induced therapy in late stroke with fMRI studies pre and post therapy. In: *27th Annual International Conference of the IEEE Engineering in Medicine and Biology Society (EMBS '05)*, pp.3695-3698, ISBN 0-7803-8741-4, Shanghai, China, September 1-4, 2005

Baron, J.C., Cohen, L., Cramer, S., Dobkin, B., Johansen-Berg, H., Loubinoux, I., Marshall, R.S., & Ward, N.S. (2004). Neuroimaging in stroke recovery: a position paper from the first international workshop on neuroimaging and stroke recovery. *Cerebrovascular diseases*, Vol. 18, No. 3, (September 2004), pp. 260-267, ISSN 0146-6917

Basmajian, J.V., Gowland, C.A., Brandstater, M.E., Swanson, L., & Trotter, J. (1982). EMG feedback treatment of upper limb in hemiplegic stroke patients: a pilot study. *Archives of Physical Medicine and Rehabilitation*, Vol. 63, No. 12, (December 1982), pp. 613-616, ISSN 0003-9993

Blanton, S., Wilsey, H., & Wolf, S.L. (2008). Constraint-induced movement therapy in stroke rehabilitation: perspectives on future clinical applications. *NeuroRehabilitation*, Vol. 23, No. 1, (2008), pp. 15-28, ISSN 1053-8135

Buterfisch, C., Hummelsheim, H., & Mauritz, K.H. (1995). Repetitive training of isolated movements improves the outcome of motor rehabilitation of the centrally paretic hand. *Journal of the neurological sciences*, Vol. 130, No. 1, (May 1995), pp. 59-68, ISSN 0022-510X

Butler, A.J., & Page, S.J. (2006). Mental practice with motor imagery: evidence for motor recovery and cortical reorganization after stroke. *Archives of Physical Medicine and Rehabilitation*, Vol. 87, No. 12, Suppl. 2, (December 2006), pp. S2-11, ISSN 0003-9993

Calautti, C., & Baron, J.C. (2003). Functional neuroimaging studies of motor recovery after stroke in adults: a review. *Stroke*, Vol. 34, No. 6, (June 2003), pp. 1553-1566, ISSN 1524-4628

Carey, J.R., Kimberley, T.J., Lewis, S.M., Auerbach, E.J., Dorsey, L., Rundquist, P., & Ugurbil, K. (2002). Analysis of fMRI and finger tracking training in subjects with chronic stroke. *Brain*, Vol. 125, No. 4, (April 2002), pp. 773-788, ISSN 0006-8950

Carr, J., & Shepherd, R. (2000). A motor learning model for rehabilitation. In: *Movement science: foundations for physical therapy in rehabilitation.* Carr, J., Shepherd, R., (Eds.), pp. 33-110, Aspen Publisher, ISBN 0-8342-1747-3, Gaithersburg, USA

Chollet, F., DiPiero, V., Wise, R.J.S., Brooks, D.J., Dolan, R.J., & Frackowiak, R.S.J. (1991). The functional anatomy of the motor recovery after stroke in humans: A study with positron emission tomography. *Annals of neurology*,Vol. 29, No. 1, (January 1991), pp. 63-71, ISSN 0364-5134

Clark, S.A., Alland, T., Jenkins, W.M., & Merzenich, M.M. (1988). Receptive fields in the body-surface map in adult cortex defined by temporally correlated inputs. (1988). *Nature*, Vol. 332, No. 6163, (March 1988), pp. 444-445, ISSN 0028-0836

Dean, C., & Mackey, F. (1992). Motor assessment scale scores as a measure of rehabilitation outcome following stroke. *Australian Journal of Physiotherapy*, Vol. 38, No. 1, (1992), pp. 31-35, ISSN 0004-9514

Dong, Y., Dobkin, B.H., Cen, S.Y., Wu, A.D., & Winstein, C.J. (2006). Motor cortex activation during treatment may predict therapeutic gains in paretic hand function after stroke. *Stroke*, Vol. 37, No. 6, (June 2006), pp. 1552-1555, ISSN 1524-4628

EUSI. (2003). European Stroke Initiative Recommendations for Stroke Management - update 2003. *Cerebrovascular diseases*, Vol. 16, No. 4, (2003), pp. 311-337, ISSN 1015-9770

Grotta, J.C., Noser, E.A., Ro, T., Boake, C., Levin, H., Aronowski, J., & Schallert, T. (2004). Constraint-induced movement therapy. *Stroke*, Vol. 35, No. 11, (Suppl 1), (November 2004), pp. 2699-2701, ISSN 0039-2499

Hallett, M. (2001). Plasticity of the human motor cortex and recovery from stroke. *Brain Research Reviews*, Vol. 36, No. 2-3, (October 2001), pp. 169-174, ISSN 0165-0173

Hamzei, F., Liepert, J., Dettmers, C., Weiller, C., & Rijntjes, M. (2006). Two different reorganization patterns after rehabilitative therapy: an exploratory study with fMRI and TMS. *Neuroimage*, Vol. 31, No. 2, (June 2006), pp. 710-720, ISSN 1053-8119

Hamzei, F., Dettmers, C., Rijntjes, M., & Weiller, C. (2008). The effect of cortico-spinal tract damage on primary sensorimotor cortex activation after rehabilitation therapy. *Experimental Brain Research*, Vol. 190, No. 3 (September 2008), pp. 329-336, ISSN 0014-4819

Held, J.M. (2000). Recovery of function after brain damage: theoretical and practical implications for therapeutic intervention, In: *Movement science: foundations for physical therapy in rehabilitation.* Carr, J., Shepherd, R., (Eds.), pp. 189-211, Aspen Publisher, ISBN 0-8342-1747-3, Gaithersburg, USA

Jang, S.H., Kim, Y.H., Cho, S.H., Lee, J.H., Park, J.W., & Kwon, Y.H. (2003). Cortical reorganization induced by task-oriented training in chronic hemiplegic stroke patients. *Neuroreport*, Vol. 14, No. 1, (January 2003), pp. 137-141, ISSN 0959-4965

Jenkins, W.M., Merzenich, M.M., Ochs, M.T., Allard, T., & Guíc-Robles, E. (1990). Functional reorganization of primary somatosensory cortex in adult owl monkeys after behaviorally controlled tactile stimulation. *Journal of neurophysiology*, Vol. 63, No. 1, (January 1990), pp. 82-104, ISSN 0022-3077

Johansen-Berg, H., Dawes, H., Guy, C., Smith, S.M., Wade, D.T., & Matthews, P.M. (2002). Correlation between motor improvements and altered fMRI activity after rehabilitative therapy. *Brain*, Vol. 125, No. 12, (December 2002), pp. 2731-2742, ISSN 0006-8950

Kawashima, R., Matsumura, M., Sadato, N., Naito, E., Waki, A., Nakamuram, S., Matsunami, K., Fukuda, H., & Yonekura, Y. (1998). Regional cerebral blood flow changes in human brain related to ipsilateral and contralateral complex hand movements - a PET study. *European Journal of Neuroscience*, Vol. 10, No. 7, (July 1998), pp. 2254-2260, ISSN 0953-816X

Kim, Y.H., Park, J.W., Ko, M.H., Jang, S.H., & Lee, P.K. (2004). Plastic changes of motor network after constraint-induced movement therapy. *Yonsei Medical Journal*, Vol. 45, No. 2, (April 2004), pp. 241-246, ISSN *0513-5796*

Kunkel, A., Kopp, B., Müller, G., Villringer, K., Villringer, A., Taub, E., & Flor, H. (1999). Constraint-induced movement therapy for motor recovery in chronic stroke patients. *Archives of Physical Medicine and Rehabilitation*, Vol. 80, No. 6, (June 1999), pp. 624-628, ISSN 0003-9993

Kwakkel, G., Kollen, B.J., Grond, J., & van der Prevo, A.J. (2003). Probability of regaining dexterity in the flaccid upper limb: impact of severity of paresis and time since onset in acute stroke. *Stroke*, Vol. 34, No. 9, (September 2003), pp. 2181-2186, ISSN 0039-2499

Kwakkel, G., Meskers, C.G.M., van Wegen, E.E., Lankhorst, G.J., Geurts, A.C.H., van Kuijk, A.A., Lindeman, E., Visser-Meily, A., de Vlugt, E., & Arendzen, J.H. (2008). Impact of early applied upper limb stimulation: the EXPLICIT-stroke programme design. *BioMed Central Neurology*, Vol. 8, No. 49, (December 2008), ISSN 1471-2377

Langan, J., & van Donkelaar, P. (2008). The influence of hand dominance on the response to a constraint-induced therapy program following stroke. *Neurorehabilitation and Neural Repair*, Vol. 22, No. 3, (May-June 2008), pp. 298-304, ISSN 1545-9683

Langhorne, P., Coupa, F., & Pollock, A. (2009). Motor recovery after stroke: a systematic review. *Lancet Neurology*, Vol. 8, No. 8, (August 2009), pp. 741-754, ISSN 1474-4422

Lee, R.G., & van Donkelaar, P. (1995). Mechanisms underlying functional recovery following stroke. (1995). *Canadian journal of neurological sciences*, Vol. 22, No. 4, (November 1995), pp. 257-263, ISSN 0317-1671

Levy, C.E., Nichols, D.S., Schmalbrock, P.M., Keller, P., & Chakeres, D.W. (2001). Functional MRI evidence of cortical reorganization in upper-limb stroke hemiplegia treated with constraint-induced movement therapy. *American Journal of Physical Medicine & Rehabilitation*, Vol. 80, No. 1, (January 2001), pp. 4-12, ISSN 0894-9115

Liepert, J., Uhde, I., Graf, S., Leidner, O., & Weiller, C. (2001). Motor cortex plasticity during forced-use therapy in stroke patients: a preliminary study. *Journal of neurology* Vol. 248, No. 4, (April 2001), pp. 315-321, ISSN 0340-5354

Liepert, J., Hamzei, F., & Weiller, C. (2004). Lesion-induced and training-induced brain reorganization. *Restorative neurology and neuroscience,* Vol. 22, No. 3-5, (2004), pp. 269-277, ISSN 0922-6028

Lin, K.C., Chung, H.Y., Wu, C.Y., Liu, H.L., Hsieh, Y.W., Chen, I.H., Chen, C.L., Chuang, L.L., Liu, J.S., & Wai, Y.Y. (2010). Constraint-induced therapy versus control intervention in patients with stroke: a functional magnetic resonance imaging study. *American Journal of Physical Medicine & Rehabilitation,* Vol. 89, No. 3, (March 2010), pp. 177-185, ISSN 0894-9115

Luft, A.R., McCombe-Waller, S., Whitall, J., Forrester, L.W., Macko, R., Sorkin, J.D., Schulz, J.B., Goldberg, A.P., & Hanley, D.F. (2004). Repetitive bilateral arm training and motor cortex activation in chronic stroke: a randomized controlled trial. *JAMA,* Vol. 292, No. 15, (October 2004), pp. 1853-1861, ISSN 0098-7484

Mark, V.W., Taub, E., & Morris, D.M. (2006). Neuroplasticity and constraint-induced movement therapy: Review. *Europa Medicophysica,* Vol. 42, No. 3, (September 2006), pp. 269-284, ISSN 0014-2573

Marshall, R.S., Perera, G.M., Lazar, R.M., Krakauer, J.W., Constantine, R.C., & DeLaPaz, R.L. (2000). Evolution of cortical activation during recovery from corticospinal tract infarction. *Stroke,* Vol. 31, No. 3, (March 2000), pp. 656-661, ISSN 1524-4628

Mudie, M.H., & Matyas, T.A. (1996). Upper extremity retraining following stroke: effects of bilateral practice. *Neurorehabilitation and neural repair,* Vol. 10, No. 3, (September 1996), pp. 167-184, ISSN 1545-9683

Nakayama, H., Jorgensen, H.S., Raaschou, H.O., & Olsen, T.S. (1994). Recovery of upper extremity function in stroke patients: the Copenhagen stroke study. *Archives of Physical Medicine and Rehabilitation,* Vol. 75, No. 4, (April 1994), pp. 394-398, ISSN 0003-9993

Nelles, G., Jentzen, W., Jueptner, M., Muller, S., & Diener, C. (2001). Arm training induced brain plasticity in stroke studied with serial positron emission tomography. *Neuroimage,* Vol. 13, No. 1, (June 2001), pp. 1146-1154, ISSN 1053-8119

Netz, J., Lammers, T., & Hömberg, V. (1997). Reorganization of motor output in the non-affected hemisphere after stroke. *Brain,* Vol. 120, No. 9, (September 1997), pp. 1579-1586, ISSN 0006-8950

Nudo, R.J., Miliken, G.W., Jenkins, W.M., & Merzenich, M.M. Use-dependent alterations of movement representations in primary motor cortex of adult squirrel monkeys. (1996). *Journal of Neuroscience,* Vol. 16, No. 2, (January 1996), pp. 785-807, ISSN 0270-6474

Parker, V.M., Wade, D.T., & Langton Hewer, R. (1986). Loss of arm function after stroke: measurement, frequency and recovery. *International Rehabilitation Medicine,* Vol. 8, No. 2, (1986), pp. 69-73, ISSN 0379-0797

Puh, U., Vovk, A., Sevšek, F., & Šuput, D. (2007) Increased cognitive load during simple and complex motor tasks in acute stage after stroke. *International Journal of Psychophysiology,* Vol. 63, No. 2, (February 2007), pp. 173-80, ISSN 0167-8760

Puh, U., Vovk, A., & Šuput, D. (in publication).

Salmelin, R., Forss, N., Knuutila, J., & Hari, R. (1995). Bilateral activation of the human somatomotor cortex by distal hand movements. *Electroencephalography and clinical neurophysiology,* Vol. 95, No. 6, (December 1995), pp. 444-452, ISSN 0013-4694

Schaechter, J.D., Kraft, E., Hilliard, T.S., Dijkhuizen, R.M., Benner, T., Finklestein, S.P., Rosen, B.R., Cramer, S.C. (2002). Motor recovery and cortical reorganization after constraint-induced movement therapy in stroke patients: a preliminary study. *Neurorehabilitation and Neural Repair*, Vol. 16, No. 4, (December 2002), pp. 326-338, ISSN 1545-9683

Schaechter, J.D. (2004). Motor rehabilitation and brain plasticity after hemiparetic stroke. *Progress in neurobiology*, Vol. 73, No. 1, (May 2004), pp. 61-72, ISSN 0555-4047

Sheng, B., & Lin, M. (2009). A longitudinal study of functional magnetic resonance imaging in upper-limb hemiplegia after stroke treated with constraint-induced movement therapy. *Brain Injury*, Vol. 23, No. 1, (January 2009), pp. 65-70, ISSN 0269-9052

Shumway-Cook, A., & Woollacott, M.H. (2007). *Motor control: translating research into clinical practice* (3rd ed.). Lippincott Williams & Wilkins, ISBN 0-7817-6691-5, Philadelphia, USA

Sirtori, S., Corbetta, D., Moja, L., & Gatti, R. (2009). Constraint-induced movement therapy for upper extremities in stroke patients. *Cochrane Database of Systematic Reviews*, Issue 4, No. CD004433, (October 2009), ISSN 1469-493X

Sterr, A., Elbert, T., Berthold, I., Kolbel, S., Rockstroh, B., & Taub, E. (2002). Longer versus shorter daily constraint-induced movement therapy of chronic hemiparesis: an exploratory study. *Archives of Physical Medicine and Rehabilitation*, Vol. 83, No. 10, (October 2002), pp. 1374-1377, ISSN 0003-9993

Szaflarski, J.P., Page, S.J., Kissela, B.M., Lee, J.H., Levine, P., & Strakowski, S.M. (2006). Cortical reorganization following modified constraint-induced movement therapy: a study of 4 patients with chronic stroke. *Archives of Physical Medicine and Rehabilitation*, Vol. 87, No. 8, (August 2006), pp. 1052-1058, ISSN 0003-9993

Taub, E., Uswatte, G., King, D.K., Morris, D., Crago, J.E., & Chatterjee, A. (2006). A placebo-controlled trial of constraint-induced movement therapy for upper extremity after stroke. *Stroke*, Vol. 37, No. 4, (April 2006), pp. 1045-1049, ISSN 0039-2499

Turton, A., Wroe, S., Trepte, N., Fraser, C., & Lemon, R.N. (1996). Contralateral and ipsilateral EMG responses to transcranial magnetic stimulation during recovery of arm and hand function after stroke. *Electroencephalography and clinical neurophysiology*, Vol. 101, No. 4, (August 1996), pp. 316-328, ISSN 0013-4694

Van der Lee, J.H. (2001). Constraint-induced therapy for stroke: more of the same or something complitely different? *Current opinion in neurology*,Vol. 14, No. 6, (December 2001), pp. 741-744, ISSN 1350-7540

van Peppen, R.P.S., Kwakel, G., Wood-Dauphinee, S.W., Hendriks, H.J., Van der Wees, P.J., & Dekker, J. (2004). The impact of physiotherapy on functional outcome after stroke: What's the evidence? *Clinical Rehabilitation*, Vol. 18, No. 8, (December 2004), pp. 833-862, ISSN 0269-2155

Wade, D.T., Langton Hewer, R., Wood, V.A., Skilbeck, C.E., & Ismail, H.M. (1983). The hemiplegic arm after stroke: measurement and recovery. *Journal of neurology, neurosurgery, and psychiatry*, Vol. 46, No. 6, (June 1983), pp. 521-524, ISSN 0022-3050

Wittenberg, G.F., Chen, R., Ishii, K., Bushara, K.O., Eckloff, S., Croarkin, E., Taub, E., Gerber, L.H., Hallett, M., & Cohen, L.G. (2003). Constraint-induced therapy in stroke: magnetic-stimulation motor maps and cerebral activation. Neurorehabilitati*on and Neural Repair*, Vol. 17, No. 3, (September 2003), pp. 48-57, ISSN 1545-9683

Wolf, S.L., Lecraw, D.E., Barton, L.A., & Jann, B.B. (1989). Forced use of hemiplegic upper extremities to reverse the effect of learned nonuse among chronic stroke and head-injured patients. *Experimental neurology*, Vol. 104, No. 2, (May 1989), pp. 125-132, ISSN 0014-4886

Wu, C.Y., Hsieh, Y.W., Lin, K.C., Chuang LL, Chang YF, Liu HL, Chen CL, Lin KH, & Wai YY. (2010). Brain reorganization after bilateral arm training and distributed constraint-induced therapy in stroke patients: a preliminary functional magnetic resonance imaging study. *Chang Gung Medical Journal*, Vol. 33, No. 6, (November-December 2010), pp. 628-638, ISSN 2072-0939

7

Reliability Maps in Event Related Functional MRI Experiments

Aleksandr A. Simak[1,2], Michelle Liou[*,1], Alexander Yu. Zhigalov[1], Jiun-Wei Liou[2] and Phillip E. Cheng[1]
[1]*Institute of Statistical Science, Academia Sinica*
[2]*Department of Computer Science and Information Engineering, National Taiwan University*
Taiwan, R.O.C.

1. Introduction

In functional magnetic resonance imaging (fMRI) studies, the blood oxygen level-dependent (BOLD) signal change, in contrast to noise, is typically small (< 5%; e.g., Chen & Small, 2007). Although the quality of acquired image data may be improved by pre-processing images with low- or high-pass filters, classification of voxels into the active/inactive status could vary from one study to the next even when the same experimental paradigm is implemented (Maitra, 2009). Reliability assessment would contribute significantly to the knowledge on noise structures in image data, as a function of stimulus sequences, ethnic groups, imaging techniques and scanner differences (Biswal et al., 1996; Genovese et al., 1997; Maitra et al., 2002).

In the literature, there have been two main approaches to quantifying reliability of activation. The first involves the analysis of fMRI data acquired in a group of subjects (or more than one group) performing the same task in different days under multiple experimental conditions. The noise structure can be assessed by the intra-class correlation (ICC) analysis (Brennan, 2001; McGraw & Wong, 1996), which provides individual sources of noise associated with experiment-specific conditions (Aron et al., 2006; Fernandez et al., 2003; Franco et al., 2009; Friedman et al., 2008; Manoach et al., 2001; Miezin et al., 2000; Raemaekers et al., 2007; Specht et al., 2003; Zuo et al., 2010). The second approach considers the same group of subjects in multiple experimental replications, and evaluates test-retest reliability by modeling the number of times out of all replications, that a voxel is consistently classified as active given a decision threshold, as a mixture of binomial random variables (Genovese et al., 1997; Noll et al., 1997). This statistical approach has been extended by incorporating more accurate mixtures distributions and optimization procedure for estimating test-retest reliability (Gullapalli et al., 2005; Maitra et al., 2002).

Other than studying noise structures, reliability analysis would also provide information on invariant brain activity during the experimental session as a useful addition to the conventional measurement of response amplitudes. In a study using the forward-backward viewing movies paradigm, for instance, Hasson et al. (2010) have shown that brain responses in the visual cortex are highly reliable between subjects for both forward and backward presentations; responses in other cortical regions such as the precuneus, lateral sulcus, temporal-parietal junction tend to be less reliable in the backward presentation. However, disrupting the viewing order has no effect on response amplitudes in major cortical regions; markedly though, reliability magnitude varies in these regions. This type of studies has introduced dissociation between persistency and amplitude in brain activity.

The event-related paradigm was originally proposed for detecting transient BOLD responses to brief stimuli or tasks, but its potential use is not limited to short-term stimulation (Josephs et al., 1997). In statistical analysis of event-related fMRI data, a few design contrasts must be specified to estimate stimulus and task effects (Friston et al., 2002; Strother et al., 2004; Worsley et al., 2002). Conventionally, the ICC or test-retest reliability indices have been computed across experimental replicates using the t- or F-values, which are standardized parameter estimates in a linear model with BOLD responses as the dependent variable and a few design contrasts as regressors. The design contrast constitutes a hypothesis on temporal behavior in the brain following the stimulus or task onset.

In this chapter, we outline a reliability analysis procedure applicable directly to BOLD responses (i.e., image intensity) without a prior specification of design contrasts. In a sense, the procedure assesses the persistency in BOLD responses during the experimental session. Nonpersistency implies that a brain region is either heavily contaminated by noise or possibly contains a transient response, the onset of which is not reproducible between replicates. In applications, the procedure would suggest a collection of stable brain responses and their spatial distributions that may or may not be easily modeled or detected by using a weighted linear sum of a few basis functions (Lindquist et al., 2009). For instance, it might not be immediately clear how to specify design contrasts for a relatively longer duration of stimuli (> 40 sec per event) or for analysis of spontaneous brain activity under the eyes-closed and -open states. Stable BOLD responses can be further classified into distinct types featuring the time to response peak, amplitude, duration and sign (increased or decreased responses).

In the method section, we will elaborate the step-by-step procedure for assessing reliability of BOLD responses, testing reliability indices for statistical significance, and constructing reliability maps. For illustration, the method will be applied to an empirical dataset collected in a change detection task using the event-related paradigm (Huettel et al., 2001). Empirical results will show that the criterion of persistency is more sensitive to activity in the grey matter in contrast to that in the white matter. Finally, we will discuss the neurophysiological basis and clinical usage of reliability maps.

2. Hemodynamic response functions

In statistical analysis of fMRI data, it is important to model the BOLD responses as a function of the external stimulus (Buxton et al., 1997; Friston et al., 2000; Obata et al., 2004). By convention, a canonical hemodynamic response function (HRF) can be convolved with the external stimulus function to estimate the responses. The HRF can be formulated using one or two gamma functions to model a slight intensity dip after the response has fallen back to zero (Friston et al., 1998; Lange & Zeger, 1997). The estimated response at a particular scan is then subsampled from the response function specified at the scan acquisition time (Bandettini et al., 1993; Worsley et al., 2002). Canonical HRF assumes an instantaneous short stimulus with a few parameters determined by empirically observing activity in the primary visual cortex (Boynton et al., 1996; Glover, 1999); the function has been well fitted to experimental data in many fMRI studies involving healthy subjects, and is suitable for testing hypotheses on the strength and location of brain activation. However, the function may be ineffectual with experiments involving younger children or clinical patients.

There is an increasing amount of literature showing significant variability in HRFs between brain regions and subjects (Aguirre et al., 1998; Handwerker et al., 2004). The HRF variability also appears between experimental sessions recorded in different days on the same subject (Neumann et al., 2003). If variability in HRFs is known to be quite large, an empirically derived HRF can be used instead of the theoretical one in the generalized linear model (GLM) analysis of fMRI data (Handwerker et al., 2004). However, the variability problem cannot be precisely resolved by inserting an empirical HRF into the GLM because the HRF onset time and latency also varies seriously between brain regions especially in event-related experiments with long-term stimuli. In addition to microvasculature disturbances to variability in HRFs, the temporal behavior of BOLD signal has been found stable in repeated trials recorded in a single session (Aguirre et al., 1998; Miezin et al., 2000; de Zwart et al., 2005). Conditional on a fixed brain region, the HRF shape and amplitude can be highly reproducible within a subject.

Numerous studies in recent years have reported the relative efficiency of different HRF models, including finite impulse response models using basis functions and extension of the canonical HRF to more complicated situations with possible temporal and dispersion derivatives (Lindquist et al., 2009; Stephan et al., 2007). On the other hand, localization of brain activity can be done by data driven methods such as independent component analysis (ICA) or group ICA methods (Gu & Pagnoni, 2008; Varoquaux et al., 2010), which can extract reproducible components between experimental trials or between subjects. Most data driven methods assume non-Gaussian distributions for unknown temporal behaviors, which would make thresholding more difficult in constructing activation maps based on voxel-wise component scores. As was mentioned, BOLD responses can be highly reproducible in a fixed brain region within each subject. In this chapter we introduce a simple procedure for research into stable temporal behaviors in the brain, which can be further classified into different response patterns for selecting regions of interest (ROIs) or for GLM analysis.

3. Measures of reliability

Reliability analysis requires assessment data to be structured in similar events or replicates. Event-related fMRI experiments are normally conducted over a period of time which is split into smaller segments or experimental runs to allow subjects to rest. Different runs can be considered as experimental replicates implemented under the same condition for evaluation of between-run reliability. Although the notation used in this section has been designed for between-run reliability analysis, a generalization of the method to other types of situations can be easily made by analogy (e.g., between trials or between subjects). The ICC index is a prominent statistic for measuring reliability of image data between runs. Here we specify the assumption used for computing the index, and its potential competitors. Let S denote the variance–covariance matrix of image data between M runs in a single voxel. The ICC index can be expressed as

$$\mathrm{ICC} = \frac{M}{M-1}\left[1 - tr(\mathbf{S})(\underline{1}'\mathbf{S}\underline{1})^{-1}\right], \tag{1}$$

where $\underline{1}$ is the summing vector of order M, and *tr*(*S*) is the trace of *S*. The index has additionally assumed that the assessment data between replicates can be expressed as an additive equation except for random measurement errors.

The index is particularly sensitive to the variance within each run; if variances of image intensity vary from one run to the next, the size of ICC becomes smaller. However, the index is unaffected by adding a constant to image intensity within each run. As an alternative to ICC, the agreement index is sensitive to all aspects of between-run variation including the mean image intensity. An interested reader may refer to McGraw & Wong (1996) for a detailed comparison between the ICC and agreement index. In general, the two indices give comparable results when the number of scan volumes increases in each run. In some experimental paradigms, the scale of image intensity is allowed to vary between runs, and the additive assumption could be too restrictive for general applications. For example, tasks with high and low working memory loads are implemented in different runs. There are also reliability indices robust to scale changes; that is, image data in one run can be expressed as a linear combination of those in another run.

In our empirical studies, reliability indices with lesser restrictive assumptions always yield greater index values, but the ordering of voxels according to index values remains unchanged especially with fMRI data. Interested readers may refer to Liou (1989) for a review on robust reliability indices. An alternative approach is to specify a common factor model underlying image data and to compute the reliability index based on factor loadings (McDonald, 1999). If the common factor model is misspecified, the reliability estimate using factor loadings could be seriously biased (Yang & Green, 2010). An empirical comparison between the ICC and factor analysis models for estimating reliability can be found in Lucke (2005).

We now assume that the maximum autocorrelation coefficient in a fMRI time series decreases toward zero as the time-lag between the correlated observations increases toward infinity. It follows from a standard result for a weakly dependent sequence of random variables (Peligrad, 1996, Theorem 2.1) that the asymptotic distribution of elements in *S* can be assumed to be multivariate Gaussian as the number of scan volumes $n \to \infty$,

$$\sqrt{n}(\mathrm{vech}\boldsymbol{S} - \mathrm{vech}\boldsymbol{\Phi}) \to \mathrm{N}(0, 2\mathrm{H_M}(\boldsymbol{\Phi}\otimes\boldsymbol{\Phi})\mathrm{H_M'}),$$

where $\otimes$ is the Kronecker product and $\boldsymbol{\Phi}$ is the population counterpart of *S*; vech*S* denotes the vector of those non-duplicated elements in *S*, and the operational matrix $\mathrm{H_M}$ satisfies the identity vech$S$ $=\mathrm{H_M}$vec$S$ (Henderson & Searle, 1979). Because ICC is a differentiable function of a multivariate Gaussian vector, the asymptotic variance of ICC can be derived as follows

$$\mathrm{Var(ICC)} \approx 2\mathrm{n}^{-1}\mathrm{d}'\mathrm{H_M}(\boldsymbol{\Phi}\otimes\boldsymbol{\Phi})\mathrm{H_M'}\mathrm{d}, \tag{2}$$

where d′ is the derivative of ICC with respect to vech′*S* as follows:

$$d' = \frac{M}{(M-1)(\underline{1}'\Phi\underline{1})^2}\left[-(1'\Phi 1)\text{vec}'IM + tr(\mathbf{\Phi})(\underline{1}'\otimes\underline{1}')\right]G_M$$

and vec$\boldsymbol{S}$ = $G_M$vech$\boldsymbol{S}$. With a moderate size of n (> 100), it is reasonable to assume that

$$Z = (\text{ICC} - \mu_{\text{ICC}})/\text{Std(ICC)} \tag{3}$$

is distributed as a standard Gaussian distribution with mean 0 and variance 1, where μ_{ICC} is the mean value in the population and Std(ICC) denotes the square root of Var(ICC) in (2). In applications, one may hypothesize that $\mu_{\text{ICC}} = 0$ and test an observed ICC for statistical significance against this hypothesis.

4. Multiple testing

The ICC value is computed by using temporal information within each individual voxel, and the resulting Z value in (3) can be tested against a nominal Type-I error rate α. In this chapter, we assume that only positive ICC values are acceptable. With $\alpha = 0.05$ for a one-tailed test, for example, voxels with $Z \geq 1.64$ can be selected for constructing reliability maps. As the number of voxels to be evaluated increases, the likelihood of having at least one Type-I error out of all tests also increases in the experiment. By the Bonferroni inequality, $p_B \leq \alpha/\text{V}$, where V is the total number of voxels with positive Z values, the familywise error (FWE) rate can be controlled at α by selecting error rate at p_B for each test. Because of the spatial dependence among image voxels, the Bonferroni procedure tends to be too conservative in general (Nichols & Hayasaka, 2003).

Alternatively, the multistep test uses a sequence of ordered p-values which are compared against different thresholds. The false discovery rate (FDR) is a step-up test widely applied in neuroimaging studies (Chumbley et al., 2010; Genovese et al., 2002; Langers et al., 2007). The FDR procedure considers $p_{\text{FDR}} \leq (i/\text{V})[\alpha/\text{C(V)}]$ as the critical value for the i-th test in the ordered sequence to control the false positive rate at α, where C(V) is a predetermined constant. The choice of the constant depends on the joint distribution of p-values in the sequence. For instance, $\text{C(V)} = 1$, in case of the Gaussian noise with nonnegative correlation across voxels, and $\text{C(V)} = \sum_{i=1}^{V} i^{-1}$, in case of no assumption on dependence (Genovese et al., 2002). The FDR procedure is easily implemented even for large data sets, and more powerful than the Bonferroni procedure (Langers et al., 2007; McNamee & Lazar, 2004; Nichols & Hayasaka, 2003).

The random field theory (RFT) methods account for spatial dependence in the data, as captured by the maximum of a random field (Nichols & Hayasaka, 2003; Worsley, 1996). It has been shown that the probability of observing a cluster of voxels exceeding a threshold in a smooth Gaussian RF can be approximated by the expected Euler characteristic (EC). The EC counts the number of clusters above a sufficiently high threshold in a smoothed Gaussian RF. Methods based on the RFT comprise a flexible framework for neuroimaging inference, but RFT relies on the assumptions of stationarity and smoothness (Nichols & Hayasaka, 2003). Without spatial smoothing on ICC values, the RFT methods yield similar results to the Bonferroni procedure in our applications. In the empirical example, we will only present results based on the FDR procedure with C(V) = 1. An interested reader may refer to Nichols and Hayasaka (2003) for a detailed comparison between different approaches to controlling the FWE.

5. Reliability maps

In fMRI experiments, it is reasonable to assume that environmental, physiological, and psychological factors fluctuate randomly throughout the experimental period on a moment-by-moment basis, and these random effects occur equally likely in all runs. Imaging techniques, such as pulse sequences, imaging parameters and scanner performance, also affect the quality of observations. Those artifacts, however, may be systematic and non-random as long as the same scanners, sequences, and parameters are implemented in the experiments. In addition to regular prewhitening procedures (i.e., slice timing, motion correction, and adjustment for autocorrelation), the fMRI time series in reliability analysis must be corrected for major trend effects in order to account for magnetic field drifts.

There are qualitative descriptions of reliability indices, for instance, poor (<0.00), slight (0.00-0.20), fair (0.21-0.40), moderate (0.41-0.60), substantial (0.61-0.80), and almost perfect (0.81-1.00) (Landis & Koch, 1977). The size of ICC also depends on the number of runs and number of scan volumes. However, the standardized ICC in (3) can take into account the sample size effects. In order to construct the reliability maps, the Z value is computed by substituting sample estimate S for population $\boldsymbol{\Phi}$ in (3) for each individual voxel using the preprocessed fMRI time series. Voxels with Z values significantly greater than zero can be selected to construct the reliability maps (e.g., $Z \geq 1.64$ with Type I error controlled at $\alpha = 0.05$). In order to control the FWE, the Bonforroni correction, random field theory, and FDR control methods can be applied (Hochberg & Tamhane, 1987; Worsley et al., 1996). In the empirical example, we only present results based on the FDR method which yields most reasonable findings as compared with the other two methods.

The reliability analysis can be applied to each individual subject as well as to a group of subjects. After normalization of each subject's fMRI scans to a standard brain atlas (e.g., the MNI brain), the group standardized ICC for K subjects can be computed as follows:

$$Z_G = \left(\Sigma_j^K \mathrm{ICC}_j\right) / \sqrt{\Sigma_j^K \mathrm{Var}(\mathrm{ICC}_j)}\,, \tag{4}$$

where ICCj denotes the ICC index corresponding to the j-th subject. The Z_G values can be tested for significance against a standard Gaussian distribution with FDR control of FWE in the normalized space.

6. Empirical example

We illustrate the use of the reliability analysis procedure in an example using the long-term stimulus in the experiment (42 sec per event). The dataset was collected in an event-related fMRI experiment involving 10 subjects for investigating brain functions in a change-detection task (Huettel et al., 2001; fMRIDC Accession No: 2-2001-111T9). There were 10 stimulus trials in each run, and each subject completed 10-12 runs in his/her experimental session. In each trial, a pair of images was presented with difference in either the presence/absence of a single object or color of the object. The subjects made the behavioral response by pressing a button when they felt that there was something changing on the trial.

Each trial began with 2 sec fixation cross at the center of the screen as a warning signal, followed by the first 30 sec of the trial, during which two images were presented for 300 ms, separated by a 100-ms mask. The mask was removed during the last 10 sec of the trial, and the stimuli alternated every 400ms. During the experiment, the subjects were instructed to keep their eyes on the display at all times.

Figure 1 lists the frequency distribution of categorized trials in four response-time intervals, namely, 0-10, 10-20, 20-30 and 30-40 sec according to the time point at which a subject made the change identification responses. All distributions in the figure show two frequency peaks in the first and last bins. On the average, the between-subject variation is small by inspecting the behavioral data. Figure 2 plots the frequency distribution of voxel-wise Z values in (3) for each of the 10 subjects. Theoretically, the ICC values lie within the range of $(-\infty, 1]$, and the plots suggest that all subjects have similar ICC distributions except for Subjects 7 and 8, whose ICC values are mainly distributed in the negative direction (smaller proportions of positive ICC values). The two subjects have average shorter reaction times as compared with other subjects. During the experimental sessions, instantaneous BOLD responses could occur in the two subjects, which may or may not be related to the task. The image data of these two subjects were later eliminated from the group reliability analysis. In applications, visual inspection on the ICC distributions would suggest removing irregular subjects from the group analysis.

Reliability analysis was applied to each individual subject's data without normalization of image to the MNI template. Figure 3 shows the reliability maps for four subjects whose behavioral data and ICC values have comparable distributions in Figures 1 and 2, respectively. The maps for each subject were constructed by computing Z values in (3) for every voxel, and then testing these values for significance against a standard Gaussian distribution using the FDR control of FWE at $\alpha = 0.05$. The colored overlays in Figure 3 are those voxels exceeding the FDR threshold, and were shown by using each subject's own anatomy in the background. The time series data in the colored regions were further clustered into different patterns using the k-mean method (MacQueen, 1967). Figure 3 also plots the response patterns that are reproducible between the four subjects derived from the k-mean method.

The response functions in Figure 3 suggest that there are at least two types of increased BOLD responses (blue and yellow) time locked to the stimulus onset, and one type of decreased responses (green) also time locked to the stimulus onset. The onset time of one increased response (red) is earlier than the stimulus onset. The time to the response peak varies between the three increased BOLD responses and between the four subjects. The time to the dip in the decreased response also varies between the four subjects. The response function in yellow in the figure shows a minor peak in the last 10 sec of the trial during which the mask was removed between images in the change detection task. In applications, these response functions can be smoothed and inserted into the design matrix of GLM in SPM or FSL for advanced statistical analysis, such as comparing stimulus or task effects in different groups.

In order to illustrate group reliability maps, functional and anatomical images of eight subjects (1, 2, 3, 4, 5, 6, 9 and 10) with more reliable data were normalized to the MNI template. The ICC values corresponding to the same voxel in the normalized brain were computed for each of the eight subjects. The average ICCs across the eight subjects and Z_G values were computed for all voxels in the normalized brain. Figure 4 shows the group reliability maps in different brain regions. Brain regions with higher Z_G values imply that there were stable temporal behaviors during the experimental session in these regions. The reliability maps might suggest potential ROIs for probing high-level brain functions.

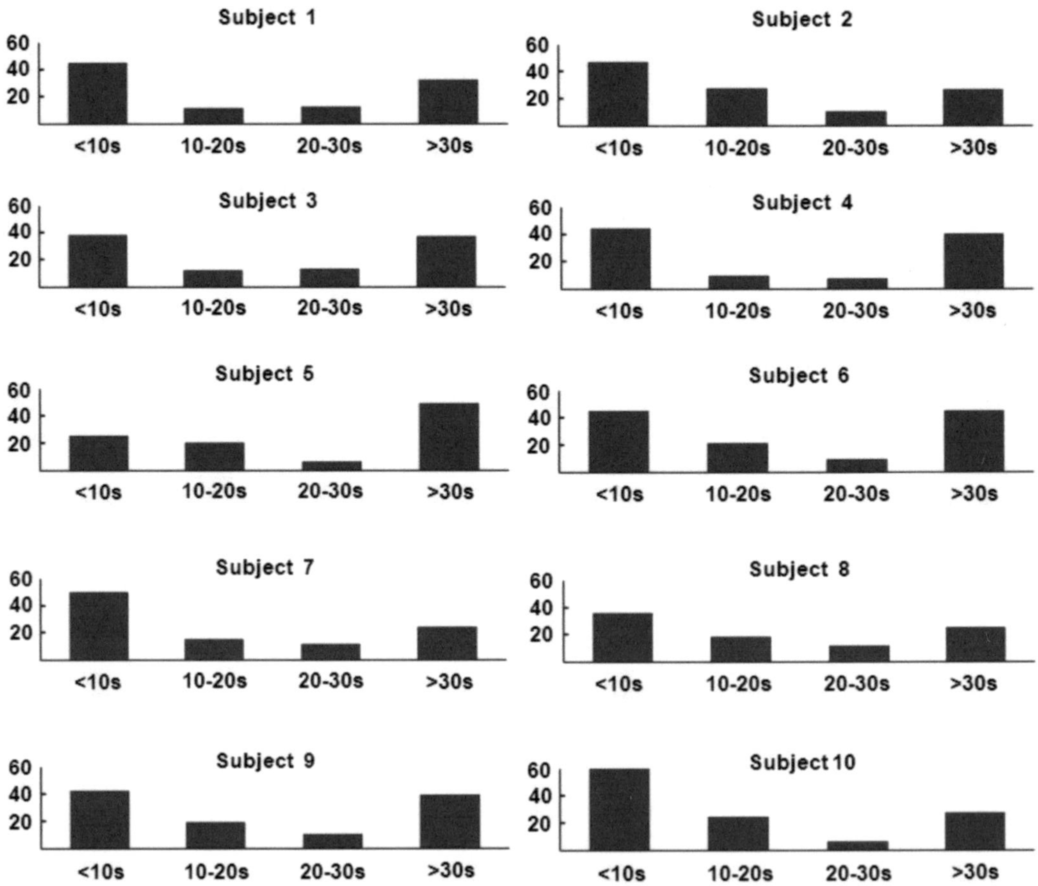

Fig. 1. The frequency distribution of categorized trials in four response-time intervals, namely 0-10, 10-20, 20-30 and 30-40 sec, according to the time point at which a subject made the change identification responses.

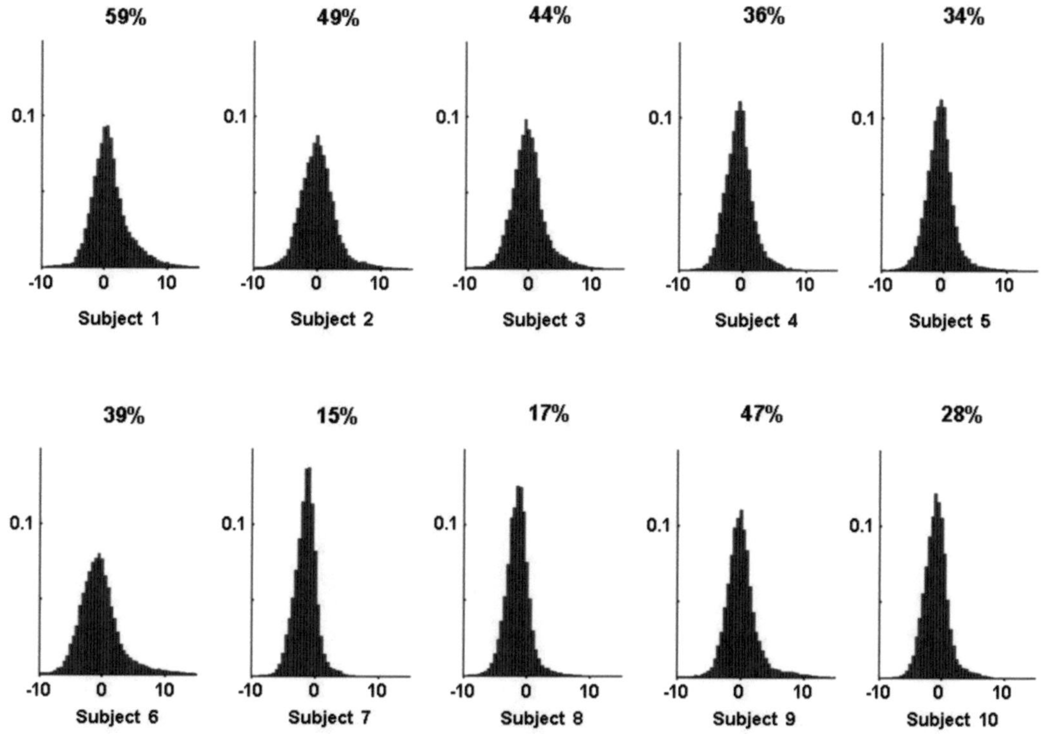

Fig. 2. The frequency distributions of standardized ICC values for each of the 10 subjects. The percentage above each individual's histogram shows the proportion of voxels with positive ICC values.

The average time series across the eight subjects in different voxels with significant Z_G values were clustered using the k-mean method. Figure 5 shows the BOLD responses based on the average time series. According to the figure, there are at least two types of decreased responses (green and brown) in the group reliability maps. Figure 6 shows the brain regions corresponding to different BOLD response patterns in Figure 5. The color overlays in Figure 4 and 6 have the same spatial locations with the normalized anatomy in the background. It is interesting to note that the onset time of responses in the parahippocampal gyrus, posterior cingulate and precuneus (the red plot) is slightly earlier than the stimulus onset. This suggest that a mechanism could be carried over from the previous trial to a new trial. The parahippocampal gyrus participates in novelty perception, and the posterior cingulate and precuneus, in attentional shift. The early-onset response could be induced by a preparatory mechanism in anticipation of an expected task (Sirotin & Das, 2009).

Responses in the parahippocampal gyrus, middle frontal gyrus, precuneus and superior/inferior parietal lobule (the yellow plot) show a second peak in the last 10 sec of each trial during which the mask was removed between two images. The second peak could be induced by the task change (with/without the mask). The early decreased responses (in green) in the insula, supramarginal, angular gyrus and precuneus could be coupled with the early increased responses (in red) carried over from the previous trial. The late decreased responses (in brown) in the cingulate gyrus, superior temporal gyrus and medial frontal gyrus could be coupled with increased responses (blue and yellow) for performing the change detection task.

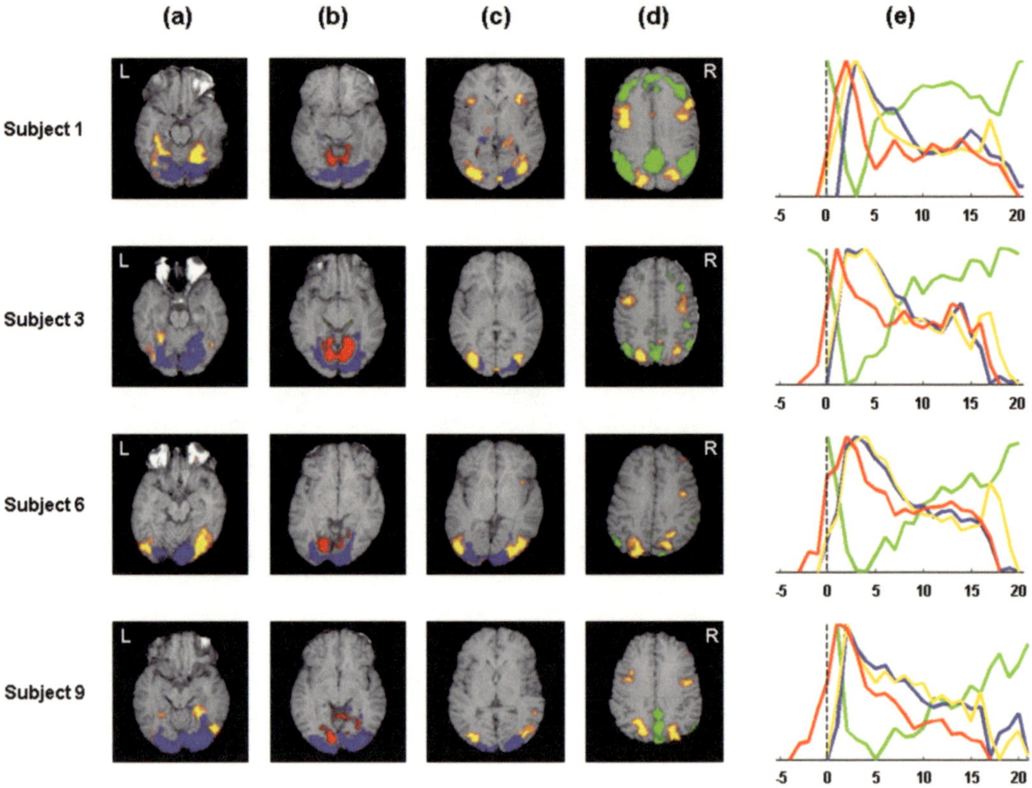

Fig. 3. The reliability maps of four subjects participating in the change detection task. The colored voxels have ICC values that are significantly greater than zero by a standard Gaussian test with the FDR control of FWE at $\alpha = 0.05$. The selected slices are all in the axial sections; the slices in columns (a), (b), (c) and (d) locate approximately at z = -9, -4, +5 and +33, respectively. The BOLD response plots in column (e) are those stable response patterns associated with each subject from the k-mean method. The spatial distribution of each response pattern in the brain is highlighted using the same color. The reliability maps are reported by showing in a subject's own anatomy in the background with colored overlays indicating those voxels with Z values exceeding the FDR thresholds.

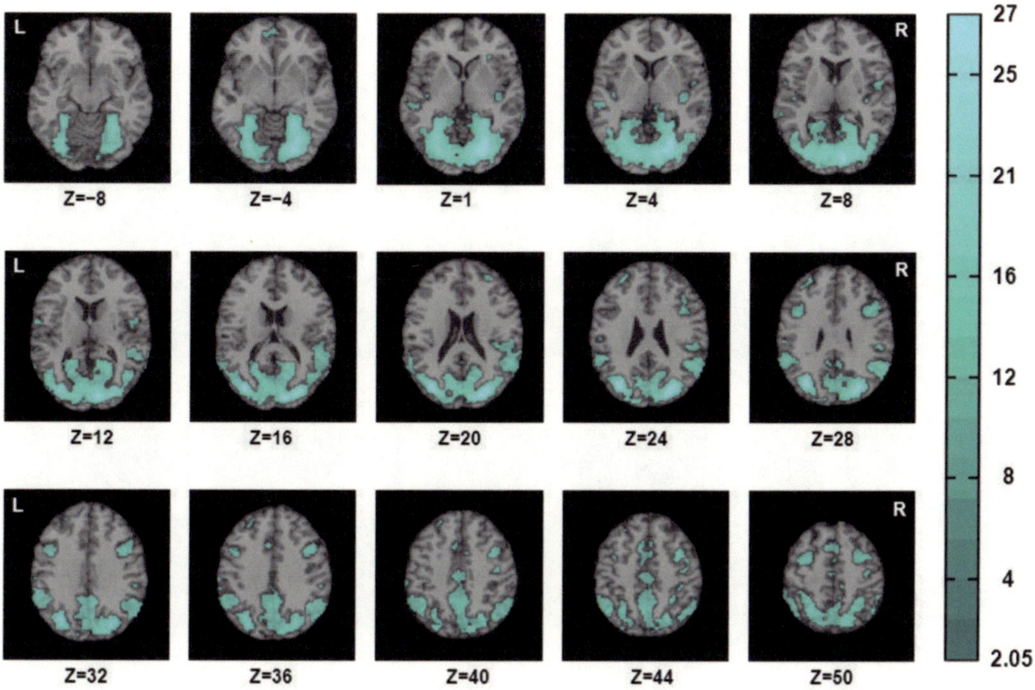

Fig. 4. The group reliability maps for eight subjects participating in the change detection task. The colored voxels have Z_G values significantly greater than zero by a standard Gaussian test with the FDR control of FWE at $\alpha = 0.05$. Coordinates are in the normalized space of the Talairach and Tournoux 1988 brain atlas. The intensity of the color indicates the size of Z_G values.

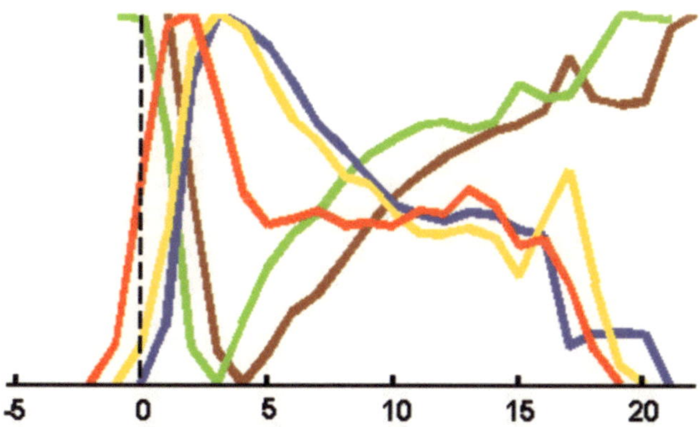

Fig. 5. Stable response patterns from the k-mean method; the patterns are found by averaging time series across 8 subjects in each voxel in the normalized space.

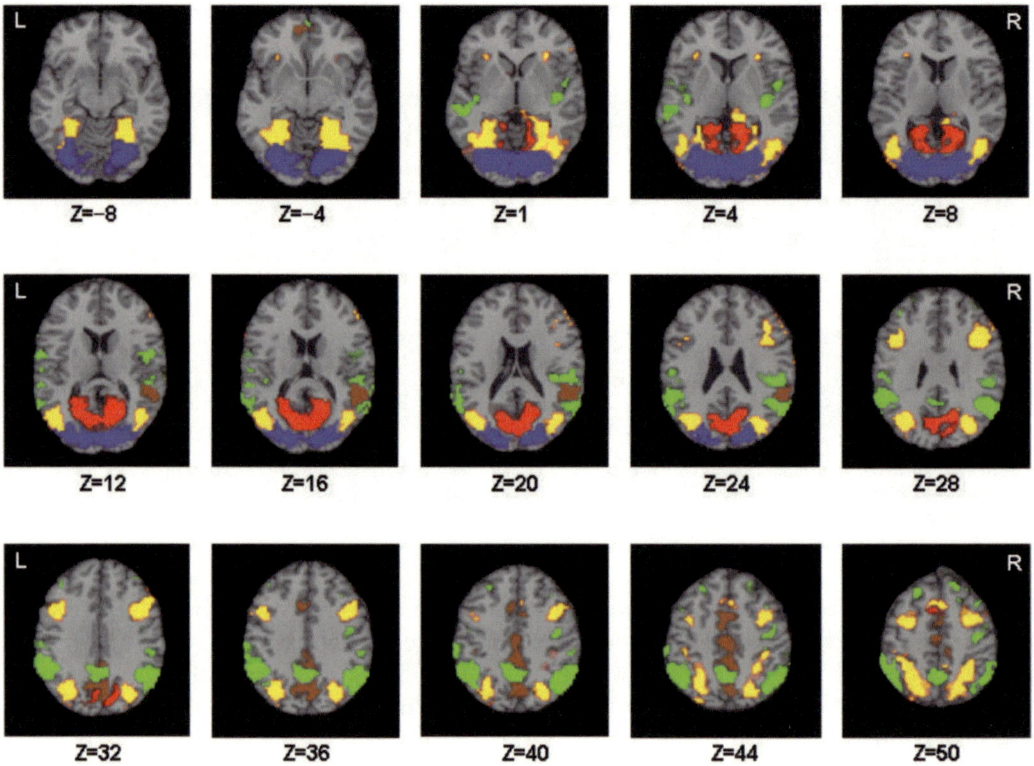

Fig. 6. The group reliability maps for eight subjects using the same colors corresponding to the response plots in Figure 5. The increased responses in blue are mainly distributed in the fusiform gyrus, lingual gyrus, middle occipital gyrus and cuneus; those in yellow are distributed in the parahippocampal gyrus, middle frontal gyrus, precuneus, and superior/inferior parietal lobule; those in red are distributed in the parahippocampal gyrus, posterior cingulate and precuneus. The decreased responses in green are distributed in the insula, precuneus, and inferior parietal lobule; those in brown are distributed in the cingulate gyrus, superior temporal gyrus and medial frontal gyrus.

7. Discussion

Comparing with other existing methods, reliability maps are simple in construction, and offer rich information on temporal behaviors of different brain regions. The method is applicable to each individual subject as well as to a group of subjects, and has potential use for investigating the HRF variability between subjects and between brain regions. Without reliability assessment, some functional mechanisms could be overlooked in the analysis such as novelty perception in the last few seconds of each trial in the change detection task. One restriction of reliability assessment is that the fMRI time series must be partitioned into replicates (e.g., experimental runs). This might not pose difficulty in applications. For instance, we applied the same procedure to the resting state fMRI with alternate eyes-closed and -open periods (3 min per state with two replications). It was found that the thalamus showed most reliable results, but BOLD responses in this region were quite different from those in other regions. Regions located in the default mode network (e.g., precuneus) also had moderate sizes of reliability. By the conventional approaches to analyzing resting state data (e.g., independent component analysis, and the seed correlation approach), one would mainly find those regions located in the default mode network. We conclude that persistency in BOLD responses as measured by the ICC index is an important indicator of temporal behaviors in fMRI experiments.

The asymptotic theory supporting reliability maps need not require a large number of scan volumes or any stationarity assumption. In our experience, the procedure works well in datasets involving two runs with 160 scan volumes each. In clinical studies involving patients, the number of experimental replicates might be small (a few runs), and the reliability maps would support information on functional distortions in task execution, especially for those decreased responses in Figure 5. Although the k-mean methods can be applied directly to image data without using reliability maps, those clusters of larger size may give ambiguous response patterns for each subject. As was mentioned, nonpersistency might suggest random noise or transient BOLD responses. In event-related experiments with long-term stimuli, there might be several kinds of transient responses occurring in each trial with different onset times. For example, novelty in perceived images may depend on the order of stimulus presentation. The proposed reliability analysis procedure can only assess those temporal behaviors that regularly occur across trials and runs, which could be the major limitation of the procedure.

8. Conclusion

There have been an increasing number of event-related fMRI studies in cognitive, psychological, and medical research. The procedure for constructing reliability maps is proposed mainly for experiments using event-related designs involving a relatively longer stimulus trial. Its potential use is not limited to event-related designs, however. The method had successfully identified reliable regions in a block-design experiment with two runs involving alternate blocks of high- and low-load working memory tasks. Reliability maps suggest stable temporal behaviors in the experimental session that vary between brain regions among individual subjects. Reliability maps would assist researchers to select ROIs for further analysis, or to insert the obtained response functions into GLM for testing stimulus and task effects. In clinical studies with a small number of replicates, reliability maps can assist for detecting functional disorders in the brain for each individual patient. We conclude that the proposed procedure would support a stream of research probing more complicated BOLD responses in fMRI studies such as the early-onset mechanism in the change detection task.

9. Acknowledgment

The authors are indebted to the fMRIDC at the University of California, Santa Barbara for supporting the data sets analyzed in this study. This research was supported by grants NSC98-2410-H-001-012-MY3 and NSC099-2811-H-001-004 from the National Science Council, Taiwan.

10. References

Aguirre, G. K.; Zarahn, E. & D'Esposito, M. (1998). The variability of human BOLD hemodynamic responses. *NeuroImage*, Vol.8, No.4, (November 1998), pp. 360-369, ISSN 1053-8119

Aron, A. R.; Gluck, M. A. & Poldrack, R. A. (2006). Long-term test-retest reliability of functional MRI in a classification learning task. *NeuroImage*, Vol.29, No.3, (February 2006), pp. 1000-1006, ISSN 1053-8119

Bandettini, P. A.; Jesmanowicz A.; Wong E. C. & Hyde J. S. (1993). Processing strategies for time-course data sets in functional MRI of the human brain. *Magnetic Resonance in Medicine*, Vol.30, No.2, (August 1993), pp. 161 - 173, ISSN 1522-2594

Biswal, B.; DeYoe, E. & Hyde, J. (1996). Reduction of physiological fluctuations in fMRI using digital filters. *Magnetic Resonance in Medicine*, Vol.35, No.1, (January 1996), pp. 107-113, ISSN 1522-2594

Boynton, G. M.; Engel, S. A.; Glover, G. H. & Heeger, D. J. (1996). Linear systems analysis of fMRI in human V1. *Journal of Neuroscience*, Vol.16, No.13, (July 1996), pp. 4207-4221, ISSN 0270-6474

Brennan, R. L. (2001). Generalizability theory. New York: *Springer Verlag*

Buxton, R. B. & Frank, L. R. (1997). A model for the coupling between cerebral blood flow and oxygen metabolism during neural stimulation. *Journal of Cerebral Blood Flow Metabolism*, Vol.17, pp. 64–72, ISSN 0271-678X

Chen, E. E. & Small, S. L. (2007). Test–retest reliability in fMRI of language: group and task effects. *Brain and Language*, Vol.102, No.2, (August 2007), 176–185, ISSN 0093-934X

Chumbley, J.; Worsley, K. J.; Flandin, G. & Friston, K. J. (2010). Topological FDR for neuroimaging. *NeuroImage*, Vol.49, No.4, (February 2010), pp. 3057-3064, ISSN 1053-8119

de Zwart, J. A.; Silva, A. C.; van Gelderen, P.; Kellman, P.; Fukunaga, M.; Chu, R.; Koretsky, A. P.; Frank, J. A. & Duyn, J. H. (2005). Temporal dynamics of the BOLD fMRI impulse response. *NeuroImage*, Vol.24, No.3, (February 2005), pp. 667–677, ISSN 1053-8119

Fernandez, G.; Specht, K.; Weis, S.; Tendolkar, I.; Reuber, M.; Fell, J.; Klaver, P.; Ruhlmann, J.; Reul, J. & Elger, C. E. (2003). Intrasubject reproducibility of presurgical language lateralization and mapping using fMRI. *Neurology*, Vol.60, No.6, (March 2003), pp. 969– 975, ISSN 0028-3878

Franco, A. R.; Pritchard, A.; Calhoun, V. D. & Mayer, A. R. (2009). Interrater and intermethod reliability of default mode network selection. *Human Brain Mapping*, Vol.30, No.7, (July 2009), pp. 2293–2303, ISSN 1097-0193

Friedman, L.; Stern, H.; Brown, G. G.; Mathalon, D. H.; Turner, J.; Glover, G. H.; Gollub, R. L.; Lauriello, J.; Lim, K. O.; Cannon, T.; Greve, D. N.; Bockholt, H. J.; Belger, A.; Mueller, B.; Doty, M. J.; He, J.; Wells, W.; Smyth, P.; Pieper, S.; Kim, S.; Kubicki, M.; Vangel, M. & Potkin, S. G. (2008). Test-retest and between-site reliability in a multicenter fMRI study. *Human Brain Mapping*, Vol.29, No.8, (August 2008), pp. 958-972, ISSN 1097-0193

Friston, K. J.; Josephs, O.; Rees, G. & Turner, R. (1998). Nonlinear event-related responses in fMRI. *Magnetic Resonance in Medicine*, Vol.39, No.1, (January 1998), pp. 41-52, ISSN 1522-2594

Friston, K. J.; Mechelli, A.; Turner, R. & Price, C. J. (2000). Nonlinear responses in fMRI: The Balloon model, Volterra kernels and other hemodynamics. *NeuroImage*, Vol.12, No.4, (October 2000), pp. 466-477, ISSN 1053-8119

Friston, K. J.; Penny, W.; Phillips, C.; Kiebel, S.; Hinton, G. & Ashburner, J. (2002). Classical and Bayesian inference in neuroimaging: Theory. *NeuroImage*, Vol.16, No.2, (June 2002), pp. 465-483, ISSN 1053-8119

Genovese, C. R.; Noll, D. C. & Eddy, W. F. (1997). Estimating test-retest reliability in functional MR imaging I: Statistical methodology. *Magnetic Resonance in Medicine*, Vol.38, No.3, pp. 497-507, ISSN 1053-8119

Genovese, C. R.; Lazar, N. A. & Nichols, T. (2002). Thresholding of statistical maps in functional neuroimaging using the false discovery rate. *NeuroImage*, Vol.15, No.4, (April 2002), pp. 870-878, ISSN 1053-8119

Glover, G. H. (1999). Deconvolution of impulse response in event-related BOLD fMRI. *NeuroImage*, Vol.9, No.4, (April 1999), pp. 416–29, ISSN 1053-8119

Gu, Y. & Pagnoni, G. (2008). A unified framework for group independent component analysis for multi-subject fMRI data. *NeuroImage*, Vol.42, No.3, (September 2008), pp. 1078-1093, ISSN 1053-8119

Gullapalli, R. P.; Maitra, R.; Roys, S.; Smith, G.; Alon, G., & Greenspan, J. (2005). Reliability Estimation of grouped functional imaging data using penalized maximum likelihood. *Magnetic Resonance in Medicine*, Vol.53, No.5, (May 2005), pp. 1126–1134, ISSN 1053-8119

Handwerker, D.; Ollinger, J. & D'Esposito M. (2004). Variation of BOLD hemodynamic responses across subjects and brain regions and their effects on statistical analyses. *NeuroImage*, Vol.21, No.4, (April 2004), pp. 1639–1651, ISSN 1053-8119

Hasson, U.; Malach, R. & Heeger, D. J. (2010). Reliability of cortical activity during natural stimulation. *Trends in Cognitive Sciences*, Vol.14, No.1, (December 2009), pp. 40-48, ISSN 1364-6613

Henderson, H. V. & Searle, S. R. (1979). Vec and Vech operators for matrices, with some uses in Jacobians and multivariate statistics. *The Canadian Journal of Statistics*, Vol.7, No.1, pp. 65-81, ISSN 0319-5724

Hochberg, Y. & Tamhane, A. C. (1987). Multiple Comparison Procedures. New York: *John Wiley*, ISBN 978-0471470151

Huettel, S. A., Guzeldere, G., & McCarthy, G. (2001). Dissociating neural mechanisms of visual attention in change detection using functional MRI. *Journal of Cognitive Neuroscience*, Vol.13, No.7, (October 2001), pp. 1006-1018, ISSN 0898-929X

Josephs, O.; Turner, R. & Friston, K. J. (1997). Event-Related fMRI, *Human Brain Mapping*, Vol.5, No.4, pp. 243-248, ISSN 1097-0193

Landis, J. R. & Koch, G. G. (1977). The measurement of observer agreement for categorical data. *Biometrics*, Vol.33, No.1, (March 1977), pp. 159-174, ISSN 0006-341X

Lange, N. & Zeger, S. L. (1997). Non-linear fourier time series analysis for human brain mapping by functional magnetic resonance imaging (with discussion). *Applied Statistics*, Vol.46, No.1, pp. 1-29, ISSN 1467-9876

Langers, D. R.; Jansen, J. F. & Backes, W. H. (2007). Enhanced signal detection in neuroimaging by means of regional control of the global false discovery rate. *NeuroImage*, Vol.38, No.1, (October 2007), pp. 43-56, ISSN 1053-8119

Lindquist, M. A.; Meng Loh J.; Atlas, L. Y. & Wager, T. D. (2009). Modeling the hemodynamic response function in fMRI: efficiency, bias and mis-modeling. *NeuroImage*, Vol.45, No.1, Suppl.1, (March 2009), pp. S187-198, ISSN 1053-8119

Liou M. (1989). A note on reliability estimation for a test with components of unknown functional length. *Psychometrika*, Vol.54, No.1, (March 1989), pp. 153-163, ISSN 0033-3123

Lucke, J. F. (2005). The α and the ω of congeneric test theory: An extension of reliability and internal consistency to heterogeneous tests. *Applied Psychological Measurement*, Vol.29, No.1, (January 2005), pp. 65-81, ISSN 1552-3888

MacQueen, J. (1967). Some methods for classification and analysis of multivariate observations. *Proceedings of 5th Berkeley Symposium on Mathematical Statistics and Probability*, Vol.1, pp. 281-297, Berkeley, Calif.: University of California Press, 1967, ISSN 0097-0433

Maitra, R. (2009). Assessing certainty of activation or inactivation in test-retest fMRI studies. NeuroImage, Vol.47, No.1, (August 2009), pp. 88-97, ISSN 1053-8119.

Maitra, R.; Roys, S. R. & Gullapalli, R. P. (2002). Test–retest reliability estimation of functional MRI data. *Magnetic Resonance in Medicine*, Vol.48, No.1, (July 2002), pp. 62–70, ISSN 1053-8119

Manoach, D. S.; Halpern, E. F.; Kramer, T. S.; Chang, Y.; Goff, D. C. & Rauch, S. L. (2001). Test–retest reliability of a functional MRI working memory paradigm in normal and schizophrenic subjects. *American Journal of Psychiatry*, Vol.158, No.6, (June 2001), pp. 955–958, ISSN 1535-7228

McDonald, R. P. (1999). Test theory: A unified approach. Mahwah, NJ: Lawrence Erlbaum, ISBN 0805830758

McGraw, K. & Wong, S. (1996). Forming inferences about some intraclass correlation coefficients. *Psychological Methods*, Vol.1, No.1, (March 1996), pp. 30–46, ISSN 1082-989X

McNamee, R. L. & Lazar, N. A. (2004). Assessing the sensitivity of fMRI group maps. *NeuroImage*, Vol.22, No.2, (June 2004), pp. 920-931, ISSN 1053-8119

Miezin, F. M.; Maccotta, L.; Ollinger, J. M.; Petersen, S. E. & Buckner, R. L. (2000). Characterizing the hemodynamic response: Effects of presentation rate, sampling procedure, and the possibility of ordering brain activity based on relative timing. *NeuroImage*, Vol.11, No.6, (June 2000), pp. 735-759, ISSN 1053-8119

Neumann, J.; Lohmann, G.; Zysset, S. & von Cramon, D. Y. (2003). Within-subject variability of BOLD response dynamics. *NeuroImage*, Vol.19, No.3, (July 2003), pp. 784-796, ISSN 1053-8119

Nichols, T. & Hayasaka, S. (2003). Controlling the familywise error rate in functional neuroimaging: a comparative review. *Statistical Methods in Medical Research*, Vol.12, No.5, (October 2003), pp. 419-446, ISSN 0962-2802

Noll, D. C.; Genovese, C. R.; Nystrom, L. E.; Vazquez, A. L.; Forman, S. D.; Eddy, W. F. & Cohen, J. D. (1997). Estimating test–retest reliability in functional MR imaging: II. Application to motor and cognitive activation studies. *Magnetic Resonance in Medicine*, Vol.38, No.3, (September 1997), pp. 508–517, ISSN 1053-8119

Obata, T.; Liu, T. T.; Miller, K. L.; Luh, W. M.; Wong, E. C.; Frank, L. R. & Buxton, R. B. (2004). Discrepancies between BOLD and flow dynamics in primary and supplementary motor areas: Application of the Balloon model to the interpretation of BOLD transients. *NeuroImage*, Vol.21, No.1, (January 2004), pp. 144–153, ISSN 1053-8119

Peligrad, M. (1996). On the asymptotic normality of sequences of weak dependent random variables. *Journal of Theoretical Probability*, Vol.9, No.3, (July 1996), 703-715, ISSN 1572-9230

Raemaekers, M.; Vink, M.; Zandbelt, B.; van Wezel, R. J. A.; Kahn, R. S. & Ramsey, N. F. (2007). Test–retest reliability of fMRI activation during prosaccades and antisaccades. *NeuroImage*, Vol.36, No.3, (July 2007), pp. 532–542, ISSN 1053-8119

Sirotin, Y. B.; Das, A. (2009). Anticipatory haemodynamic signals in sensory cortex not predicted by local neuronal activity. Nature, 457, (January 2009), pp. 475-479, ISSN 0028-0836

Specht, K.; Willmes, K.; Shah, N. J. & Jancke, L. (2003). Assessment of Reliability in functional imaging studies. *Journal of Magnetic Resonance Imaging*, Vol.17, No.4, (April 2003), pp. 463–471, ISSN 1522-2586

Stephan, K. E.; Weiskopf, N.; Drysdale, P. M.; Robinson, P. A. & Friston, K. J. (2007). Comparing hemodynamic models with DCM. *NeuroImage*, Vol.38, No.3, (November 2007), pp. 387–401, ISSN 1053-8119

Strother, S.; LaConte, S.; Hansen, L. K.; Anderson, J.; Zhang, J.; Pulapura, S. & Rottenberg, D. (2004). Optimizing the fMRI data-processing pipeline using prediction and reproducibility performance metrices: I. A preliminary group analysis. *NeuroImage*, Vol.23, Suppl.1, (2004), pp. S196-S207, ISSN 1053-8119

Varoquaux, G.; Sadaghiani, S.; Pinel, P.; Kleinschmidt, A.; Poline, J. B. & Thirion, B. (2010). A group model for stable multi-subject ICA on fMRI datasets. *NeuroImage*, Vol.51, No.1, (May 2010), pp. 288-299, ISSN 1053-8119

Worsley, K. J. (1996). The geometry of random images, *Chance*, Vol.9, No.1, pp. 27-40, ISSN 0933-2480

Worsley, K. J.; Liao, C. H.; Aston, J.; Petre, V.; Duncan, G. H.; Morales, F. & Evans, A. C. (2002). A general statistical analysis for fMRI data. *NeuroImage*, Vol.15, No.1, (January 2002), pp. 1-15, ISSN 1053-8119

Worsley, K. J.; Marrett, S.; Neelin, P.; Vandal, A. C.; Friston, K. J. & Evans, A. C. (1996). A unified statistical approach for determining significant signals in images of cerebral activation. *Human Brain Mapping*, Vol.4, No.1, 58–73, ISSN 1097-0193

Yang, Y. & Green, S. B. (2010). A note on structural equation modeling estimates of reliability. *Structural Equation Modeling*, Vol.17, No.1, (January 2010), pp. 66-81, ISSN 1070-5511

Zuo, X. N.; Kelly, C.; Adelstein, J. S.; Klein, D. F.; Castellanos, F. X. & Milham, M. P. (2010). Reliable intrinsic connectivity networks: Test-retest evaluation using ICA and dual regression approach. *NeuroImage*, Vol.49, No.3, (February 2010), pp. 2163-2177, ISSN 1053-8119

8

Language Reorganization After Stroke: Insights from fMRI

Vanja Kljajevic
Instituto Gerontológico Matia
Spain

1. Introduction

As one of the most complex brain functions and a uniquely human mental faculty, language has a special status in brain sciences. Issues on language functioning have been investigated from various perspectives, including language acquisition in a developing brain, language dissolution in damaged brain, language processing in neurologically healthy adult speakers of one, two, or more languages, and so on. However, the neural substrates of language were not investigated in a great detail until the recent advancement of neuroimaging techniques. One reason for this situation is the fact that animal studies, which have considerably contributed to the growth of knowledge in other domains of brain sciences, are not an option when studying language. Until recently, most of our knowledge on the language-brain relationship came from lesion-deficit studies. Since naturally occurring focal cortical lesions, such as those found in stroke patients, rarely affect a single brain function and—in addition to cortically often run cortico-subcortically, it was difficult before the advancement of neuroimaging technologies to determine how the complex functionality of language relates with brain structures. Nevertheless, studying the neural underpinnings of language in patients with language disorders caused by illness or brain injury resulted in important observations and development of a theoretical framework in the 19th century (e.g., Broca, 1861) that led to a formulation of the fundamental research questions in this field that are still object of scientific inquiry. The lesion-deficit approach originated in the work of Broca, Wernicke, and Leichtheim in the 19th century, and was re-established and further developed by Geschwind, Galaburda, Goodglass, Kaplan, Kertesz and their students in the 20th century. This neurological or aphasiological model correlated language disorders and brain lesions, with the goal of explaining the effects of lesion on language performance and by extension the neural basis of language. In general, it mostly employed crude language concepts, such as speech production, comprehension, fluent vs. non-fluent speech, etc., without considering insights from linguistics. The situation dramatically changed with the development of generative grammar (Chomsky, 1957, and subsequent work) which postulates that language is a *mental organ* and that grammar is a theory of language, which is structured in a modular way and *somehow* instantiated in the brain (Chomsky, 1986). The generative paradigm turned out to be a productive theoretical approach in linguistics that has led to development of sophisticated theories, motivating a great deal of neuroimaging research on language.

Some basic ideas of the lesion-deficit approach have been questioned in light of new evidence from neuroimaging. For instance, the idea that there exist specific language-dedicated areas, such as Broca's area (Brodmann areas (BAs) 44, 45) and Wernicke's area (BA 22) that support language production and comprehension respectively, and that damage to either area, or to the white matter fibre tract that connects them—the arcuate fasciculus—, leads to specific aphasic syndromes (Ardilla, 2010) turned out to be at best an oversimplification (Hickok & Poeppel, 2004). The causal link between a lesion and specific behaviour, which has often been pointed out as the key feature of the model, appears to be misleading, because it is not possible to establish only on the bases of lesion whether the deficit is due to damage to a mechanism housed at the lesion site or due to damage to the connections passing through the site (Green & Price, 2001). Further complication of this issue is brought about by the facts that lesioned area may retain some functional capacity, that sometimes areas that are not close to the lesion site react to lesion by producing abnormal responses, and that "redundant" areas may take over the function that was previously supported by the lesioned area. In addition, this approach misses a difference between the areas that have a better blood supply and thus may be more resilient to damage, and other areas. It appears that we cannot specify all the areas supporting a specific task based on a lesion in the brain (Price, 2000; Green & Price, 2001). Regardless, lesion-deficit studies have enabled valuable insights into the brain-behavior relationship that secured this method a unique status in brain sciences. The basic framework has been modified over time to include methods, models, and formalities from other disciplines, such as experimental psychology, cognitive science, computational approaches (Chatterjee, 2005), and since recently it has been strongly affected by neuroimaging.

Functional neuroimaging techniques such as Positron Emission Tomography (PET) and functional Magnetic Resonance Imaging (fMRI) have the capacity to fully specify areas supporting a specific task with a spatial resolution of 5-10 mm, revealing (relative) functional specializations of particular brain areas. The main contribution of functional neuroimaging to studying language is the insight that language is not a unified phenomenon and that in fact it is supported by many brain areas (Kutas et al., 2000; Price, 2010). A "single" language function, such as auditory comprehension, typically involves a complex of linguistic computations and representations that are carried out by cognitive subsystems supported by an extensive network of cortical brain areas and white matter pathways. For instance, the phonological subsystem supporting auditory comprehension activates certain temporal areas as well as the dorsal region of Brodmann area (BA) 44. The semantic level of auditory comprehension is also distributed; e.g., passive listening activates temporal region BA 22/42 bilaterally, while other semantic tasks may activate left BA 47, BA 45/46 and BA 44 (Friederici, 1998). The syntactic subsystem, which too contributes to auditory comprehension, is supported by Broca's area (BAs 44, 45), the angular gyrus (BA 39), the supramarginal gyrus (BA 40), the superior temporal gyrus (BA 22), involving also the white matter structures, such as the basal ganglia (Kutas et al., 2000; Caplan et al., 2000). The auditory language comprehension network further depends on the functional connectivity between the areas, in particular the white matter pathways such as the inferior occipito-frontal fasciculus, the arcuate fasciculus, and the middle and inferior longitudinal fasciculi (Turken & Dronkers, 2011). Since auditory sentence comprehension depends on memory and attention, the hippocampal, medial temporal, and frontal lobe structures that support memory, and the parietal lobe, which is implicated in attention, also contribute to language processing (Kutas et al., 2000).

However, language is even more complex than what postulating the basic linguistic levels such as phonetics/phonology, morphology, syntax, semantics and discourse typically entails. Evidence from aphasia suggests that, for instance, certain aspects of syntax may be impaired with other syntactic aspects being spared in the same patient, which indicates that analyses of language at a much finer level of granularity are needed. In order to investigate language in the brain at a finer level, researchers used a variety of methodologies to study components of the linguistic levels, such as processing of syntactic movement of sentential elements, and storage and manipulation of traces left behind the moved elements (e.g., Grodzinsky, 2000; Fiebach et al., 2001, 2002). Activation in the left inferior frontal gyrus, for example, was reported for both a specific syntactic operation that moves elements in a sentence, *syntactic movement* (Grodzinsky, 2000; Ben-Shachar et al., 2003, 2004), and for an aspect of working memory (WM) that has been claimed to support exclusively syntactic processing, *syntactic WM* (Fiebach et al., 2001). Intra- and inter-sentential processes are so intricate that it may not be possible for neuroimaging or as a matter of fact any other current method in the brain sciences to fully capture their temporal and spatial dynamics at the level of analysis they require, allowing reliable conclusions on the principles of cerebral organization of language (Poeppel & Embick, 2005; Pulvermüller, 2010). Thus, methodological refinements that will better align research on the neural basis of language with the developments in theoretical linguistics are much needed.

Following the realization that language is more distributed in the brain than previously thought and that there may not be one-to-one mappings between specific brain areas and language tasks (e.g., speech production, comprehension), the focus has recently shifted from the search for highly specialized "language areas" to efforts to capture the spatial and temporal dynamics of language as a distributed function. An example of model that is anchored in this view, which incorporates insights from lesion-deficit studies, neuroimaging, and electrophysiological studies, is the dual-stream model of speech production and comprehension (Hickok & Poeppel, 2000, 2007). According to this model, language is functionally realized via two broad *streams of processing*, the dorsal and ventral streams. Namely, cortical speech processing begins with a spectrotemporal analysis supported by auditory cortices in both hemispheres. Thus computed information moves to the phonological network in the middle to posterior portion of the superior temporal sulcus, where there is a slight left hemisphere (LH) bias for processing involving phonological processes and representations. From this point, information moves via the dorsal stream, which is strongly left-lateralized and supports auditory-motor integration in speech processing, and the ventral stream, which is bilateral with a slight LH bias and supports auditory comprehension. In other words, the dorsal stream maps phonological representations onto articulatory motor representations, and the ventral stream maps them onto lexical conceptual representations. The dorsal stream in its posterior part involves a portion of the Sylvian fissure at the parietal-temporal boundary, supporting the sensory-motor interface; its anterior portion in the frontal lobe includes Broca's area and its vicinity, while its more dorsal premotor component "corresponds to the portions of the articulatory network" (Hickok & Poeppel, 2007, p. 395). The ventral stream in its posterior portion (posterior middle and inferior portions of the temporal lobes) supports linking of phonological and semantic information (the lexical interface), while its more anterior areas support the combinatorial network.

In addition to capturing the differences in the respective functional anatomies of the two processing streams, the dual-stream model also aligns research on language with the recent developments in cognitive neuroscience that seek to establish a broader understanding of *what* and *where* of the processes in the brain. For instance, according to recent research on vision, audition, and the visuomotor system, sensory-motor integration and spatial stimuli processing are carried by a dorsal stream, while stimuli perception and recognition are carried by the ventral stream (Saur et al., 2008). To put it differently, the two processing streams support different types of computations in the brain regardless of the domain, including language. What is in particular interesting about this model is not only its distributed and dynamic nature, but also its ability to incorporate *interface* components of language functioning. This is an important feature that brings the model closer to the theories on human cognitive architecture that postulate existence of *integrative* and *interface* modules (e.g., Jackendoff, 1997, 2002), providing the neural basis to cognitive interface modules. More importantly for our purposes, the two pathways for language postulated by the dual stream model capture language processing in neurologically intact brain—at least in tasks prototypical for each of the streams (Saur et al., 2008) and account for aphasic syndromes (Hickok & Poeppel, 2004).

In order to further illustrate the role of fMRI in language research, with a particular regard to language reorganization after stroke, we will next address the concept of explanatorily significant progress in cognitive neuroscience, against which contribution of fMRI to post-stroke aphasia research will be discussed. Then, we will focus on issues such as aphasia, patterns of aphasic deficits, and the brain's potential to adapt to lesions causing aphasia. We will conclude the chapter discussing some methodological challenges in using fMRI to study post-stroke aphasia and questions for future research.

1.1 Neuroimaging: Towards *explanatorily significant progress*?

The impact of neuroimaging on language studies and its contribution to our understanding of the language-brain relationship has recently been challenged in light of the findings indicating that in addition to supporting a particular language function, a single brain area may be activated in tasks that are not language related (Hickok & Poeppel, 2005; Fedorenko & Kanwisher, 2009; Pulvermüller, 2010). Hickok and Poeppel (2005) argue that, despite the large number of published neuroimaging studies that address various aspects of the question of how language is instantiated in the brain, the progress has not been *explanatorily significant*. For instance, neuroimaging reveals that Broca's area, which was traditionally defined as a "classical language area", supports various tasks related to memory, music (e.g., Maess et al., 2001; Patel, 2003), calculation, object manipulation (Binkofski et al., 2004), motor imagery (Binkofski et al., 2000), perception of meaningful but not meaningless sequences of hand and mouth actions (Fadiga et al., 2006a, Fadiga et al., 2006b), time perception, rhythmic perception, processing of complex geometric patterns (Fink et al., 2006), prediction of sequential patterns, and so on.

When a single area is associated with a variety of tasks, it is important to understand whether the activation of that area during a specific task reflects that the area in question is necessary for the task or whether it perhaps reflects strategies used to optimize performance on the task (Price, 2000). In case of Broca's area, growing number of neuroimaging studies report activation in this area, without providing a principal explanation of how it contributes to the functionality across domains. Several proposals have been put forth to explain the rich functionality of Broca's area. For example, it has been proposed that it supports: (a) selection of information from competing sources (Thompson-Schill, 2005), (b) a broader cognitive control function (Novick et al., 2005, 2010), (c) language specific linearization of hierarchical language dependencies (Grewe et al., 2005), (d) processing of hierarchical dependencies like those found in language and musical syntax (Opitz & Friederici, 2007), to mention a few.

Despite the current lack of consensus on the role of Broca's area in a variety of tasks involving cognition, perception, and action, the fact is that evidence from neuroimaging has enabled insights about the involvement of this area in various types of processing, helping to reveal some widely accepted misconceptions on this intriguing brain area. As an example, building on some earlier CT findings, structural MRI has established that the brain area that Pierre Paul Broca pointed out as probably responsible for the speech loss in his historic patients Leborne and Lelong in the 1860s does not actually coincide with what we call today "Broca's area" (Dronkers et al., 2007). Together with structural and other functional neuroimaging methods as well as with new observer-independent methods of cytoarchitectonic analysis (Amunts et al, 1999, 2003), fMRI has created a new picture of this area. Further, functional MRI and PET evidence supports the view that damage to Broca's area is neither sufficient nor necessary to induce Broca's aphasia and that, in contrast to the previously held belief on the existence of functionally highly-specialized language areas, there may be no brain areas that are dedicated *exclusively* to specific language functions.

When it comes to the fact that an impressive amount of data on a specific brain area does not necessarily translate into explanatorily significant progress, Broca's area is not an exception. A large body of evidence indicates that the extrastriate body area (EBA) and the fusiform body area (FBA) also support variety of tasks (Downing & Peelen, *in press*). There is currently little understanding of their roles in these tasks, and in particular their roles in across-domains information binding remains unclear. Downing & Peelen (*in press*) have proposed that the body areas in the occipitotemporal cortex (OTC) do not actually support processing of the body itself (as a category), but rather its shape and posture (that is, its features), forming a perceptual network that supports processing in other cortical systems. Further examples of relative functional specialization of brain areas and distribution of function pertain to the case of action and action words. For instance, verbs *lick*, *pick*, and *kick* activate not only the brain areas that are typically engaged in processing of words and concepts; they also activate the areas that support realization of actions to which these words refer. In a recent fMRI study Hauk and colleagues (2004) have shown that tongue movements were associated with the activation of the premotor areas posterior to the inferior frontal area typically activated by face-related words, and overlapping activations in the motor cortex were found for arm-related words and finger movements, and for leg-related words and foot movements. In another fMRI study, Orlov and colleagues (2010) found consistent segregated activations within the OTC for five different visually presented categories of body parts, such as the upper face, lower face, upper limbs, trunk, and the lower limbs. More importantly, the OTC was a site where the visual information converged with the information on these categories from the motor domain. What is interesting about these findings is not only the triple dissociation in the neural support of the mentioned cases of verb category (Hauk et al., 2004), or the evidence on which particular area of OTC supports which body-part category (Orlov et al., 2010), but rather the insight on how the cortical language and action systems in the former case, and vision and the motor system in the latter case, contribute to the human conceptual combinatorics. It appears that regardless of the domain (e.g., words vs. actions, visual perception vs. movement) certain features of an object are selected, combined, and arranged into configurations that can be accessed by mechanisms supported by different brain areas. Furthermore, activations in the OTC have also been reported in congenitally blind participants in tasks involving tactile stimuli, Braille reading, and imagery of object shapes when canonical sounds of these objects were presented (Mahon et al., 2009).

Another interesting finding comes from Chen and Zeki's (2011) fMRI study in which, adopting Kant's distinction between inherited concepts, such as time and space, and acquired ones, such as artifacts, the authors investigated whether different brain mechanisms support processing of inherited (e.g., faces) versus acquired concepts (e.g., chairs). In addition to the evidence for an "overlapping and segregated system for object representation" (p. 9) in the ventral visual cortex, they also found a fronto-parietal activation associated with violation of the inherited concepts that was not found when deformed artifacts were presented. Based on these findings, they conclude that the distinction between the two categories is neurally supported and that there may exist a hard-wired preference for processing of certain features of objects. Taking these findings into account, one could wonder whether features associated with body shape and posture could also be hard-wired in some sense. Bodies and faces provide important cues on identity of others (Peelen & Downing, 2007). Given that meaning in humans is highly systemic, it is possible that selection and extraction of such specific cues from the visual stimuli is neurally specified to the OTC areas. Thus, the body areas in OTC may form a part of an *interface* which, by extracting information on specific features of stimuli, enables the conceptual network to select, combine, and arrange these features into interpretable configurations. An important step towards explanatorily significant progress in this research area will be to explain how the perceptual network interfaces with a distributed conceptual network.

We can conclude that, although a principled explanation of brain areas with rich functionality, such as Broca's area and OTC, is currently lacking, the accumulating knowledge about these areas is valuable in itself as it continues to clarify issues on the brain-behaviour relationship. It has led to a revision of the traditional conceptualization of an intriguing area, such as Broca's, as well as to appreciation of the complex nature of functional segregations within OTC. Research on both brain areas also exemplifies how methodological advancements in neuroimaging have contributed to the growth of knowledge on brain's functionality.

Debates among researchers who study the neural correlates of language go beyond the functionality of Broca's area and the question of existence of brain areas supporting exclusively language vs. possibly having multiple relative specializations (e.g., Fedorenko and Kanwisher, 2009; Grodzinsky, 2010; Pulvermüller, 2010), and extend to issues such as neuroplasticity in developing and injured brains, brain's potential for language reorganization after injury, and the role of hemispheric specialization in such processes. Studying these issues holds a key to better understanding of not only language in the brain, but also human cognitive architecture more generally.

2. fMRI of post-stroke aphasia

Establishing potential for long-term recovery of language in post-stroke patients requires information on which neuroanatomical areas are damaged by a stroke, what the extent of damage is (Naeser & Palumbo, 1994), and with which areas is the remaining functionality associated (Price, 2000). Having this information as early as possible allows patients with poor prediction of recovery to sooner enroll in non-verbal treatment programs that may improve their communication abilities, and patients with good prediction of recovery to early begin intensive behavioral or stimulation interventions specifically designed to optimize their recovery of language.

While structural neuroimaging can provide important insights on changes in the brain structures after a stroke, functional neuroimaging is essential in deriving predictions on recovery based on the remaining functionality. As a matter of fact, one critical aspect of the progress in language-brain research enabled by neuroimaging methods pertains to the insights on neuroplasticity and the brain's ability to reorganize the function after injury. Neuroplasticity—or brain plasticity—is a term that refers to the brain's ability to adapt to change, be it environmental pressure, learning experience, or brain damage (Johansson, 2011). The ability of damaged brain to recover language depends on the type of damage, lesion site and size. Individual brain dynamics and factors such as intensity of speech therapy, involvement in social interaction and verbal communication outside the speech therapy setting, concomitant diagnoses such as depression as well as age, sex, and so on also affect one person's potential for recovery, leading to different individual results in recovery of stroke patients with similar lesions. These factors add up to such a large variability in recovery that a recent follow up study with first-ever stroke patients up to 90 days after stroke onset "failed to identify any prognostic factors" (Johansson, 2011, p. 152.).

A classic example of the brain differently adapting to different types of lesion is represented by low-grade gliomas vs. stroke. In the former case, the functionality is typically taken over by the surrounding areas (Desmurget et al., 2007), while in the latter case activations have been reported in both perilesional and contralesional areas. fMRI evidence also shows that smaller stroke lesions are typically associated with activations of perilesional areas, while larger stroke lesions induce activation of the homologue areas in the opposite hemisphere (Cao et al, 1999). Aligned with these findings are insights that a better language recovery is associated with the activations in the original network (Karbe et al., 1998). Functional language reorganization after stroke – and in particular the role of the right hemisphere (RH) in it – has been debated in the literature for several decades. Curiously, until recently the patterns of language recovery after stroke were typically studied in chronic aphasia (Cramer & Riley, 2008), where in fact reorganization has already taken place. In order to understand better the post-stroke reorganization of language processes, we need to study acute and subacute aphasia, focusing on the remaining functionality of the lesioned area(s) and new functionality of areas not typically recruited by a certain language task. Before we review the dynamics of language reorganization and recovery from aphasia, few remarks on aphasic language are in order.

2.1 Becoming a structure: Patterns of aphasic language

Aphasia is a language disorder caused by brain damage due to a stroke, traumatic brain injury, tumour, atrophy and other neurological conditions. Patterns of language deficits differ across various types of aphasia, depending mostly on the size and location of brain lesion. While there are numerous classifications of aphasias, all aphasic types can be roughly divided into non-fluent (such as Broca's aphasia, transcortical motor or global aphasia) and fluent aphasias (e.g., Wernicke's aphasia, anomic and transcortical sensory aphasia). Regardless of the type of aphasia or language of aphasic person, all aphasic speech is characterized by errors in use of grammar. As a general principle, more complex elements of a language paradigm are more vulnerable, while more frequent elements are more resistant to impairment (Paradis, 2001; Ulatowska et al., 2001). One way in which complexity may affect aphasic language abilities is reflected in these patients' efforts to simplify their speech output by choosing short, simple sentences, as found in non-fluent, agrammatic speakers, or by choosing random substitutions of items within a paradigm, as found in fluent, paragrammatic aphasic speakers. Further, agrammatic Broca's aphasics typically perform better on tasks involving nouns than on tasks involving verbs, which are grammatically more complex than nouns. In fact, verb deficit is among the main defining features of this type of aphasia: only a small number of verbs is typically found in spontaneous speech of these patients regardless of language. They typically omit auxiliaries (such as *is, will*), and either omit or substitute inflectional affixes (such as *–ed* in *walked*) (Miceli, Silveri, Villa & Caramazza, 1984; Menn & Obler, 1990; Hagiwara, 1995, Friedmann & Grodzinsky, 1997; Bastiaanse & Thompson, 2003; Burchert et al., 2005; Druks & Carroll, 2005; Diouny, 2007; Bastiaanse, 2008). It has been claimed that paragrammatic speakers, on the other hand, exhibit the opposite pattern, performing better on tasks involving verbs than those with nouns, and making semantic errors and circumlocutions in production of critical forms (Druks, 2002).

Another often reported feature of Broca's aphasia is a specific pattern of sentence comprehension: these patients comprehend sentences such as (1)-(3) above chance, while their comprehension of noncanonical sentences, such as (4)-(6), is at chance (Caramazza & Zurif, 1976; Hickok et al., 1993; Mauner et al., 1993; Grodzinsky et al., 1999, Grodzinsky, 2000).

Canonical sentences:

1. The girl kissed the boy (active),
2. The girl that kissed the boy is tall (subject-relative),
3. It was the girl that kissed the boy (subject cleft).

Non-canonical sentences:

4. The boy was kissed by the girl (passive),
5. The boy that the girl kissed is shy (relative),
6. It was the boy that the girl kissed (cleft).

Apart from these general features, patterns of impairment of aphasic speech production and comprehension differ in structurally different languages in ways that reflect specific features of particular languages. Better understanding of cross-linguistic differences in patterns of aphasic language is important for development of theories capable of accounting for data across languages as well as for designing treatments usable in languages that are less studied than English. For instance, omission of articles (*a, an, the*) is typical for English speaking aphasics, whereas this is not an option in languages that do not have articles, such as Croatian. Similarly, in highly inflected languages such as Slavic, bound morphemes (e.g. *-ed* in *walked*) cannot be omitted, because that would result in nonwords; instead, bound morphemes are substituted. Since languages such as English allow omission of bound morphemes, patterns of aphasic deficit in English-speaking aphasics differ from patterns of aphasic speakers of languages structurally different from English.

Cross-linguistic differences in aphasic patterns are found not only at the word level, but also at the sentence-level. As an example, Ardila (2001) found that the comprehension strategies in Spanish speaking Broca's aphasics differed from the patterns found in English speaking Broca's aphasics. The reported differences in the patterns of aphasic performance reflect structural differences between the two languages, with English-speaking aphasics relying on word-order strategies, and Spanish-speaking aphasics relying on morphosyntactic markers with high cue validity in this language. Similarly, Kljajevic and Murasugi (2010) have shown that, unlike English speaking Broca's aphasics, whose strategy was based on word order, Croatian aphasic speakers relied on case cueing as a strategy in comprehension of wh-structures when their comprehension was compromised. Case cueing as a strategy in Croatian is language-specific: Croatian has a free word order and marks semantic roles of elements in a sentence by morphological cases. In contrast, English has a strict word order and these roles are assigned to a word's position in a sentence. Thus, highly inflectional languages appear to support strategies that are not available in languages without rich morphology. More importantly for our purposes is that when different strategies are used in a particular task, the areas activated by the task may differ in patients with a lesion in the same brain area. This complicates interpretation of findings and prediction of recovery, making it difficult to understand whether such activations reflect language processes or compensation strategies (Sidtis, 2007). Differences in cognitive strategies used in a particular task represent a difficulty of the same order in fMRI research as individual anatomical and functional variability among aphasic patients (Zahn et al., 2006).

In addition to cross-linguistic variability in patterns of aphasia, individual differences in reacting to lesion, differences in speed of recovery, intensity and length of speech therapy, the degree of social involvement and communication outside speech therapy and so on also affect patterns of recovery in aphasic patients. Thus, it is important to study aphasia not only across structurally different languages, but also individually, taking into account individual differences in patients' potential for recovery and strategies enabled by the structural peculiarities of a particular language. In both cases, fMRI is an indispensible tool of investigation, neuroimaging assessment and neuroimaging-guided rehabilitation.

2.2 Grammatical category as the main organizing principle of language in the brain?

It has often been claimed that one hallmark of aphasic language is a double dissociation between verb and noun production in non-fluent vs. fluent aphasia, with a better production of verbs than nouns in fluent, and better production of nouns than verbs in non-fluent aphasia. The dissociation is interpreted as evidence of two different mechanisms supporting the two grammatical categories, with the left frontal lobe supporting verb production and the left temporal lobe supporting production of nouns. However, neuroimaging evidence on the neural substrates of verbs and nouns is heterogeneous (Perani et al, 1999; Tyler et al., 2001; Shapiro et al, 2006; Arévalo et al., 2007; Luzzatti et al., 2006), and even suggests that BAs 45 and 9 may support encoding of grammatical properties of words, regardless of the grammatical category. One could object that the heterogeneity of neuroimaging evidence may be due to the fact that verb processing is not a monolithic task, reflecting different aspects of verb processing. More direct evidence on a network of areas supporting verb category comes from research by Luzzatti and colleagues (2006): verb deficit in their aphasic participants was associated with the posterior temporo-parietal, fronto-temporal perisylvian, insular and basal ganglia lesions in the left hemisphere.

Luzzati et al.'s (2006) finding is consistent with the evidence that shows that an aphasia syndrome can have different localizations (Ardilla, 2010) as well as with the growing cross-linguistic evidence obtained in a variety of tasks that indicate that fluent aphasic speakers, too, have difficulty with verbs. Namely, fluent aphasic patients produce fewer verbs in spontaneous speech than neurologically intact speakers (Bastiaanse et al., 1996; Edwards, 2002; Kim & Leach, 2004) and exhibit problems with verb retrieval (Bastiaanse & Jonkers, 1998; Kambanaros, 2008), access to argument structure and thematic representation of verbs (Russo et al., 1998), finite verb inflection (Varlakosta et al., 2006), and time reference through verb forms (Kljajevic & Bastiaanse, 2011). Thus, verb deficit is present in aphasia regardless of whether the lesion causing the disorder is located in the anterior vs. posterior cortical areas, or whether it runs cortically or cortico-subcortically.

These findings indicate the need to focus on analysis of features, instead of grammatical categories as such, and the importance of considering findings from both lesion-deficit studies and functional MR imaging. Combining the two methods is crucial when studying aphasia, because each method has unique strengths and weaknesses. As pointed out in section 1, lesion-deficit studies may contribute information on which area is necessary for a specific function. However, they cannot tell us whether a deficit is caused by lesion to that specific site or to a network to which the area belongs (Price, 2000; Turken & Dronkers, 2011). Naturally occurring lesions are typically large, rarely affecting a single area, and complex in the sense that they affect more than one function. On the other hand, fMRI provides information on the remaining functionality of the injured tissue, involvement of other brain areas "taking over" the function, and the reorganization processes at work. However, due to the correlational nature of fMRI evidence, combining this method with lesion-deficit studies leads to strong evidence that a specific brain area supports a particular function.

2.3 fMRI of language deficits

One example of language deficits that occur in all types of aphasia is naming deficit. This deficit is typically tested in a naming task, where a patient is required to name visually presented objects or pictures of objects. While imaging overt speech is crucial for assessment of speech recovery in aphasic individuals, important insights on language recovery processes were obtained in fMRI studies that used the silent paradigm (Davies et al., 2006; Harnish et al., 2008). One problem related to using covert speech is that it prevents monitoring of task performance (Peck et al., 2004). In contrast, imaging overt speech allows analysis of accuracy and reaction times, which are important indicators of treatment effects in aphasia (Thompson & van Ouden, 2008). However, unlike silent paradigm, neuroimaging of overt aphasic speech is associated with challenges. Some of them are artifacts due to speaking and head movement and artifacts caused by jaw and tongue movements during articulation. Hearing and speech recording may also be difficult in such experiments, because of the scanner noise. In addition, non-fluent aphasic patients' speech may be difficult to transcribe, because it is typically hesitant, effortful, and characterized by many false starts. It is precisely the hesitant nature of aphasic speech and differences in timing of response output that make the block design a preferred choice over the event related design when assessing overt aphasic speech (Martin et al., 2005). The main advantage of using the block design is the possibility of collecting data during the silent period, which is enabled by the hemodynamic response delay. Using the block design during blood oxygenation level-dependent (BOLD) fMRI relies on "the temporal dynamics of the hemodynamic response delay where increased blood flow remains 4 or 8 seconds after the response", allowing data collection after the task and "during the silent period of no speech, minimizing motion artifact from overt speech" (Martin et al., 2005, p. 195).

The main assumption when choosing this method is that the hemodynamic response in aphasia patients is similar to that in controls. However, it has been pointed out in the literature that stroke affects blood flow, thereby affecting performance on cognitive tasks, even in patients whose infarcts were not in the cortex (Pineiro et al., 2002). Bonakdarpur and colleagues (2007) studied differences in a hemodynamic response function (HRF) in 5 post-stroke aphasic patients and 4 healthy individuals, focusing on Broca's area and the posterior perisylvian network (including Wernicke's area, the angular and supramarginal gyri), and RH homologues of these regions, plus the occipital area as a control area. The main finding of their study is a delay in time to peak in the left perisylvian area in 3 aphasic patients (up to 20 seconds after stimulus) that were not found in their left visual cortex, or in the same areas in the control subjects. This is an important finding, because "many fMRI studies with stroke patients use a canonical HRF for data analysis, peaking at about 6 seconds following a cognitive event", which makes it possible that these studies actually missed or underestimated activations (Thompson & den Ouden, 2008, p. 476). However, Peck and colleagues (2004) report decrease in TTP of the hemodynamic response in right auditory cortex, homologue of Broca's area, motor cortex and pre-suplementary motor area associated with improved performance on overt word generation tasks after a treatment of 3 aphasic patients. This indicates that TTP data contain valuable information on patients' response to treatment, because changes in TTP reflect changes in the amount of time that a patient spends on a task from presentation of stimulus to verbal response. Thus, fMRI can be used to evaluate speed of processing in perilesional areas and other areas of the brain that take over the function of injured area(s) (Peck et al., 2004). Additional challenges are fMRI signal variability in general (Bandettini, 2009) and possibly insufficient signal to noise ratio for BOLD signal detection in damaged areas in aphasic patients in particular (e.g., Bonakdarpour et al., 2007).

Since naming difficulties occur in all types of aphasia, they are in the focus of rehabilitation as well as neuroimaging research on recovery of language in aphasic patients. Other types of aphasic deficits have also been investigated by fMRI. In a recent study, Thompson et al. (2010) studied brain correlates of verb argument structure processing in aphasic patients and healthy elderly people. Verb processing critically depends on verb's argument structure. Aphasic patients, in particular non-fluent aphasics, have difficulty producing verbs with more complex argument structure. In an fMRI study with event-related design Thompson et al. (2010) have shown that aphasic patients exhibited the right hemispheric preference in processing verb argument structure while recruiting the spared tissue in the posterior language network. The activated brain areas were the same as those in the non-brain damaged control subjects; that is, argument structure processing typically activates bilateral posterior perisylvian region in healthy young and elderly subjects. Thus, activations in the RH in aphasic patients reflect recruitment of the spared tissue in this network.

Recently, Saur and colleagues (2006) have shown that the patterns of reorganization differ at distinct phases of language post-stroke recovery. They studied sentence comprehension in aphasic patients at three different time points: acute, subacute and chronic phase. The main finding of their study is that the acute phase is associated with little perilesional activation, the subacute phase is associated with activation of the right hemisphere homologous areas, while in the chronic phase a re-shifting of function to the left hemisphere language areas is associated with further language improvement. According to this model, activation of the right hemisphere areas in a chronic aphasic patient would indicate poor recovery. Saur et al.'s model of temporal dynamics of post-stroke language recovery opens some important questions: For instance, Why progress in language recovery after stroke seems to require changes in lateralization? Does this hold for both small and large lesions? Will the same pattern emerge when patients are tested on a different task?

Another recent functional MR imaging study focused on the brain's potential to reorganize syntax in post-stroke patients (Tyler et al., 2010). Syntax is believed to be strongly left-lateralized and the study set out to investigate the RH's capacity to take over syntactic processing following damage to the LH. The main finding of the study is that lesion in left BA 47/45 impaired syntax and resulted in decreased activity, while increased activation in the homologous RH areas did not result in better syntactic performance in their aphasic participants. Their findings indicate that the brain cannot reorganize syntax after injury to left BA 45/47 and that the capacity of RH to take over function critically depends on the type of language function. This is an important finding that sheds new light on the debate on the role of the non-dominant hemisphere in language recovery in damaged brain.

Hemispheric differences in specialization for language were first observed in the 1850s, when Broca and his contemporaries reported that LH damage was associated with aphasia more often than RH damage. This insight led to the conclusion that the LH is dominant or specialized for language (Josse & Tzourio-Mazoyer, 2004). Neuroimaging obviously opened new possibilities for investigation of hemispheric specialization for language—an issue of high importance for work with patients who suffered unilateral brain lesions. Functional neuroimaging methods including fMRI have recorded activations across different brain areas in both hemispheres associated with a variety of language tasks in patients ranging from mild to severe aphasia and at different temporal post-stroke points (acute, subacute, chronic), resulting in controversial evidence. Future research needs to address in more detail the role of contralesional areas in language recovery, in particular in acute and subacute phases, in studies with large number of patients and including variety of language tasks.

2.3.1 Imaging the bilingual post-stroke brain

With at least 50% of the world's population being bilingual (Weeks, 2010) and stroke as one of leading causes of disability worldwide, the issue of how brain damage affects patterns of aphasia in those who speak more than one language receives increasing attention among researchers. The term "bilingual aphasia" currently refers to aphasic speakers who were fluent in two languages (or dialects) before they had a stroke. Since bilingual aphasics do not necessarily exhibit the same type and extent of language deficit in both languages, researchers now agree that these patients should be assessed in both languages (Fabro, 2001). However, they do not agree on the question of in which language the patient should receive speech therapy (Abutalebi et al., 2009). Another hotly debated issue related to this topic is the cortical organization of two languages in a bilingual brain: Are different languages supported by different brain areas? Or are they supported by the same brain areas, sharing processing resources?

The neural basis of bilingual aphasia and its recovery patterns are still largely unknown (Paradis, 1987), which is not surprising given that it is not clear whether two languages of a healthy bilingual speaker are supported by the same or different brain areas. Research so far indicates that the most common patterns of recovery in bilingual aphasia are: (a) parallel recovery in both languages, (b) selective recovery, in which one language recovers over time while the other does not, and (c) successive recovery, in which both languages recover, with one of them improving before the other (Paradis, 1985). Variations within these patterns have also been observed, such as so-called alternating recovery (in which recovery of language A is followed by recovery of language B, which is associated with the loss of language A), alternating antagonistic recovery (in which alternations between spared A-lost B vs. lost A-spared B happen day after day), mixing of the two languages in speech production, etc. (Green, 2001). The variability in recovery patterns is so great that bilingual aphasia represents one point of research where progress was remarkably limited: "No correlation has been found between pattern of recovery and neurological, etiological, experiential or linguistic parameters: not site, size or origin of lesion, type or severity of aphasia, type of bilingualism, language structure type or factors related to acquisition or habitual use" (Paradis (1995, p. 211), cited in Green & Price (2001, p. 191)). Obviously, much more work needs to be done in this area in order to establish how the brain accommodates more than one language and how it mediates bilingual recovery.

Investigation of neural correlates of treatment by using functional neuroimaging is an important new perspective in research on bilingual aphasia. Functional neuroimaging is critical in this type of research, because it can provide information on functional reorganization in the brain that is not available through other methods (Meinzer et al., 2007; Green, 2008). For instance, in a longitudinal single case study, Abutalebi and colleagues (2009) used fMRI and dynamic causal modelling to investigate recovery of language in a Spanish-Italian bilingual aphasic speaker. They designed a treatment for naming deficit in their patient, JRC, who suffered from global aphasia, with anomia affecting equally both languages. Testing was done before a picture naming-based speech therapy, specifically designed to improve JRC's naming abilities, after the specific speech therapy, which took 6 weeks, and after the global speech therapy, which was administered over 4 months. The patient chose to rehabilitate his second language, Italian. The authors report improvement in picture naming, increased activations in the brain areas supporting naming as well as in the areas supporting language control processes, but no generalization of improvement to the language that was not treated—Spanish. Following the initial better L1 than L2 pattern, a reverse patter of better L2 than L1 due to speech therapy in L2 was observed, which was associated with worsening of performance on naming tasks in L1. Similarly, while in early post-stroke phase activations associated with performance in L1 and L2 were similar in location and extension, the specific speech in L2 was associated with language reorganization only on tasks in L2, which JRC fully recovered. Interestingly, the activation pattern reflecting behavioural improvement was similar to the language activation pattern in healthy bilinguals, with the left inferior frontal gyrus and the left fusiform gyrus supporting picture naming. Their findings on the role of control processes in recovery of language open the question of how to best manipulate these processes in neuroimaging-guided treatment of language disorders in bilingual speakers. Theoretically, the findings are relevant for the debate on whether treatment in one language inhibits overall recovery of both languages.

2.3.2 Imaging the impact of language training on post-stroke brain

After a stroke, spontaneous language recovery takes places during the first 6 to 12 months. It has been pointed out in the literature that it is difficult to disentangle whether changes in language behaviour result from the healing processes (diaschisis) or neuronal reorganization (Pulvermüller et al., 2005; Hillis, 2006). fMRI is an important research tool not only in investigation of spontaneous language recovery, but also in treatment-induced recovery (Crosson et al., 2010). For instance, it can map changes in brain functionality following a treatment to assess its effectiveness (Menzer et al., 2011). However, even though the field of rehabilitation neuroscience is growing, current understanding of how therapy affects language recovery is still limited (Cherney & Small, 2006), regardless of the importance of treatment effectiveness assessments in the acute and subacute post-stroke phases (Cramer & Riley, 2008). Research so far has shown that longitudinal fMRI of aphasic language is an effective tool for detection of changes in activation patterns (Saur et al., 2006) and activation magnitude (Meltzer et al., 2009) over time.

For instance, Vitali and colleagues (2007) used event-related fMRI design in a single-case study of two severe, chronic aphasic patients. They studied picture-naming performance before and after a phonological cueing training, and found improvement in naming of the trained sets of items, which did not generalize to the untrained materials. The neuroimaging findings from this study confirm that both types of processes are associated with improvement of the naming function: activations of the perilesional areas indicating restitution of function in the original network, and activations of the contralateral homologue areas, indicating compensation strategies at work. More importantly, the study indicates that improvement of function is possible even in chronic patients. One can hope that neuroimaging-guided rehabilitation practices represent a transition to a new paradigm of language rehabilitation that will become increasingly available in hospitals.

An important aspect of the use of fMRI in treatment-induced recovery of aphasia pertains to combining this method with transcranial magnetic and electrical stimulation to guide rehabilitation and enhance recovery (Devlin & Watkins, 2007; Naeser et al., 2005). As an electrical organ, the brain is susceptible to modification of function via electromagnetic stimulation. Studies using repetitive TMS and transcranial Direct Current Stimulation (tDCS) in combination with fMRI and EEG have shown that targeting specific brain areas may improve naming abilities not only in aphasic but also in patients with Alzheimer's dementia (AD). For instance, repetitive TMS can increase or decrease cortical excitability, inducing inhibition at frequencies ≤1 Hz or facilitation at ≥ 5 Hz. Cotelli et al. (2006) found that administering an rTMS intervention during which both the left and right dorsolateral prefrontal cortex was stimulated in 15 patients diagnosed with mild to moderate AD significantly improved these patients' ability to name actions. In another study, Cotelli et al. (2008) have shown that rTMS improved naming of actions and objects in 24 patients in the advanced stage of AD. Interventions such as rTMS are warranted in patients with AD, because evidence suggests some functional deficits in AD are associated with damage to specific brain areas (Horasty et al., 1999). For instance, Apostolova and colleagues (2008) have shown that language function in AD patients correlated with gray matter atrophy in specific brain areas, and that, overall, language performance of AD patients critically depended on the integrity of the perisylvian cortical regions. Further, it has been shown that although cortical atrophy is relatively widespread in early AD and affects both hemispheres, the LH regions seem to be affected earlier and more severely than the RH areas, with the latter areas taking about two years to reach the level of atrophy of the LH areas, establishing atrophic symmetry (Toga & Thompson, 2003).

Evidence on improvement of naming due to stimulation is even more robust in aphasic patients (e.g., Naeser et al., 2005; Martin et al., 2009), where lesions are focal, and treatment is intended to encourage *recovery* of function instead of enhancement of *compensation*, as in AD patients. TMS nicely complements fMRI because it can be used to test the hypotheses on the retained functionality of the lesioned area or newly acquired functionality of activated areas not typically involved in a specific language function. Such treatments are often based on the assumption that brain areas that assume functionality of the damaged areas may be temporarily disrupted by stimulation, which then forces the original areas to take over the function. A treatment of aphasia that is based on this principle is known as *constraint induced aphasia therapy* (Pulvermüller et al., 2001).

The above examples from naming tasks show that improvement of language performance is possible even in chronic aphasic and AD patients. The role of fMRI is likely to grow with further developments of research in this area, improvement of stimulation methods and their increasing contribution to rehabilitation practices.

3. Challenges and limitations

The main goal of this chapter was to discuss the increasing role of fMRI in current research on language in post-stroke brain. While fMRI has become an essential tool for research on brain's functionality, some challenges make it difficult to justify the overwhelming enthusiasm of the research community regarding this method. Several influential publications reviewed challenges in conducting functional MR imaging in general (e.g., Utall, 2001; Devlin & Poldrack, 2007; Bandettini, 2009, among others) and in research on language in particular (e.g., Sidtis, 2006). Among the problems associated with the use of fMRI to study language are: processes at the macroscopic level that fMRI records may not reflect the processes at microscopic level, lack of consensus among researchers on localization practices, differences in practices in dealing with individual neuroanatomical variability, the fMRI signal variability, the correlational nature of fMRI evidence and its interpretation with regard to cognitive processes, and limited temporal resolution (Utall, 2001; Devlin & Poldrack, 2007; Bandettini, 2009). In addition, there are some challenges specific to using fMRI in research with post-stroke patients, such as artifacts due to production of overt speech, individual variability in functional recovery and use of cognitive strategies, small number of aphasic participants in studies, and the issue of choosing an appropriate method of analysis (e.g., choosing specific ROIs may leave out some areas that may turn out to be important). Furthermore, lesions typically have different extent and lack of an overlap of lesions may lead to missing activations in perilesional areas (Zahn et al., 2006). Neural substrates of language recovery after stroke and functional reorganization involve networks supported by connections that enable interactions among regions. Thus, more research is needed on how disruption of white matter pathways affects recovery of function and how they contribute to initiation of functionality in areas previously not implicated in the function at question (Turken & Dronkers, 2011).

4. Conclusion

In conclusion, the impact of neuroimaging on studying language has been profound. Methods such as fMRI have shown that the traditional concept that language is "located" in specific brain areas such as Broca's and Wernicke's is oversimplified and that the brain supports language processing via complex, sophisticated networks. The growing number of fMRI studies on language in neurologically intact and injured brains has enabled arriving at neurally relevant linguistic generalizations and deepened our understanding of possible principles of the neural organization of language, post-lesional neuroplasticity and recovery processes, revealing also that some previously widely held assumptions do not hold. Still, some specific questions on where in the brain certain linguistic representations are formed, where in the brain specific linguistic computations take place, how the non-dominant hemisphere supports recovery of language in injured brain, or how bilingual brain recovers language functionality—will probably have to wait for answers for some time.

5. Acknowledgement

The main ideas developed in this chapter were first presented in an invited talk "Language and neuroscience: Can studying language reveal how the brain works?" that I gave at BioDonostia, San Sebastian, Spain, on March 14, 2011, and were further refined in my talk given at the Department of Speech and Hearing Sciences, University College Cork, Cork, Ireland, on June 17, 2011.

6. References

Abutalebi, J., Della Rosa, P.A., Tettamanti, M., Green, D.W. & Cappa, S.F. (2009). Bilingual aphasia and language control: A follow-up fMRI and intrinsic connectivity study. *Brain and Language, 109,* 141-156.

Amunts, K., Schleicher, A., Bürgel, U., Mohlberg, H., Uylings, H.B.M. & Zilles, K. (1999). Broca's Region Revisited: Cytoarchitecture and Intersubject Variability. *The Journal of Comparative Neurology,* 412, 319-341.

Amunts, K., Schleicher, A., Ditterich, A. & Zilles, K. (2003). Broca's region: Cytoarchitectonic Asymmetry and Developmental Changes. *The Journal of Comparative Neurology,* 465, 72-89.

Apostolova, L.G., Lu, P., Rogers, S., Dutton, R.A., Hayashi, K.M., Toga, A.W., Cummings, J.L. & Thompson, P.M. (2008). 3D mapping of language networks in clinical and pre-clinical Alzheimer's disease. *Brain and Language,* 104, 33-41.

Arévalo, A., Perani, D., Cappa, S.F., Butler, A., Bates, E., Dronkers, N. (2007). Action and object processing in aphasia: From nouns and verbs to the effect of manipulability. *Brain and Language,* 100, 79–94.

Ardila, A. (2010). A Proposed Reinterpretation and Reclassification of Aphasic Syndromes. *Aphasiology,* 24, 363-394.

Bandettini, P.A. (2009). What's New in Neuroimaging Methods? *Ann. N.Y. Acad. Sci.,* 1156, 260-293.

Bastiaanse, R. (2011). The retrieval and inflection of verbs in the spontaneous speech of fluent aphasic speakers. *Journal of Neurolinguistics,* 24, 163-172.

Bastiaanse, R., Edwards, S., Kiss, K. (1996). Fluent aphasia in three languages: Aspects of spontaneous speech. *Aphasiology,* 10, 561-575.

Bastiaanse, R. & Jonkers, R. (1998). Verb retrieval in action naming and spontaneous speech in agrammatic and anomic aphasia. *Aphasiology,* 12, 951-969.

Bastiaanse, R. (2008). Production of verbs in base position by Dutch agrammatic speakers: Inflection versus finiteness. *Journal of Neurolinguistics,* 21, 104–119.

Ben-Shachar, M., Hendler, T., Kahn, I., Ben-Bashat, D. & Grodzinsky, Y. (2003). The neural reality of syntactic transformations: evidence from functional magnetic resonsance imaging. *Psychological science,* 14, 433-440.

Ben-Shachar, M., Palti, D. & Grodzinsky, Y. (2004). Neural correlates of syntactic movement : converging evidence from two fMRI experiments. *NeuroImage,* 21, 1320-1336.

Benedet, M., Christiansen, J. & Goodglass, H. (1998). A cross-linguistic study of grammatical morphology in Spanish and English speaking agrammatic patients. *Cortex,* 34, 309–336.

Binkofski, F., Amunts, K., Stephen, K.M., Posse, S., Schormann, T., Freund, H.J., Zilles, K. & Seitz, R.J. (2000). Broca's Region Subserves Imagery of Motion: A Combined Cytoarchitectonic and fMRI Study. *Human Brain Mapping*, 11, 273-285.

Binkofski, F. & Buccino, G. (2004). Motor functions of the Brocas region'. *Brain and Language*, 89, 362-369.

Bonakdarpour, B., Parrish, T.B. & Thompson, C.K. (2007). Hemodynamic response function in patients with stroke-induced aphasia: Implications for fMRI data analysis. *NeuroImage*, 36, 322-331.

Broca P. Remarks on the Seat of the Faculty of Articulate Language, Followed by an Observation of Aphemia [1861]. In: *Philosophy and the Neurosciences: A Reader.* (2001). Bechtel R, Stffleabeam S, Mundale J, Manic, P. (Eds.), (87-99), Blackwell Publishers, Oxford.

Burchert, F., Swoboda-Moll, M. & De Bleser, R. (2005). Tense and agreement dissociations in German agrammatic speakers: Underspecification versus hierarchy. *Brain and Language*, 94, 188–199.

Cao, Y., Vikingstad, E. M., George, P. K., Johnson, A. F., & Welch, K. M. A. (1999). Cortical Language Activation in Stroke Patients Recovering From Aphasia With Functional MRI. *Stroke, 30,* 2331-2340.

Caplan, D., Alpert, N., Waters, G. & Olivieri, A. (2000). Activation of Broca's Area by Syntactic Processing Under Conditions of Concurrent Articulation. *Human Brain Mapping*, 9, 65–71.

Caramazza, A., Zurif, E. (1976). Dissociation of Algorithmic and Heuristic Processes in Language Comprehension: Evidence from Aphasia. *Brain and Language*, 3, 572-582.

Chatterjee, A. (2005). A Madness to the Methods in Cognitive Neuroscience. *Journal of Cognitive Neuroscience, 17,* 847-849.

Chen, C-H. & Zeki, S. (2011). Fronto-parietal Activation Distinguishes Face and Space from Artifact Concepts. *Journal of Cognitive Neuroscience,* doi:10.1162/jocn.2011.21617, 1-11.

Chenery, L.R. & Small, S.L. (2006). Task-dependent changes in brain activation following therapy for non-fluent aphasia: Discussion of two individual cases. *Journal of International Neuropsychological Society*, 12, 828-842.

Chomsky, N. 1957. *Syntactic Structures*. Janua Linguarum IV. The Hague: Mouton.

Chomsky, N. 1986. *Knowledge of Language: Its Nature, Origin and Use*. Praeger, New York.

Cotelli, M., Manenti, R., Cappa, S. F., Geroldi, C., Zanetti, O., Rossini, P.M. & Miniussi, C. (2006). *Arch Neurology, 63,* 1602-1604.

Cotelli, M., Manenti, R., Cappa, S. F., Zanetti, O. & Miniussi, C. (2008). Transcranial magnetic stimulation improves naming in Alzheimer's disease patients at different stages of cognitive decline. *European Journal of Neurology, 15,* 1286-1292.

Cramer, S.C. & Riley, J.D. (2008). Neuroplasticity and brain repair after stroke. *Current Opinion in Neurology*, 21, 76-82.

Crosson, B., McGregor, K., Gopinath, K.S., Conway, T.W., Benjamin, M., Chang, Y.L., Moore, A.B., Raymer, A.M., Briggs, R.W., Sherod, M.G., Wierenga, C.E. & White, K.D. (2007). Functional MRI of Language in Aphasia: A Review of the Literature and the Methodological Challenges. *Neuropsychol Rev*, 17(2), 157-177.

Davis, C.H., Harrington, G. & Baynes, K. (2006). Intensive semantic intervention in fluent aphasia: A pilot study with fMRI. Aphasiology, 20(1), 59-83.

Desmurget, M., Bonnetblanc, F. & Duffau, H. (2007). Contrasting acute and slow-growing lesions: a new door to brain plasticity. *Brain, 130,* 898-914.

Devlin, J.T. & Poldrack, R.A. (2007). In praise of tedious anatomy. *Neuroimage,* 37(4), 1033-41

Devlin, J. T. & Watkins, K. E. (2007). Stimulating language: insights from TMS. *Brain, 130,* 610-622.

Diouny, S. (2007). Tense/agreement in Moroccan Arabic: The Tree-Pruning Hypothesis. *SKY Journal of Linguistics,* 20, 141–169.

Dronkers, N,F., Plaisant, O., Iba-Zizen, M.T. & Cabanis, E.A. (2007). Paul Broca's historic cases: high resolution MR imaging of the brains of Leborgne and Lelong. *Brain,* 130, 1432-1441.

Druks, J. (2002). Verbs and nouns—a review of the literature. *Journal of Neurolinguistics,* 15, 289-315.

Druks, J. & Caroll, E. (2005). The crucial role of tense for verb production. *Brain and Language,* 94,1–18.

Eaton, K.P., Szaflarski, P., Altaye, M., Ball, A.L., Kissela, B.M et al. (2008). Reliability of fMRI for studies of language in post-stroke aphasia subjects. *NeuroImage, 41,* 311-322.

Edwards, S. (2002). Grammar and fluent aphasia. In: Fava, E. (ed.). *Clinical linguistic theory and applications in speech pathology and therapy* (pp. 249-266). John Benjamins, Amsterdam/ Philadelphia.

Fabbro, F. (2001). The Bilingual Brain: Bilingual Aphasia. *Brain and Language, 79,* 201-210.

Fadiga, L. & Craighero, L. (2006a). Hand actions and speech representation in Broca's area. *Cortex,* 42, 486–490.

Fadiga, L., Craighero, L., Desto, M. F., Finos, L., Cotillon-Williams, N. et al. (2006b). Language in shadow, *Social Neuroscience,* 1, 77–89.

Fedorenko, E. & Kanwisher, N. (2009). Neuroimaging of Language: Why Hasn't a Clearer Picture Emerged? *Language and Linguistics Compass, 3(4),* 839-865.

Fiebach, C.J., Schlesewsky, M. & Friederici, A.D. (2001). Syntactic Working memory and the Establishment of Filler-Gap Dependencies: Insights from ERPs and fMRI. *Journal of Psycholinguistic Research,* 30, 321-338.

Fiebach, C.J., Schlesewsky, M., Friederici, A. (2002). Separating Syntactic memory Costs and Syntactic Integration Costs during Parsing: the Processing of German Wh-questions. *Journal of Memory and Language,* 47, 250-272.

Fink, G.R., Manjaly, Z.M., Stephen, K.E., Gurd, J.M., Zilles, K., Amunts K., Marshall, J.C. (2006). A Role for Broca's Are Beyond Language Processing: Evidence from Neuropsychology and fMRI. In: *Broca's Region.* Amunts, K. & Grodzinsky, Y. (Eds). Oxford University Press, Oxford.

Friederici, A. (1998). The neurobiology of language comprehension, In: *Language Comprehension: A Biological Perspective,* Friederici, A.D. (Ed.), (pp. 263-301). Springer, Berlin/Heidelberg/New York.

Friedmann, N. & Grodzinsky, Y. (1997). Tense and agreement in agrammatic production: pruning the syntactic tree. *Brain and Language,* 56, 397–425.

Green, D.W. (2008). Bilingual aphasia: adapted language networks and their control. *Annual Review of Applied Linguistics,* 28, 25-48.

Green, D.W. & Price, C.J. (2001). Functional imaging in the study of recovery patterns in bilingual aphasia. *Bilingualism: Language and Cognition,* 4(2), 191-201.

Greewe, T., Bornkessel, I., Zysset, S., Wiese, R., von Cramon, Y.D., Schlesewsky, M. (2005). The Reemergence of the Unmarked: A New Perspective on the Language-Specific Function of Broca's Area. *Human Brain Mapping,* 26, 178–190.

Grodzinsky, Y. (2000). The Neurology of Syntax: Language Use without Broca's Area. *Behavioral and Brain Sciences,* 23, 1-71.

Grodzinsky, Y. (2010). The Picture of the Linguistic Brain: How Sharp Can It Be? Reply to Fedorenko & Kanwisher. *Language and Linguistics Compass 4/8,* 605-622.

Grodzinsky, Y., Pinango, M.M., Zurif, E. & Drai, D. (1999). The critical role of group studies in neuropsychology: Comprehension regularities in Broca's aphasia. *Brain and Language,* 67, 134-147.

Hagiwara, H. (1995). The breakdown of functional categories and the economy of derivation. *Brain and Language,* 50, 92–116.

Harasty, J.A., Halliday, G.M., Kril, J.J., Code, C. (1999). Specific temporoparietal gyral atrophy reflects the pattern of language dissolution in Alzheimer's disease. *Brain,* 122, 675-686.

Harasty, J. A., Halliday, G. M., Kril, J. J. & Code, C. (1999). Specific temporoparietal gyral atrophy reflects the pattern of language dissolution in Alzheimer's disease. *Brain, 122,* 675-686.

Harnish, S., Neils-Strunjas, J., Lamy, M. & Eliassen, J. (2008). Use of fMRI in the Study of Chronic Aphasia recovery After Therapy: A Case Study. *Top Stroke Rehabil, 15,* 468-483.

Hauk, O., Johnsrude, I. & Pulvermüller, F. (2004). Somatotopic Representation of Action Words in Human Motor and Premotor Cortex. *Neuron,* 41, 301-307.

Hickok, G., Zurrif, E. & Canseco-Gonzales, E. (1993). Structural Description of Agrammatic Comprehension. *Brain and Language,* 45, 371-395.

Hickok, G. & Poeppel, D. (2000). Towards a Functional Anatomy of Speech Perception. *Trends in Cognitive Sciences, 4,* 131-138.

Hickok, G. & Poeppel, D.(2004). Dorsal and ventral streams: a framework for understanding aspects of the functional anatomy of language. *Cognition,* 92, 67-99.

Hickok, G. & Poeppel, D.(2007).The cortical organization of speech processing. *Nature Reviews Neuroscience,* 8, 393-402.

Hillis, A. (2006). The right place at the right time? *Brain,* 129, 1351-1356.

Jackendoff, R. (1997). *The Architecture of the Language Faculty.* The MIT Press, Cambridge, MA.

Jackendoff, R. (2002). *Foundations of Language. Brain, Meaning, Grammar, Evolution*. Oxford University Press, Oxford.

Johansson, B.B. (2011). Current trends in stroke rehabilitation. A review with focus on brain plasticity. *Acta Neurol Scand, 123,* 147-159.

Josse, G. & Tzourio-Mazoyer, N. (2004). Hemispheric specialization for languge. *Brain Research Reviews, 44,* 1-12.

Kambanaros, M. (2008). The trouble with nouns and verbs in Greek fluent aphasia. *Journal of Communication Disorders,* 44, 1-19.

Karbe, H., Thiel, A., Weber-Luxenburger, G., Herholz, K., Kessler, J. & Heiss, W.-D. (1998). Brain Plasticity in Poststroke Aphasia: What Is the Contribution of the Right Hemisphere? *Brain and Language, 64,* 215-230.

Kim, M. & Leach, T. (2004). Verb retrieval in fluent aphasia in two elicitation contexts. *Clinical Aphasiology Conference,* Park City, UT: (May, 2004)

Kljajevic, V. (2009). fMRI in Language Recovery after Stroke. *Acta Fac. Med. Naiss,* 26(4), 217-223.

Kljajevic, V. & Murasugi, K. (2010). The role of morphology in the comprehension of wh-dependencies in Croatian aphasic speakers. *Aphasiology,* 24, 1354-1376.

Kljajevic, V. & Bastiaanse, R. (2011). Time reference in fluent aphasia: Evidence from Serbian. In: *Multidisciplinary Aspects of Time and Time Perception,* Vatakis, A., Cumminis, F., Esposito, A., Papadelis, G. & Giagkou, M. (Eds.), (pp. 258-274). Springer, Berlin.

Kutas, M., Federmeier, K.D., Coulson, S., King, J.W. & Münte, T.F. (2000). Language. In: *Handbook of Psychophysiology,* Cacioppo, J.T., Tassinary, L.G. & Berntson, G. (Eds). (576-601). Cambridge University Press, Cambridge.

Lee, A., Kannan, V., & Hillis, A.E. (2006). The Contribution of Neuroimaging to the Study of Language in Aphasia. *Neuropsychol Rev, 16,* 171-183.

Luzzatti, C., Aggujaro, S., Crepaldi, D. (2006). Verb-Noun Double Dissociation in Aphasia: Theoretical and Neuroanatomical Foundations. *Cortex,* 42, 875-883.

Maess, B., Koelsch, S., Gunter, T., Friederici, A. (2001). Musical syntax is processed in Broca's area: an MEG study. *Nature Neuroscience,* 4, 540-545.

Mahon, B.Z., Anzellotti, S., Schwarzbach, J., Zampini, M. & Caramazza, A. (2009). Category-Specific Organizatin in the Human Brain Does not Require Visual Experience. *Neuron,* 63, 397-405.

Martin, P.I., Naeser, M.A., Doron, K.W., Bogdan, A., Baker, E.H., Kurland, J., Renshaw, P. & Yurgelun-Todd, D. (2005). Overt naming in aphasia studied with functional MRI hemodynamic delay design. *NeuroImage, 28,* 194-204.

Martin, P.I., Naeser, M., Ho, M., Treglia, E., Kapplan, E., Baker, E. & Pascual-Leone, A. (2009). Research with Transcranial Magnetic Stimulation in the Treatment of Aphasia. *Curr Neurol Neurosci Rep,* 9, 451-458.

Mauner, G., Fromkin, V. A., & Cornell, T. L. (1993). Comprehension of acceptability judgment in agrammatism: Disruption in the syntax of referential dependency. *Brain and Language,* 45, 340–370.

Meinzer, M., Flaisch, T., Breitenstein, C., Wienbruch, C., Elbert, T. & Rockstroh, B. (2008). Functional re-recruitment of dysfunctional brain areas predicts language recovery in chronic aphasia. *NeuroImage*, 39, 2038-2046.

Meinzer, M., Harnish, S., Conway, T. & Crosson, B. (2011). Recent developments in functional and structural imaging of aphasia recovery after stroke. *Aphasiology*, 25(3), 271-290.

Meltzer, J.A., Postman-Caucheteux, W.A., McArdle, J.J. & Braun, A.R. (2009). Strategies for longitudinal neuroimaging studies of overt language production. *NeuroImage*, 47, 745-755.

Menn, L. & Obler, L.K. (1990). Cross-language data and theories of agrammatism. In: *Agrammatic aphasia: A Cross-language Narrative Sourcebook* (pp. 1369–1389), Menn, L., Obler, L.K. (eds.). John Benjamins Publishing Co., Amsterdam.

Miceli, G., Silveri, C.M., Villa, G. & Caramazza, A. (1984). On the basis for the agrammatic's difficulty in producing main verbs. *Cortex*, 20, 207–220.

Naeser, M. & Palumbo, C.L. (1994). Neuroimaging and Language Recovery in Stroke. *Journal of Clinical Neurophysiology*, 11, 150-174.

Naeser, M.A., Martin, P., Nicholas, M., Baker, E.H., Seekins, H., Helm-Estabrooks, N. et al. (2005). Improved naming after TMS treatments in a chronic, global aphasia patient—case report. *Neurocase, 11(3)*, 182–193.

Novick, J.M., Trueswell, J.C. & Thompson-Schill, S.L. (2005). Cognitive control and parsing: Reexamining the role of Broca's area in sentence comprehension. *Cognitive Affective, & Behavioral Neuroscience*, 5(3):263-281.

Novick, J.M, Trueswell, J.C. & Thompson-Schill, S.L. (2010). Broca's Area and Language Processing: Evidence for the Cognitive Control Connection, *Language and Linguistics Compass*, 4(10): 906-924.

Optiz, B. & Friederici, A.D. (2007). Neural Basis of Processing Sequential and Hierarchical Syntactic Structures. *Human Brain Mapping*, 28, 585-592.

Orlov, T., Makin, Tamar, R. & Zohary, E. (2010). Topographic representation of the Human Body in the Occipitotemporal Cortex. *Neuron*, 68, 586-600.

Paradis, M. (1987). *The assessment of bilingual aphasia*. Psychology Press, New York.

Paradis, M. (2001). The need for awareness of aphasia symptoms in different languages. *Journal of Neurolinguistics*, 14, 85–91.

Patel, A. (2003). Language, music, syntax and the brain. *Nature Neuroscience*, 7, 674–681.

Peelen, M.V. & Downing, P.E. (2007). The neural basis of visual body perception. *Nature Reviews Neuroscience*, 8, 636-643.

Peelen, M.V. & Downing, P.E. (in press). The role of occipitotemporal body-selective regions in person perception. *Cognitive Neuroscience*. Retrieved in May, 2011. Available from : http://mc.manuscriptcentral.com/pcns.

Peck, K.K., Moore, A.B., Crosson, B.A., Gaiefsky, M., Gopinath, K.S., White, K. & Briggs, R.W. (2004). Functional Magnetic Resonance Imaging Before and After Aphasia Therapy. *Stroke*, 35, 554-559.

Perani, D., Cappa, S.F., Schnur, T., Tettamanti, M., Collina, S., Rosa, M.M., Fazio, F. (1999). The neural correlates of verb and noun processing. A PET Study. *Brain*, 122, 2337–2344.

Pineiro, P., Pendlebury, H., Johansen-Berg, H. & Matthews, P.M. (2002). Altered Hemodynamic Responses in Patients After Subcortical Stroke measured by Functional MRI. *Stroke,* 33, 103-109.

Poeppel, D. & Embick, D. (2005). Defining the relation between linguistics and neuroscience. In: *Twenty-First Century Psycholinguistics. Four Cornerstones.* (pp. 103-120), Cutler, A. (Ed.). Lawrence Erlbaum Associates, Mahwah, NJ.

Price, C.J. (2000). Functional Imaging Studies of Aphasia. In : *Brain Mapping: The Disorders,* J.C. Mazziotta, A.W. Toga & R.S.J. Frackowiak (Eds.), (181-199), Academic Press, San Diego.

Price, C.J. (2010). The anatomy of language: a review of 100 fMRI studies published in 2009. *Ann. N.Y. Acad. Sci. 1191,* 62-88.

Pulvermüller, F. (2010). Brain-Language Research: Where is the Progress? *Biolinguistics, 4(2-3),* 255-288.

Pulvermüller, F., Neininger, B., Elbert, T., Mohr, B., Rockstroh, B., Koebbel, P. & Taub, E. (2001). Constraint-Induced Therapy of Chronic Aphasia After Stroke. *Stroke, 32,*1621-1626.

Pulvermüller, F., Hauk, O., Zohsel, K., Neininger, B. & Mohr, B. (2005). Therapy-related reorganization of language in both hemispheres of patients with chronic aphasia. *NeuroImage, 28,* 481-489.

Russo, K.D., Peach, P. & Shapiro, L.S. (1998). Verb preference effects in the sentence comprehension of fluent aphasic individuals, *Aphasiology,* 12, 537-545.

Saur, D., Lange, R., Baumgaertner, A., Schraknepper, V., Willmes, K., et al. (2006). Dynamics of language reorganization after stroke. *Brain, 129,* 1371-1384.

Saur, D., Kreher, B.W., Schnell, S., Kümmerer, D., Kellmeyer, P. et al. (2008). Ventral and dorsal pathways for language. *PNAS,* 105, 18035-18040.

Shapiro, K.A., Moo, L.R., Carmazza, A. (2006). Cortical signatures of noun and verb production. *PNAS,* 103, 1644–1649.

Smits, M., Visch-Brink, E., Schraa-Tam, C., Koudstaal, P.J. & van der Lugt, A. (2006). Functional MR Imaging of Language Processing: An Overview of Easy-to-Implement Paradigms for Patient care and Clinical research. *RadioGraphics, 26,* S 145-S 158.

Spironelli, C., Angrilli, A. & Pertile, M. (2008). Language plasticity in aphasics after recovery : Evidence from slow evoked potential. *NeuroImage, 40,* 912-922.

Thompson, C.K. & den Ouden, D.B. (2008). Neuroimaging and Recovery of Language in Aphasia. *Current Neurology and Neuroscience Reports,* 8, 475-483.

Thompson-Schill, S.L. (2005). Dissecting the Language Organ: A new Look at the Role of Broca's Area in Language Processing. In: *Twenty-First Century Psycholinguistics. Four Cornerstones,* Cutler A, (Ed.), (173-190), Lawrence Erlbaum Associates, Mahwah, NJ.

Toga, A.W. & Thompson P.M. (2003). Mapping brain asymmetry. *Nature Reviews Neuroscience,* 4, 37-48.

Turken, A.U. & Dronkers, N.F. (2011). The neural architecture of the language comprehension network: converging evidence from lesion and conncetivity analysis. *Frontiers in Systems Neuroscience,* 5, 1-20.

Tyler, L.K., Russell, R., Fadili, J. & Moss, H.E. (2001). The neural representation of nouns and verbs: PET study. *Brain*, 124, 1619–1634.
Tyler, L.K., Wright, P., Rendall, B., Marslen-Wilson, W.D. & Stamatakis, E.A. (2010). Reorganization of syntactic processing following left-hemisphere brain damage: does right-hemisphere activity preserve function ? *Brain, 133,* 3396-3408.
Ulatowska, H.K., Sadowska, D. & Kądzielawa, D. (2001). A longitudinal study of agrammatism in Polish : A case study. *Journal of Neurolinguistics*, 14, 321-336.
Uttal WR. (2001). *The New Phrenology.* The Limits of Localizing Cognitive Processes in the Brain. A Bradford Book, Cambridge, MA.
Van Lancker Sidtis, D. (2006). Does functional neuroimaging solve the questions of neurolinguistics? *Brain and Language,* 98, 276—290.
Varlakosta, S., Valeonti, N., Kakavoulia, M., Lazaridou, M., Economou, A., Protopapas, A. (2006). The breakdown of functional categories in Greek aphasia: Evidence from agreement, tense, and aspect. *Aphasiology,* 20, 723-743.
Vitali, P., Abutalebi, J., Tettamanti, M., Danna, M., Ansaldo, A.-I., Perani, D., Joanette, Y. & Cappa, S.F. (2007). Training-Induced Brain Remapping in Chronic Aphasia: A Pilot Study. *Neurorehabil Neural Repair,* 21, 152-160.
Weeks, B.S. (2010). Issues in bilingual aphasia : An introduction. *Aphasiology, 24,* 123-125.
Zahn, R., Schwarz, M. & Huber, W. (2006). Functional activation studies of word processing in the recovery from aphasia. *Journal of Physiology – Paris,* 99, 370-385.

Section 3

Multimodal Approaches

9

The Brain Metabolites Within Cerebellum of Native Chinese Speakers Who Are Using the Traditional Logographic Reading and Writing Systems – A Magnetic Resonance Spectroscopy Approach to Dyslexia*

Ying-Fang Sun[1], Ralph Kirby[2] and Chun-Wei Li[3]
[1]*Department of Biomedical Imaging and Radiological Sciences, National Yang-Ming University No.155, Sec 2, Linong Street, Taipei,*
[2]*Department of Life Sciences and Institute of Genome Sciences, National Yang-Ming University No.155, Sec 2, Linong Street, Taipei,*
[3]*Chairman, Department of Medical Imaging and Radiological Sciences, Kaohsiung Medical University No.100, Shih-Chuan 1st Road, Kaohsiung, Taiwan, R.O.C.*

1. Introduction

Dyslexia is a term for persons who are suffering from difficulties in learning to read, write and spell, but who have a normal or even higher intelligence quotient (Hsiung, Kaplan, Petryshen, Lu, & Field, 2004). In addition to linguistic difficulties, deficits in non-linguistic domains, such as automatization, time estimation (Nicolson RI, Fawcett AJ, & Dean, P., 1996), and motor skills (Wilsher, et al., 1987) are also documented. However, not a single hypothesis is able to yet account for all the behavioural symptoms of dyslexia (Pernet, Andersson, Paulesu, & Demonet, 2009). The definition used for dyslexia depends on the research teams and varies significantly (Gersons-Wolfensberger & Ruijssenaars, 1997; Habib, 2000; Lyon, Shaywitz, & Shaywitz, 2003 ; Tunmer & Greaney, 2010). The estimates of prevalence for dyslexia in the West have ranged from 5% (Deffenbacher, et al., 2004) to 15% (Stoodley, Fawcett, Nicolson, & Stein, 2006). In addition, the gifted talents associated with dyslexia are usually neglected (Chakravarty, 2009; Everatt, Weeks, & Brooks, 2008; Levy, 1983; von Karolyi, Winner, Gray, & Sherman, 2003). Although linguistic interventions (Breteler, Arns, Peters, Giepmans, & Verhoeven, 2010; Penolazzi, Spironelli, Vio, & Angrilli, 2010) and pharmaceutical drugs (Wilsher, et al., 1987; Zavadenko, Rumiantseva, & Tolstova, 2009) might assist the reading and spelling performance of the dyslexics, some of the disadvantages are persistent, such as the difficulties in reciting multiplication tables (Miles, 1993). Gregorenko claimed that dyslexia is one of the most important public health problems (Grigorenko, et al., 2003) and despite intensive studies for more than a hundred

* Part of the work was posted in the XXIVth International Conference on Magnetic Resonance in Biological Systems, Aug 2010 Carins, Australia

years in the Western world, the exact mechanism(s) causing these difficulties is still not yet clear. The World Health Organization (WHO) recognizes dyslexia as a disease and it has ICD-10 code for R48.0, (WHO, July 2011). Many researchers believed that dyslexia has a universal biological basis (Demonet, Taylor, & Chaix, 2004; Schulte-Korne, et al., 2007; Ziegler, Perry, Ma-Wyatt, Ladner, & Schulte-Korne, 2003). In addition to behavioural (Eden, Wood, & Stein, 2003) and cognitive information on dyslexia, post-mortem studies by Galaburda et al. have shown that the dyslexics have unusual brains (Galaburda & Cestnick, 2003). Twin studies have also indicated that genes are very likely to be involved (Olson, 2002). However, the genetic transmission mode is not known. The advent of brain imaging tools permits us to undertake exploration of the brain's structure and function *in vivo*. However, due to the various subtypes of the subjects (Ho, Chan, Chung, Lee, & Tsang, 2007; King, Giess, & Lombardino, 2007; Spinelli, et al., 2010; Tree, 2008) and the different parameters applied in the various studies carried out, no consensus has been reached as yet (Sun, Lee, & Kirby, 2010). *In silico* cloning for gene prediction is still challenging and only ten candidate genes are found up to the present (Sun, Lee, & Kirby, 2009).

There are no standard tests for adult dyslexia (Brachacki, Nicolson, & Fawcett, 1995), not even a formal medical diagnosis (Demonet, et al., 2004). This is particularly true for dyslexics with Chinese ethnicity, specifically the members of communities that use the traditional Chinese logographic reading and writing systems. Therefore, an objective means that assists with diagnosis is needed. Reading performance is related to balance and involves of cerebellum (Lonnemanna, Linkersdörfera, Heselhausa, Hasselhorn & Lindberg S., 2011). Recently, the right cerebellar hemisphere has become a target for study (Pernet, Poline, Demonet, & Rousselet, 2009) and has been pinpointed as a possible biomarker for dyslexics. We have followed this trend and concentrated our efforts on the relationship between dyslexia and cerebellum (Stoodley & Stein, 2011).

2. The MRS studies on dyslexia using Caucasian subjects

The application of magnetic resonance spectroscopy (MRS) on the live human brain chemistry studies has involved Caucasians as research subjects for the most part. Specifically, the available articles on dyslexia include only volunteers that are Westerners, see Table 1. The brain metabolites in these studies could be further grouped into three categories. Firstly, ^{31}P-MRS technology that is used to assess brain metabolite ratios, namely, phosphomonoester, phosphodiester and ßNTP, which are changed in the basal ganglia of the dyslexics compared to the controls (Richardson, Cox, Sargentoni & Puri, 1997). Another study (Rae, et al., 1998) also used ^{31}P-MRS, but did not find any significant differences in the frontal lobe region. Secondly, the study used proton-MRS to detect the lactate during phonologic linguistic tasks that require extra mental efforts, which were compared to lactate levels during the passive listening. Higher levels of lactate were detected during the formal task in right handed male dyslexics but such an increase was not found with the controls (Richards, et al., 1999). Intensive linguistic training for the dyslexics was found to reduce the elevation of the lactate peak (Richards, et al., 2000) in the left anterior quadrant. This was further confirmed by using right handed female subjects and it is the morphological component (Richards, et al., 2002) of the treatments that causes the therapeutic effects, but not the phonological one. Lastly, the measurements of N-acetylaspartate (NAA), choline (Cho) and creatine (Cr) ratio in the cerebellar hemispheres have been examined (Rae, et al., 1998) and the findings suggest that there is a lowered Cho/NAA ratio in the right cerebellum and left temporo-parietal lobe of the dyslexic males.

Authors/ Reference	Metabolites/ Brain regions	Parameters for MRS	Subjects	Findings
Richardson et al. NMR in Biomedicine 1997	PME/ ßNTP PME/PDE PDE/ ßNTP **Basal ganglia**	1.5 T, ^{31}P-MRS, 4D CSI TR=5000ms T_1-weighted multi-slice transverse images	**Caucasians** 12 dyslexics (7 male, 5 females) 34.1±9.5 yr 10 controls (5 male, 5 females) 28.3± 7.2 yr No current or previous reading difficulties	The PME peak area was significantly elevated in the dyslexic group, this reflects the reduced incorporation of phospholipids into cell membranes
Rae et al. Lancet 1998	Cho, NAA, Cr **Temporo-parietal Cerebellum** ***Frontal lobe***	^{1}H-MRS T_1-weighted, multi-slice images 5 mm thickness axial view 3x3x3 cm single voxel Birdcage coil STEAM ***^{31}P-MRS***	**Caucasians** 20-41yr male 14 dyslexics 15 controls Discrepancy between reading and spelling achievement	Altered patterns of cell density in the cerebellum of the dyslexic individuals ***No significance was found***
Richards et al. J Neuroradiol. 1999	Lactate **Left anterior quadrant**	1.5T GE ^{1}H- MRS, PEPSI 1 cm^3 voxel 20mm thickness TR=4000ms TE=272ms	**Caucasians** Right handed, age, IQ, head size matched boy 6 dyslexics (124.3±1 1.1 month), 7 controls (127.3 ±10.8 months) Discrepancy in reading skills	The dyslexics have a greater area of lactate elevation in the left anterior quadrant than that of the controls during a phonological task stimulus
Richards et al. J Neuroradiol. 2000	Lactate **Left anterior quadrant**	^{1}H-MRS, PEPSI 1 cm^3 voxel TR=4000ms TE=272ms	**Caucasians** 10-13 yr right handed boy Head size (number of total voxels) matched 8 dyslexics, 7 controls	Reduced elevation of lactate level after reading/science workshop treatment in the left anterior quadrant of the dyslexics
Richards et al. Am J Neuroradiol. 2002	Lactate **Left anterior quadrant**	1.5T GE ^{1}H-MRS, PEPSI 1 cm^3 voxel TR=4000ms TE=144ms	**Caucasians** 9-12 yr 10 dyslexics (6 boys, 4 girls) 8 controls (6 boys, 2 girls)	The morphological component of language treatment reduces activation of lactate in the left frontal region in dyslexics
Rae et al. Neuropsychologia 2002	Cho, NAA, Cr **Cerebellum**	85.2MHz, Bruker ^{1}H-MRS T_1-weighted coronal images TR=803ms TE=13ms	**Caucasians** 20-41yr Handedness controlled 11 male dyslexics 9 similarly-aged controls	There are alterations in the neurological organization of the cerebellum in dyslexics
Laycock et al. Ann.N.Y. Acad.Sci.2008	Cho, NAA, Cr **Cerebellum**	3T Philip Intera ^{1}H-MRS, PRESS 1.5x1.5x1.5 cm single voxel TR=1600ms TE=144ms	**Caucasians** 20-21yrs right handed Male 6 dyslexics 6 controls	A smaller NAA/Cho ratio in right cerebellum, higher Cho/Cr in left cerebellum of the dyslexics Indicative of excessive connectivity and abnormal mylination

Table 1. The Application of Magnetic Resonance Spectroscopy (MRS) to the Study of Dyslexia

By using male subjects with handedness information and proton-MRS, the same team indicated the brain metabolites do not differ between the left and right cerebellar hemispheres of the control subjects (Rae, et al., 2002). In contrast, it is the Cho/NAA ratio in the right cerebellar hemisphere of the dyslexics that differs significantly to the controls (Rae, et al., 1998). However, in 2008, another study (Laycock, et al., 2008) found a lower NAA/Cho in the right cerebellar hemisphere and a higher Cho/Cr in the left cerebellar hemisphere of the dyslexics compared to the controls. This conflicts with the previous results (Rae, et al., 1998). The discrepancy probably comes from the differences of the voxel size, the parameters used for conducting proton-MRS and the age of the subjects, see Table 2.

Author	Brain Metabolite Ratio within Right Cerebellar Hemisphere							
Rae et al. 1998	Control N=15, 20-41 yrs, male			Dyslexic N=14, 20-41 yrs, male			Single voxel volume	Pulse sequence
	Cr/NAA	**Cho/Cr**	**Cho/NAA**	**Cr/NAA**	**Cho/Cr**	**Cho/NAA**		
	0.65±0.16	0.80±0.27	0.52±0.18	0.53±0.15	0.74±0.29	0.37±0.10	27 cm^3	STEAM
Laycock et al. 2008	Control N=6, 20-21 yrs, male			Dyslexic N=6, 20-21yrs, male			Single voxel volume	Pulse sequence
	NAA/Cr	**Cho/Cr**	**NAA/Cho**	**NAA/Cr**	**Cho/Cr**	**NAA/Cho**		
	2.01±0.33	0.9±0.18	2.30±0.50	1.94±0.25	1.10±0.20	1.78±0.12	3.75 cm^3	PRESS

Table 2. The Comparison of Brain Metabolite Ratio within Right Cerebellar Hemisphere of Two Studies Using Caucasian Subjects

3. Aims of the study

An appropriate diagnosis for dyslexic adults is lacking and has been involved to the present using behavioural or cognitive symptoms (Fawcett, 2007). We attempted to identify a more objective means for assisting dyslexic diagnosis and our aim was to test the hypothesis if the NAA/Cho ratio in the right cerebellar hemisphere of the dyslexics is lesser than that of the counterpart. It seems the right cerebellar hemisphere is the target of the dyslexic research because Pernet's group claimed that *"the best biomarker of dyslexia is the right cerebellum"* (Pernet, et al., 2009). Therefore, in this study we recruited Chinese who use the traditional Chinese logographic reading and writing systems and carried out a proton-MRS study. Specifically, we measured the NAA/Cho ratio in the cerebellum and make a comparison of the results with those obtained by other groups using Caucasians. The Institutional Review Board of National Yang-Ming University approved the study (No. 980046).

4. Materials and methods

We used a Trio Tim 3T MRI scanner from German Siemens with 12 channel head coils and Syngo MR B15 software. Water suppression was achieved with a chemically selective saturation (CHESS) pulse. A point-resolved spectroscopy sequence (PRESS) was performed for single voxel data acquisition. The parameters were similar to the ones used in Laycock's experiments, namely, TR= 2000ms, TE=135ms, single voxel size= 15X15X15mm, each voxel takes 4min 24 sec for acquisition (Laycock, et al., 2008). The placement of a single voxel within the right and left cerebellar hemispheres was achieved by using the T_1 and T_2-weighted structural images in a coronal view as described by Laycock et al.

Participants were 37 native Chinese volunteers who had given written informed consent. The including criteria for controls were healthy subjects, who enjoy reading and writing. They do not have reading or writing problems and have no history of learning disability, claustrophobia, surgical implants, pregnancy, pacemakers, psychiatric disease, neurological disease or any known medical conditions that affected brain morphology and metabolism. These controls consist of 8 right handed males aged 19-89 yrs (49.1± 22.8) and 9 right handed females aged 14-59 yrs (40.3±16.2). The potential dyslexics who joined the MRS study were self-reported from a questionnaire survey (Sun, Ting-Hsiang Lin, & Liao, 2010) conducted in July-December of year 2009.

5. Our findings and discussions

5.1 The single voxel study

5.1.1 The NAA/Cr, Cho/Cr and NAA/Cho within the cerebellar hemispheres of 37 Chinese who are using the traditional Chinese logographic reading and writing systems

Across the 19 males, the NAA/Cr ranged from 0.76-1.23 (mean ± SD 1.03±0.13) and 0.73-1.81 (1.06 ±0.26) within the right and left cerebellar hemispheres, respectively. The Cho/Cr ranged from 0.73-1.05 (0.86 ± 0.09) and 0.65-1.11 (0.91± 0.12) within the right and left cerebellar hemispheres, respectively. The NAA/Cho ranged from 0.96-1.47 (1.21 ± 0.16) and 0.81-1.69 (1.16 ± 0.22) within the right and left cerebellar hemispheres respectively.

Across the 18 females, the NAA/Cr ranged from 0.7-1.65 (mean ± SD 1.10 ± 0.21) and 0.92-1.92 (1.16 ± 0.27) within the right and left cerebellar hemispheres, respectively. The Cho/Cr ranged from 0.56-1.13 (0.91 ± 1.13) and 0.59-1.50 (0.89 ± 0.19) within the right and left cerebellar hemispheres, respectively. The NAA/Cho ranged from 0.91-1.66 (1.22 ± 0.20) and 1.08-1.89 (1.31 ± 0.23) within the right and left cerebellar hemispheres, respectively.

5.1.2 A trend toward biochemical symmetry of the cerebellar hemispheres in 37 Chinese who are using the traditional Chinese logographic reading and writing systems

The differences of the NAA/Cho between the right and left cerebellar hemispheres were determined as follows: if the NAA/Cho in the right hemisphere is greater than that of the left hemisphere, then a "+" was designated, otherwise a "-" was given; if the difference is equal to or lesser than 0.09, a "0" was assigned arbitrarily.

Across the19 males, there are 10 participants whose NAA/Cho ratio within the right cerebellar hemisphere were greater than that of the left hemisphere (designated as "+", 52.6%), 4 were about equal (designated as "0", 21.1%) and 5 had a lesser value than that of the left hemisphere (designated as "-" 26.3%). Conversely, across the 18 female subjects, there are 10 participants whose NAA/Cho ratio in the right cerebellar hemisphere were lesser than that of the left hemisphere (designated as "-", 56%), 4 were about equal (designated as "0", 22.2%) and 4 had a greater value than that of the left hemisphere (designated as "+", 22.2%).

Apparently, the NAA/Cho in the right cerebellar hemisphere of males tends to be greater than that of the left hemisphere, but this trend is absent from the female subjects that we scanned. The lateralization of NAA/Cho within the cerebellar hemispheres seems to be opposite for our Chinese male and female subjects and the percentage of biochemical symmetry is similar, namely, 21.1% and 22.2% for male and female respectively. The NAA/Cho between the right and left cerebellar hemispheres across the male control group follows the similar trend, namely, there is 1 out of 8 being symmetric (12.5%) and 7 out of 8 being rightward (87.5%). Across the female control group, there are 2 out of 9 being symmetric (22.2%), 2 out of 9 being rightward (22.2%) and 5 out of 9 being leftward (55.5%).

We further compared the ratios of NAA/Cr, Cho/Cr and NAA/Cho between the right and left cerebellar hemispheres in the control groups and designed them as NAA/Cr R/L, Cho/Cr R/L and NAA/Cr R/L respectively in Table 3. Across the 8 right handed male controls (19-89yrs), the mean of NAA/Cr R/L ratio is 1.13±0.23, with 1 out of 8 being greater than 1.5 (12.5%), 1 out 8 being lesser than 1 (12.5%), and the rest of them being slightly more than 1 (75%); the mean of Cho/Cr R/L ratio is 0.91±0.12, with 1 out of 8 being equal to 1 (12.5%), 2 out of 8 being greater than 1 (25%), and 5 out of 8 being lesser than 1 (62.5%); the mean of NAA/Cho R/L ratio is 1.25±0.21, with 1 out of 8 being greater than 1.5 (12.5%); 1 out of 8 being lesser than 1 (12.5%) and the rest of them being slightly more than 1 (75%). See Table 3.

Across the 9 right handed female controls (14-59yrs), the mean of NAA/Cr R/L ratio is 0.90±0.19, with 1 out of 9 being equal to 1 (11.1%) , 2 out of 9 being greater than 1 (22.2%) and 6 out of 9 being lesser than 1 (66.6%); the mean of Cho/Cr R/L ratio is 0.96±0.24, with 6 out of 9 being greater than 1 (66.6%), and 3 out of 9 being lesser than 1 (33.3%) ; the mean of NAA/Cho R/L ratio is 0.97± 0.26, with 4 out of 9 being greater than 1 (44.4%) and 5 out of 9 being lesser than 1 (55.5%). See Table 3.

Thus, generally speaking, the NAA/Cho R/L ratios for male controls tend to be greater than 1, while in contrast, the NAA/Cho R/L ratios for our Chinese female controls, show a trend of being lesser than 1. See Table 3.

Male ID	**Age**	**NAA/Cr R/L**	**Cho /Cr R/L**	**NAA/Cho R/L**	**Female ID**	**Age**	**NAA/Cr R/L**	**Cho/Cr R/L**	**NAA/Cho R/L**
1	19	1.15	0.96	1.20	1	14	0.53	0.49	1.08
2	23	1.19	1.01	1.18	2	23	0.88	1.01	0.88
3	43	1.62	1	1.63	3	25	0.91	1.14	0.80
4	45	1.02	0.77	1.32	4	39	1	1.21	0.83
5	52	1.15	1.07	1.08	5	43	0.90	1.21	0.75
6	53	1.05	0.81	1.30	6	51	1.17	0.77	1.52
7	69	0.81	0.86	0.95	7	53	0.75	1.04	0.73
8	89	1.09	0.79	1.38	8	56	1.09	1.03	1.06
-	-	-	-	-	9	59	0.86	0.75	1.14
Mean ±SD	49.1 ±22.8	1.13 ±0.23	0.91 ±0.11	1.25 ±0.21	Mean ±SD	40.3 ±16.2	0.90 ±0.19	0.96 ±0.24	0.97 ±0.26

Table 3. The Metabolite Lateralization in the Cerebellum of Chinese Male and Female Controls Who Are Using the Traditional Chinese Logographic Reading and Writing Systems

By using 28 right handed 20-30 yr old normal male subjects from India, Jayasundar found that there was laterization of various brain metabolites (NAA, Cr and Cho) between the interhemisphere of cerebellar regions with the following parameters: STEAM pulse, TR=6000ms, TE=135 ms, with an 8ml single voxel and a 1.5 T Siemens Helicon scanner (Jayasundar, 2002). Our results seem to agree with these earlier findings.

5.1.3 A comparison of the NAA/Cr, Cho/Cr and NAA/Cho within the cerebellar hemispheres of the controls and the potential dyslexics who are using the traditional Chinese logographic reading and writing systems

Across the 8 right handed male controls, the NAA/Cr ratio within the right and left cerebellum ranged from 0.85-1.23 and 0.76-1.18, respectively. The Cho/Cr ratio within the right and left cerebellar hemisphere ranged from 0.73-0.90 and 0.72-1.03, respectively. The NAA/Cho within the right and left cerebellar hemisphere ranged from 1.12-1.47 and 0.81-1.39, respectively. Across the 9 right handed female controls, the NAA/Cr within right and left cerebellar hemisphere ranged from 0.7-1.65 and 0.93-1.92, respectively. The Cho/Cr within right and left cerebellar hemisphere ranged from 0.56-1.13 and 0.72-1.5, respectively. The NAA/Cho within right and left cerebellar hemisphere ranged from 0.98-1.66 and 1.09-1.89, respectively.

Our results indicated that the potential dyslexics have lesser NAA/Cho within right cerebellum than the mean of 17 controls (1.29±0.19). This agrees with the findings of Laycock (Laycock, et al., 2008). Nonetheless, our sample size is too small to reach any statistical power; yet, it seems fair to suggest that these measurements might be useful for diagnosis.

Safriel et al. found the NAA/Cr, Cho/Cr and NAA/Cho in the cerebellum to be 1.51±0.26, 1.51±0.14 and 1 respectively by using 1.5T, PRESS,TR=2000 ms, TE=135ms, and an 8ml voxel. There were 10 male and 10 female normal Caucasian subjects in the age range of 22-44 years without handedness control. No specific right or left hemisphere was recorded. They concluded that sex does not seem to be a confounding factor, the NAA/Cho ratio is equal to 1 (Safriel, Pol-Rodriguez, Novotny, Rothman, & Fulbright, 2005) and the brain metabolites were equally distributed across their subjects. Rae also indicated that the bran metabolites do not differ between the left and right cerebellar hemispheres of the control subjects (Rae, et al., 2002). For our 8 right handed Chinese male controls (19-89yrs), the NAA/Cho within right cerebellar hemisphere is significantly greater than that of the left hemisphere. However, this phenomenon was not found in our female subjects.

A study by Lei et al. found that the NAA/Cho in the cerebellum to be 1.306 of 27 Chinese subjects (23-49 yrs) who are using the simplified form of Chinese characters daily. They did not specify the sex, handedness and hemispheres (Lei, et al., 2011). The parameters for the experiments are following: svs-se-135 pulse sequence, single voxel size= 15X10X15mm, TR=1500ms, TE= 1500 ms via 1.5 T German Siemens scanner. This figure is similar to the mean of NAA/Cho in the right cerebellar hemisphere of our male control group.

5.2 The chemical shift imaging study (CSI)

The comparison of metabolites in the right and left cerebellar hemispheres could be achieved more precisely by mirroring the voxels simultaneously using the chemical shift

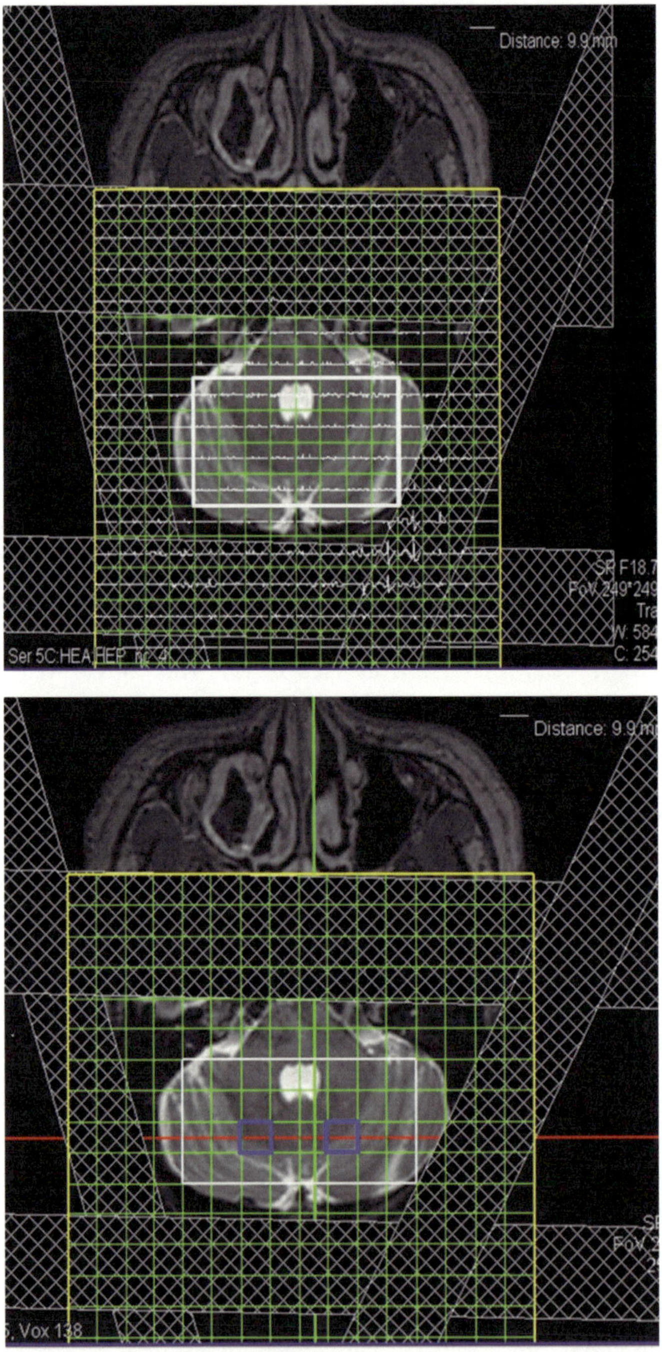

Fig. 1. Chemical shift images of the T_2-weighted axial view from a male control subject. Top: the white rectangle is the area for MRS acquiring and the yellow region with green grids shows the phase encoding steps. Four saturation bands could remove the unwanted signals from scalp and skull. Bottom: the CSI technique allows the mirror placement of a single voxel (blue square) at right and left cerebellar hemispheres simultaneously.

imaging technique with the following parameters: TR=2000ms, TE=135ms, FOV R L 160, VOL AP 160, thickness 15X15X15mm, FOV R L 60, VOL AP 40. The acquisition time is about 8 minutes. Table 4 demonstrates the NAA/Cr, Cho/Cr and NAA/Cho ratios within the right and left cerebellar hemispheres of two Chinese male controls that are using the traditional Chinese logographic reading and writing systems. Figure 1 and 2 indicated the spectra and the metabolite ratios in the specific voxels of a control subject via CSI technology.

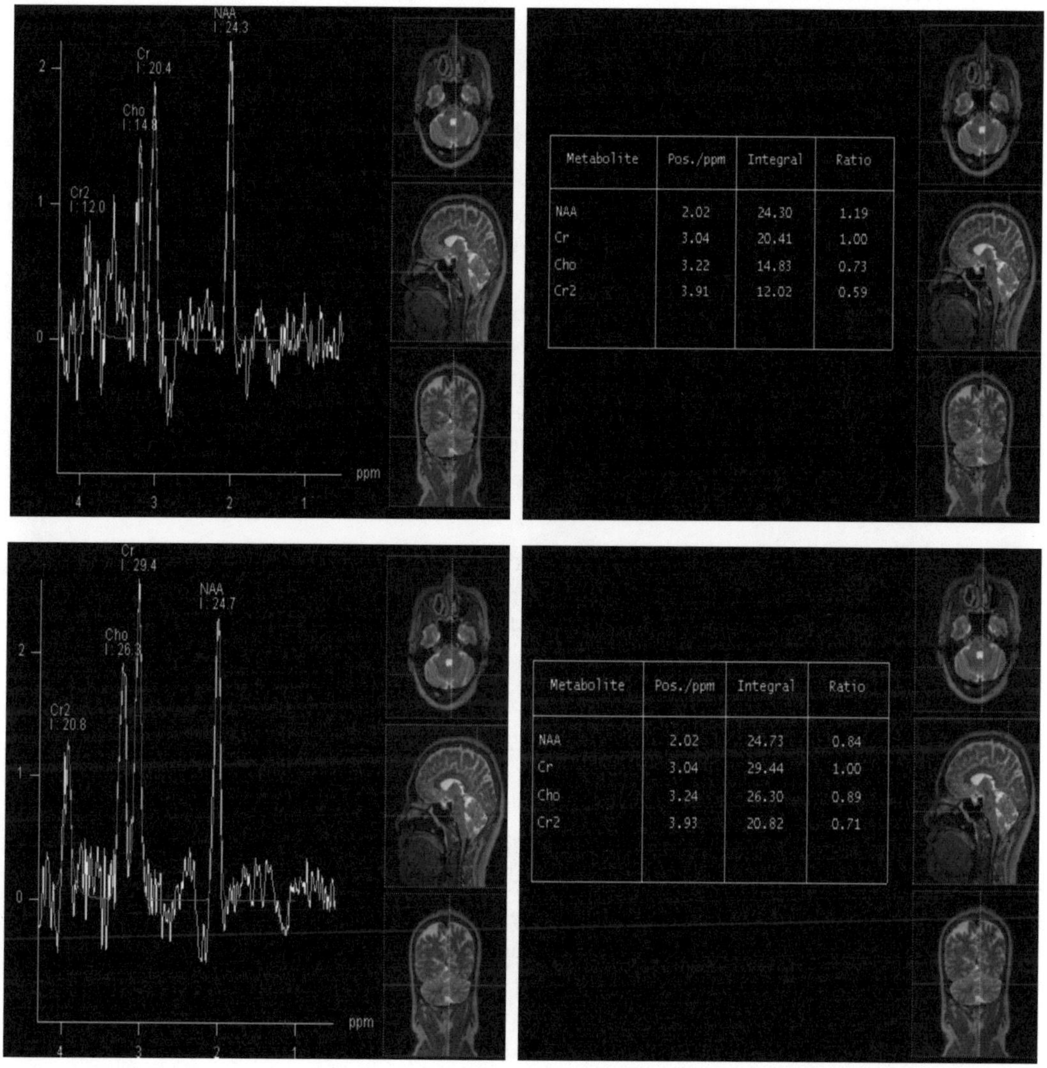

Fig. 2. The spectra and the NAA/Cr, Cho/Cr and NAA/Cho ratio of the right (up panel) and left (bottom panel) voxel in the cerebellar hemispheres corresponding to the bottom panel of Figure 1.

		NAA/Cr		Cho/Cr		NAA/Cho	
Male	Age	Right Hemi-sphere	Left Hemi-sphere	Right Hemi-sphere	Left Hemi-sphere	Right Hemi-sphere	Left Hemi-sphere
ID1	69	1.55	1.40	0.98	0.98	1.58	1.43
ID2	51	1.19	0.84	0.73	0.89	1.63	0.94

Table 4. The NAA/Cr, Cho/Cr and NAA/Cho Ratios within Cerebellum of Two Chinese Male Controls via Chemical Shift Imaging (CSI)

6. Present knowledge and future perspectives

Very few MRS studies using Chinese subjects for the measurement of brain metabolites, specifically, studies on those using traditional Chinese logographic reading and writing systems. We measured the ratios of NAA, Cr, and Cho metabolites within cerebellar cortex with handedness and sex information which offers valuable references for future studies. In addition, the chemical shift imaging technique used in a preliminary investigation here seems to be a good approach to assess the chemical lateralization of cerebellar hemispheres in future. More potential dyslexic subjects with detailed documentation in clinical features are needed for MRS experiments in order to make meaningful statistical inferences on the usefulness of this approach. Nonetheless, MRS measurement seems to be a promising approach that avoids the pitfalls of questionnaires and similar in dyslexic study.

The major limitation of the study is the difficulty in recruiting and identifying sufficient dyslexic probands, since there is no standard test for adult dyslexics. An objective reading test with an appropriate norm in traditional Chinese logographic characters might be used when screening for Chinese with dyslexia, in addition to self-reporting. A second limitation is that we were unable to examine the effect of age on the various parameters measured. To do this, it would require much larger cohorts in various age bands.

7. Summary

In this original article, we reviewed the application of magnetic resonance spectroscopy (MRS) to dyslexia. We used this non-invasive technique to measure the N-acetylaspartate (NAA) and Choline (Cho) ratio within the cerebellum of native Chinese volunteers. The aims of the experiment are, firstly, to compare the data with the results obtained from Western studies. These findings will act as a reference for longitudinal studies in future since most MRS studies have used Caucasian subjects. Secondly, we tested the hypothesis as to whether the NAA/Cho ratio within the right cerebellum is able to discriminate dyslexics from the non-dyslexics as suggested by the previous research in West. However, in contrast to the Western studies, we recruited native Chinese who use traditional Chinese characters (a logographic reading and writing linguistic system) in their daily life as subjects for our studies. Thus, this study is novel in this respect. Finally, we explored the use of the chemical shift imaging for the acquisition of data since this should yield a more precise sampling of the left and right cerebellar hemisphere simultaneously than the use of a single voxel approach.

8. Acknowledgements

We are indebted to all the volunteers who joined the study and the technician Mr. Xiang-Chen Bi for data acquisition. The study was supported by a grant (98A-C-B501 3TMRI) from National Yang-Ming University. We also acknowledge the stipend offered by the Center for Survey Research, RCHSS, Academia Sinica.

9. References

Brachacki, G. W., Nicolson, R. I., & Fawcett, A. J. (1995). Impaired recognition of traffic signs in adults with dyslexia. *J Learn Disabil, 28*(5), 297-301, 308.

Breteler, M. H., Arns, M., Peters, S., Giepmans, I., & Verhoeven, L. (2010). Improvements in spelling after QEEG-based neurofeedback in dyslexia: a randomized controlled treatment study. *Appl Psychophysiol Biofeedback, 35*(1), 5-11.

Chakravarty, A. (2009). Artistic talent in dyslexia - a hypothesis. *Med Hypotheses, 73*(4), 569-571.

Demonet, J. F., Taylor, M. J., & Chaix, Y. (2004). Developmental dyslexia. *Lancet, 363*(9419), 1451-1460.

Eden, G. F., Wood, F. B., & Stein, J. F. (2003). Clock drawing in developmental dyslexia. *J Learn Disabil, 36*(3), 216-228.

Everatt, J., Weeks, S., & Brooks, P. (2008). Profiles of strengths and weaknesses in dyslexia and other learning difficulties. *Dyslexia, 14*(1), 16-41.

Fawcett, A. J., Nicolson, RI. (2007). Dyslexia, learning and pedagogical neuroscience. *Dev Med Child Neurol, 49*(4), 306-311.

Galaburda, A. M., & Cestnick, L. (2003). Developmental dyslexia. *Rev Neurol, 36 Suppl 1*, S3-9.

Gersons-Wolfensberger, D. C., & Ruijssenaars, W. A. (1997). Definition and treatment of dyslexia: a report by the Committee on Dyslexia of the Health Council of The Netherlands. *J Learn Disabil, 30*(2), 209-213.

Grigorenko, E. L., Wood, F. B., Golovyan, L., Meyer, M., Romano, C., & Pauls, D. (2003). Continuing the search for dyslexia genes on 6p. *Am J Med Genet B Neuropsychiatr Genet, 118B*(1), 89-98.

Habib, M. (2000). The neurological basis of developmental dyslexia: an overview and working hypothesis. *Brain, 123 Pt 12*, 2373-2399.

Ho, C. S., Chan, D. W., Chung, K. K., Lee, S. H., & Tsang, S. M. (2007). In search of subtypes of Chinese developmental dyslexia. *J Exp Child Psychol, 97*(1), 61-83.

Hsiung, G. Y., Kaplan, B. J., Petryshen, T. L., Lu, S., & Field, L. L. (2004). A dyslexia susceptibility locus (DYX7) linked to dopamine D4 receptor (DRD4) region on chromosome 11p15.5. *Am J Med Genet B Neuropsychiatr Genet, 125B*(1), 112-119.

Lonnemanna, J., Linkersdörfera, J., Heselhausa, V., Hasselhorn, M., & Lindberg, S. (2011). Relations between balancing and arithmetic skills in children - evidence of cerebellar involvement? *Journal of Neurolinguistics, in press.*

Jayasundar, R. (2002). Human brain: biochemical lateralization in normal subjects. *Neurol India, 50*(3), 267-271.

King, W. M., Giess, S. A., & Lombardino, L. J. (2007). Subtyping of children with developmental dyslexia via bootstrap aggregated clustering and the gap statistic: comparison with the double-deficit hypothesis. *Int J Lang Commun Disord, 42*(1), 77-95.

Laycock, S. K., Wilkinson, I. D., Wallis, L. I., Darwent, G., Wonders, S. H., Fawcett, A. J., et al. (2008). Cerebellar volume and cerebellar metabolic characteristics in adults with dyslexia. *Ann N Y Acad Sci, 1145*, 222-236.

Lei, L., Liao, Y., Liao, W., Zhou, J., Yuan, Y., Wang, J., et al. (2011). Magnetic resonance spectroscopy of the cerebellum in patients with spinocerebellar ataxia type 3/Machado-Joseph disease. *Zhong Nan Da Xue Xue Bao Yi Xue Ban, 36*(6), 511-519.

Levy, H. B. (1983). Developmental dyslexia - a talent deficit. *Dev Med Child Neurol, 25*(6), 691-692.

Lyon, G. R., Shaywitz, S. E., & Shaywitz, B. A. (2003). Defining Dyslexia, Comorbidity, Teachers' Knowledge of Language and Reading A Definition of Dyslexia. *Annals of Dyslexia 53*, 1-14.

Miles, T. R. (1993). *Dyslexia: The Pattern of Difficulties* (2nd ed.): Whurr Publishers, London.

Nicolson, R. I., Fawcett, A. J., & Dean, P. (1996). Time estimation deficits in developmental dyslexia: evidence of cerebellar involvement. . *Proc R Soc Lond B Biol Sci 259*, 43–47.

Olson, R. K. (2002). Dyslexia: nature and nurture. *Dyslexia, 8*(3), 143-159.

Penolazzi, B., Spironelli, C., Vio, C., & Angrilli, A. (2010). Brain plasticity in developmental dyslexia after phonological treatment: a beta EEG band study. *Behav Brain Res, 209*(1), 179-182.

Pernet, C., Andersson, J., Paulesu, E., & Demonet, J. F. (2009). When all hypotheses are right: a multifocal account of dyslexia. *Hum Brain Mapp, 30*(7), 2278-2292.

Pernet, C. R., Poline, J. B., Demonet, J. F., & Rousselet, G. A. (2009). Brain classification reveals the right cerebellum as the best biomarker of dyslexia. *BMC Neurosci, 10*, 67.

Rae, C., Harasty, J. A., Dzendrowskyj, T. E., Talcott, J. B., Simpson, J. M., Blamire, A. M., et al. (2002). Cerebellar morphology in developmental dyslexia. *Neuropsychologia, 40*(8), 1285-1292.

Rae, C., Lee, M. A., Dixon, R. M., Blamire, A. M., Thompson, C. H., Styles, P., et al. (1998). Metabolic abnormalities in developmental dyslexia detected by ^{1}H magnetic resonance spectroscopy. *Lancet, 351*(9119), 1849-1852.

Richards, T. L., Berninger, V. W., Aylward, E. H., Richards, A. L., Thomson, J. B., Nagy, W. E., et al. (2002). Reproducibility of proton MR spectroscopic imaging (PEPSI):

comparison of dyslexic and normal-reading children and effects of treatment on brain lactate levels during language tasks. *AJNR 23*(10), 1678-1685.

Richards, T. L., Corina, D., Serafini, S., Steury, K., Echelard, D. R., Dager, S. R., et al. (2000). Effects of a phonologically driven treatment for dyslexia on lactate levels measured by proton MR spectroscopic imaging. *AJNR Am J Neuroradiol, 21*(5), 916-922.

Richards, T. L., Dager, S. R., Corina, D., Serafini, S., Heide, A. C., Steury, K., et al. (1999). Dyslexic children have abnormal brain lactate response to reading-related language tasks. *AJNR 20*(8), 1393-1398.

Richardson, A. J., Cox, I. J., Sargentoni, J., & Puri, B. K. (1997). Abnormal cerebral phospholipid metabolism in dyslexia indicated by phosphorus-31 magnetic resonance spectroscopy. *NMR Biomed, 10*(7), 309-314.

Safriel, Y., Pol-Rodriguez, M., Novotny, E. J., Rothman, D. L., & Fulbright, R. K. (2005). Reference values for long echo time MR spectroscopy in healthy adults. *AJNR Am J Neuroradiol, 26*(6), 1439-1445.

Schulte-Korne, G., Ziegler, A., Deimel, W., Schumacher, J., Plume, E., Bachmann, C., et al. (2007). Interrelationship and familiality of dyslexia related quantitative measures. *Ann Hum Genet, 71*(Pt 2), 160-175.

Spinelli, D., Brizzolara, D., De Luca, M., Gasperini, F., Martelli, M., & Zoccolotti, P. (2010). Subtypes of developmental dyslexia in transparent orthographies: A comment on Lachmann and Van Leeuwen (2008). *Cogn Neuropsychol*, 1-7.

Stoodley, C. J., Fawcett, A. J., Nicolson, R. I., & Stein, J. F. (2006). Balancing and pointing tasks in dyslexic and control adults. *Dyslexia, 12*(4), 276-288.

Stoodley, C. J., & Stein, J. F. (2011). The cerebellum and dyslexia. *Cortex, 47*(1), 101-116.

Sun, Y.-F., Lee, J.-S., & Kirby, R. (2009). Candidate Genes for Dyslexia by An In Silico Approach *Asian Journal of Health and Information Sciences, 4*(2-3), 81-92.

Sun, Y.-F., Lee, J. S., & Kirby, R. (2010). Brain imaging findings in dyslexia. *Pediatr Neonatol 51*(2), 83-90.

Sun, Y.-F., Ting-Hsiang Lin, & Liao, P.-S. (2010). Developing a dyslexia scale for adolescents and adults in Taiwan. *International Conference on Survey Research Methodology.*

Tree, J. J. (2008). Two types of phonological dyslexia - a contemporary review. *Cortex, 44*(6), 698-706.

Tunmer, W., & Greaney, K. (2010). Defining dyslexia. *J Learn Disabil, 43*(3), 229-243.

von Karolyi, C., Winner, E., Gray, W., & Sherman, G. F. (2003). Dyslexia linked to talent: global visual-spatial ability. *Brain Lang, 85*(3), 427-431.

WHO. (July 2011). http://apps.who.int/classifications/apps/icd/icd10online July 2011.

Wilsher, C. R., Bennett, D., Chase, C. H., Conners, C. K., DiIanni, M., Feagans, L., et al. (1987). Piracetam and dyslexia: effects on reading tests. *J Clin Psychopharmacol, 7*(4), 230-237.

Zavadenko, N. N., Rumiantseva, M. V., & Tolstova, V. A. (2009). Dyslexia: clinical, neurophysiological and neuropsychological manifestations during the treatment with nootropil. *Zh Nevrol Psikhiatr Im S S Korsakova, 109*(5), 36-42.

Ziegler, J. C., Perry, C., Ma-Wyatt, A., Ladner, D., & Schulte-Korne, G. (2003). Developmental dyslexia in different languages: language-specific or universal? *J Exp Child Psychol, 86*(3), 169-193.